GRAY MATTERS

GRAY
MATTERS

A BIOGRAPHY OF BRAIN SURGERY

THEODORE H. SCHWARTZ

DUTTON

DUTTON
An imprint of Penguin Random House LLC
penguinrandomhouse.com

Illustrations on pages 58, 59, 68, 71, 73, 93, 94, 142, 173, 176, 179, 214, 221, 234, 236, 256, 282, 301, 328, 380, 400, and 435 by Matthew Holt.

LIBRARY OF CONGRESS CATALOGING-IN-PUBLICATION DATA

Names: Schwartz, Theodore H., author.
Title: Gray matters : a biography of brain surgery / Theodore H. Schwartz.
Description: New York : Dutton, an imprint of Penguin Random House LLC, [2024] | Includes bibliographical references and index.
Identifiers: LCCN 2023051217 | ISBN 9780593474105 (hardcover) | ISBN 9780593474112 (ebook)
Subjects: MESH: Brain—surgery | Neurosurgical Procedures—history | Neurosurgery—history | Personal Narrative
Classification: LCC RD594 | NLM WL 11.1 | DDC 617.4/81—dc23/eng/20240507
LC record available at https://lccn.loc.gov/2023051217

Printed in the United States of America
3rd Printing

BOOK DESIGN BY LAURA K. CORLESS

For
Lester, Mara, Ralph,
and
Nancy, Jonathan, Benjamin, Jenna, and Alexandra

I would like to see the day when somebody would be appointed surgeon somewhere who had no hands, for the operative part is the least part of the work.

—Harvey Cushing, neurosurgeon, 1911

Brain surgery is a terrible profession. If I did not feel it will become very different in my lifetime, I should hate it.

—Wilder Penfield, neurosurgeon, 1921

I agonize over the question of which risk is greater, the disease or the operation?

—Irving S. Cooper, neurosurgeon, 1981

AUTHOR'S NOTE

The following pages contain the details of brain surgeries performed on real people: celebrities, politicians, athletes, and actual patients of mine. For those who were not my patients, no private health information has been divulged other than what is already publicly available, either through the individuals' published accounts or articles available on the internet. Regarding my own patients, their names and identifying details have been changed to conceal their identities and, whenever possible, their permission was obtained to retell their stories. I have tried as best I could to comply with the requirements of the Health Insurance Portability and Accountability Act of 1996, better known as HIPAA. In some places, this book aims to provide useful information based on my professional experience, but it is not intended to replace your doctor's medical advice. Please consult with your doctor if you believe you have any medical conditions that may require treatment.

CONTENTS

III

WHO'S IN CHARGE?

GRAY MATTERS

PROLOGUE

stare into the eyes of the patient sitting in front of me. Glassy and blood-shot, they reflect his past few sleepless nights, no doubt spent contemplating both his uncertain future and the terrifying prospect of having the hands of a relative stranger rooting around in his skull. Today my opponent is a tumor, more specifically a meningioma. It's resting at the tip of this gentleman's temporal lobe, just behind the left eye. I imagine the neurons behind those eyes firing off thought after panicked thought. How much longer until the tumor grows so large it will rob him of some essential part of himself? Has some piece already slipped away? If so, which part? And what's more terrifying: the relentless onslaught of the tumor or the anticipation of the surgery itself?

I begin the interview. My goal is to project calmness and confidence, like an airline pilot letting the passengers know they are headed into a bit of turbulence but that everything will be fine. When I'm the one in the passenger seat, I want to believe that no one better could be sitting behind the controls of that plane as it jerks and shudders, buffeted by headwinds. I tell him—metaphorically, of course—that we're in this together. This plane is *not* going down. But who am I *really* trying to convince, him or myself?

A few days later, when I arrive in the operating room, he's already under—deep in the dreamless oblivion of anesthesia. I'd stopped by the preoperative waiting area earlier that morning to say hello to him and his wife and answer all their last-minute questions. Despite his lack of sleep the night before, he didn't appear at all tired. In fact, quite the opposite: he was alert and even a bit jumpy, his body poised to engage in a battle, but not one that he will be fighting. Indeed, he'll be the battleground.

But now he is asleep, his face no longer showing the signs of worry so recently engraved upon it. This moment of peace and quiet, soon to be filled with the whir of saw penetrating skull, marks a transition, a crossroads when he still retains the vestiges of the person he once was before becoming something entirely different to me: a task I must complete.

This is when I slip under his shoulder a piece of paper, wrapped in plastic for protection. On it, a prayer has been printed in a language I cannot read: a talisman provided by his family to shepherd him through his pilgrimage and me through my campaign.

His body is now fully exposed as tubes and wires symbiotically link his organs with the anesthesiologist's machines. I take a moment to examine several markings I notice adorning his torso. Are these more benedictions? Archaic incantations? The writing is sloppy, the letters and pictures juvenile, but I gradually decipher the words. *I Love You, Daddy* is penned in blue marker down his left arm. His right arm bears a picture of a multicolored rainbow under which *Come Home Soon* is scribbled in red. On his elbow, next to a misshapen balloon heart, is a brown oval splotch atop which one of his younger children—probably the prankster of the family, not fully realizing the gravity of his father's plight—has impishly written *Poop*. Connecting the word to the blob is an arrow, a guide for me, lest there be any confusion regarding the identity of the blemish.

I am a neurosurgeon working in New York City. I've spent almost thirty years operating on people with neurological illnesses. This is my seventh surgery of the week, and today our surgical crew is a small squad of five: me, my assistant, the anesthesiologist, a scrub tech, and a circulator. The tech's job is to hand me my instruments, which often occurs before I even have time to ask. If I mistakenly ask for the wrong one, she always hands me what I need. She understands implicitly which tools I require—not from clairvoyance but from repetition. The circulator, whose job it is to set up the room before we begin and fetch anything we need as the situation arises, also doubles as our DJ.

Once the operation is underway and going smoothly, we joke around, listen to music, argue over the playlist, and tell stories about what's going on in our lives. Today we settle on Top 40. During rare moments of crisis, when an operation starts to go south, the mood changes in an instant. Music is silenced. All gossip ceases. You could hear a suture drop, should one accidentally fall to the floor. But once the storm has passed, the mood of the room quickly lifts, as if a bit of turbulence had always been expected on this flight.

Today's operation, on my patient with the poop sketch on his elbow, is far from routine. In fact, it's a procedure I've never done before. It's not that I lack the experience or missed out on the training; rather, it's an operation few neurosurgeons have ever attempted. The tumor I'm facing today rests deep in my patient's brain, surrounded by critical nerves and blood vessels, which, if damaged, could cause devastating injuries such as blindness or paralysis. Luckily, this is a benign tumor that can be cured with surgery, but it does have to be removed somehow, some way; its slow, insidious growth has brought it dangerously close to the optic nerves. If the problem isn't fixed, my patient's vision will soon begin to fade. I've removed many such tumors before but always through a more traditional approach: displacing the muscles for chewing that sit on the side of the head in the temple, removing a sizable slab of bone, and then burrowing deep inside the skull, working around and sometimes even *through* the brain.

Opening the skull in this more typical fashion—whether via the side, the top, or the back of the head, as has been done by neurosurgeons for the last hundred years—is called a craniotomy. Such operations are routine, performed at almost every hospital in the nation. Craniotomies have given brain surgeons the ability to treat a wide range of diseases of the central nervous system—tumors, blood clots, aneurysms, and infections—and this technique for opening and closing the head has been perfected over several generations through incremental improvements and modifications.

But today I'm doing something completely different. Instead of deconstructing the side of the face like a Picasso, I've asked an oculoplastic surgeon to work with me. He'll make a small incision in the eyelid and circumnavigate the eyeball, which will lead us directly to our target. It may seem impossible to imagine that there's enough room between the cup of the socket and the globe of the eye for us to do our work. But the eyeball is encased in a thick protective padding of fat, which I'm hoping to gently dislodge with my instruments to allow my scope, drill, and scissors to go in and his tumor to come out. The space will be small, our maneuverability limited, but if we're successful, the patient will be cured of his tumor without our having to reassemble the side of his head at the end of the case. His recovery should be faster and his incision will be invisible, hidden in a small crease in the eyelid.

More crucially, this approach will minimize any inadvertent damage to the brain that might occur from a standard craniotomy, which is the procedure I was taught during my training. That older, time-honored technique, while good for most tumors, in this case would mean that a few of the most fragile parts of the brain would lie directly in my path. Approaching the tumor from this new and different periorbital trajectory means—or so I hope—that I can immediately access the center of the tumor. It's more of a straight shot, if you will, unimpeded by those fragile elements—unimpeded except by the eyeball, that is. Until only a few years ago, I had previously never considered that a structure like an eyeball could be displaced en route to the brain. But that was before I began reading about a small group of surgeons scattered across the globe who'd started performing this type of surgery on a few of their patients.

I was intrigued.

First, I practiced on cadavers. I reread every word of the few published articles that described the approach. Then I waited for the right patient with the right tumor in the right location. So today's procedure is the culmination of years of preparation and anticipation.

The oculoplastic surgeon makes the incision and exposes the bone around the eye. Having an eye expert involved puts me somewhat at ease, so I can focus on what I know best. I have enough things to worry about. He retracts the orbit to give me room, if barely enough, to do my work. Into this narrow space I first pass the endoscope, essentially a long, thin telescope we use to see what we're doing. Next, with my right hand, I advance an electric-powered drill the size of a pencil. In my left hand I manipulate a curved metal suction device. The latter functions both as a retractor and a way to eliminate the bone shavings as we widen and deepen the hole.

Meanwhile my assistant, a young neurosurgeon in training, irrigates the operative field with a constant stream of saline squirted through a syringe. The three of us are crowded around the patient's head, alternately gazing both down at what we can see through the small incision and up at the multiple flat-screen displays onto which the image from the endoscope is being projected. I gently step on the foot pedal to start the drill rotating. I watch as its diamond tip begins to shave away the thin shelf of bone that separates the back of the eye from the front of the brain.

This technique—operating on the brain through the eye socket—is not a new one, having been used in a much more dubious way by Dr. Walter Jackson Freeman II, a neurologist, to perform frontal lobotomies in the 1950s. But the operation I'm performing today has about as much in common with Freeman's lobotomies as an F-16 has with Wilbur and Orville Wright's first flying machine.

As I drill, I think about how my patient obtained several opinions from other well-known neurosurgeons, all of whom recommended—no, more like insisted—that he undergo a craniotomy. What convinced him that my approach, so different from theirs, would work? I'm used to dealing with skeptics, having faced similar battles when I started operating through the nose—another of the minimally invasive surgeries I adopted early. Perhaps the success I've had with that approach—in combination with the obvious benefits of removing his tumor through the front of his head rather than the side—was enough to win the day?

After making a small hole in the bone roughly the size of a quarter, I expose a bit of the dura, the thick white covering of the brain. Using a long, thin pair of bayonetted scissors held between my thumb and forefinger, I squeeze the short, angled tips together and cut a small circle into the dura, wide enough to expose the tumor.

This approach turns out to be perfect for getting me where I need to be, and the tumor comes out quickly. I barely touch the brain. In fact, with just a few scoops of the curette, the tumor is gone. This part, the most critical move, takes ten or fifteen minutes. Dare I say it was . . . easy?

Don't get me wrong. I'm not claiming that brain surgery is easy, particularly in a world in which "It's not *brain surgery*" has become a put-down to remind everyone of their place in the pecking order of human advancement: "Oh, you swam the English Channel? Great, but it isn't brain surgery." "You wrote a novel? Cool, but it isn't brain surgery." "You solved cold fusion? Please. It isn't brain surgery."

Brain surgery is hard, for sure, but not as hard as it used to be, when the specialty was in its infancy. Surgeries back then were mostly exploratory, since surgeons had no idea where to find the problem without the benefit of MRI scans. Many patients never made it off the table, and surgeons had no semblance of a personal life, as they needed to sacrifice everything at the altar of their profession.

But much has changed over the years. New technologies, new approaches, new instruments, better training, more powerful computers, and multispecialty integrated hospital care have all transformed the modern practice of neurosurgery.

That said, people ask me all the time, "What's it *really* like to be a brain surgeon?" and I never have a good answer. *I mean, how much time have you got?* It's impossible to answer such a question over the course of a one-hour lecture, let alone during a three-minute cocktail party conversation. "Great," I usually say. "I really love my job." Then I ask about their kids or talk sports or bring up literally any other topic—because what else can I say that would even scratch the surface of describing what it's like to spend the better part of my waking hours with my hands inside someone else's skull?

On these pages, I want to tell the story of neurosurgery from its primitive beginnings, when it was mostly used to treat head trauma, to its current state as a computer-based discipline of meticulous precision.

Neurosurgery is a relatively young field, just over 120 years old, and the brave early mavericks who first ventured into the skull were as courageous as any world explorers. I will tell their tales and highlight the many ways their discoveries have rippled forward into modern practice.

Neurosurgery has also touched the lives of some of our nation's most celebrated individuals: actors, politicians, athletes, musicians. I'll explore those cases in Holmes-meets-Watson detail and reveal secrets about their treatments that are not as widely publicized. We'll also dive into some of the field's less glamorous moments, such as the era of psychosurgery and the widespread use of the frontal lobotomy as a treatment for mental illness. What is also not as well known is how this dark chapter in our specialty served to propel the field forward to what it is today.

Eventually, we will get to the philosophical implications of brain surgery: how brain surgery has contributed to our understanding of the workings of the human mind, the existence of the "self," and our illusions about being in control of our actions. Finally, we will explore the new frontier of brain-computer interfaces. Most people are vaguely aware that someday we'll be able to search the internet, drive a car, and even communicate using our minds alone, linked to a computer. But what does this really mean in practice and what is it like to have a computer interface implanted in your brain? Stay tuned.

After every operation, regardless of the results, the routine is always the same. I emerge from the operating room into the hallway, a descent from what feels to me like a holy place back into the everyday world. My aches and pains in my muscles and joints—the result of working in awkward positions for several hours—now reassert themselves. I'm aware of the slightly bitter smell of my own sweat. I rip off my paper hat and surgical mask to inhale fresh, unfiltered air instead of my own stagnating breath. Not wanting my bloodstained scrubs to alarm my patient's loved ones, I grab my white coat off its hook in the hallway and head to the family waiting room.

There they are: his wife, whom I had met in the office and seen again earlier that day before the operation, and their three children, the Magic Marker tattoo artists whose work adorned their father's torso. I see half-eaten food sitting on the table next to an open computer. Two of the three children are sleeping, having been awakened at 3:00 a.m. to reach the hospital by 5:00. It's been four hours since they last saw their father, shortly before he was wheeled into the OR.

I focus on his wife. I can sense her fear and anticipation. I know they are fearing the worst, so I immediately say out loud, but not too loud, since we're still in public, "Everything went great." Perhaps I'm violating their privacy with this public disclosure, but it seems cruel to prolong the suspense by keeping a poker face and not saying a word. Then I say, "Let's go into the private consult room." She wakes her kids and I usher them around the corner. Once behind closed doors, I say it again. "Everything went great. He's going to be fine." The news, I've learned, must first sink in before I go into the details of what I found and what to expect going forward.

This is the moment when the relief—and tears—finally hit. The wife's eyes well up and she reaches out to give me a hug as if I were her oldest and dearest friend—never mind that until very recently, we were almost complete strangers. Some family members ask my permission first: "Can I give you a hug?" But not this time. The gesture is spontaneous, genuine, and deeply human. All sense of personal boundaries collapses.

I don't mind it one bit. I live for this hug. This is the most rewarding aspect of brain surgery: the payoff, if you will, for all those years of work, all those hours—or minutes, in this case—inside the patient's skull, carefully sorting the bad cells from the good.

I

BEGINNINGS

ONE

THE MYTH

S ince its inception at around the turn of the twentieth century, brain surgery has had a reputation for complexity that has left it shrouded in an aura of mystery.

James Gaffigan, the stand-up comedian, has a bit where he asks the audience: "Can you imagine the pressure on a brain surgeon? At no point during their day can they say, 'Hey, it ain't *brain surgery!*'" Even *The Simpsons* got in on the fun. In one clip, Mr. Burns, who has just taken a saw to Homer's skull, asks Smithers for an ice-cream scoop to remove the brain. When Smithers balks, Burns cries out, "Dammit, Smithers, this isn't rocket science; it's brain surgery!"

Whatever its origin, the catchphrase misses an important fact: most of the surgeries performed by neurosurgeons take place in the spine. But, for our purposes here, we will conflate neurosurgery with brain surgery, as brain surgeons are, by definition, neurosurgeons, and all neurosurgeons are trained to do brain surgery—even those who mostly operate on the spine.

So, what *is* the genesis of the brain surgeon's pop culture reputation?

If brain surgery has a reputation for being a difficult and dangerous field requiring steely self-confidence and the highest level of technical expertise, it is due in no small part to the undisputed founding father of neurosurgery, Dr. Harvey Cushing. Cushing was arguably one of the most brilliant, hardworking, and talented surgeons ever to grace the planet. He has an almost mythological status in our field, as evidenced by the many outstanding accounts of his life and his accomplishments. As we shall see, his stature and reputation are well deserved.

Before Cushing, most of the operations now commonly performed on the brain were considered much too dangerous except in emergency situations. More than half of all patients perished merely from the undertaking. Surgeries were often slipshod, ill-conceived, and so infrequently performed as to be labeled experimental. Opening the human skull and exposing the brain was not only futile but heretical, since a doctor's guiding principle, according to the Hippocratic oath, has always been to "do no harm."

After Cushing, neurosurgery became a well-refined subspecialty of surgery whose breadth of operations was not so far off from what it is today. Patients not only survived surgery but, for the most part, were better off *after* the operation compared with before it. Because of Cushing's reputation, nearly every up-and-coming neurosurgeon living in the first third of the twentieth century made the pilgrimage to either train under him or at least observe him in action.

Cushing, the youngest of ten children, was born on April 8, 1869, into a rigidly puritanical family of doctors in Cleveland, Ohio. He was a dedicated student and athlete, passionate about baseball and gymnastics. In high school, he took an interest in woodworking, blacksmithing, and drawing, perhaps foreshadowing a career relying on dexterity. In college, he played on Yale's baseball team, which upset his father, who saw sports as a distraction from his studies. By his senior year, Cushing was the team captain.

He was a solid B student, which back then put him in the top third of his class. He joined Scroll and Key, one of Yale's all-male social clubs, and it was there that he attended a lecture by a visiting physician who made such an impression on him that he decided to follow the family tradition and become a doctor. He applied to and was accepted by Harvard Medical School, where one of his older brothers, Ned, had already studied. Most medical students in Cushing's era were admitted straight out of high

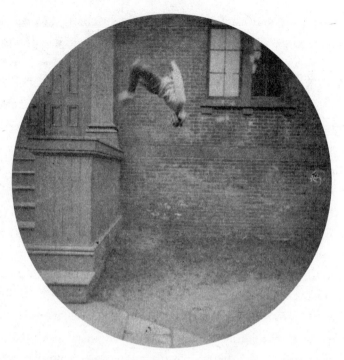

Cushing in midair executing a backflip off the steps of Yale library as an undergraduate.
*Medical Historical Library, Harvey Cushing/John Jay Whitney Medical Library,
Yale University*

school. Cushing, however, was one of only two members of his class with a college degree.

Despite his success as a student, Cushing was plagued throughout his medical school years with self-doubt and feelings of inadequacy, emotions that helped explain his unwavering drive for perfection throughout his life. In one well-documented incident, Cushing was asked to administer anesthesia to a woman about to undergo a hernia operation, which at the time consisted of a rag dipped in ether. Completely inexperienced in the task, Cushing proceeded with a beginner's trepidation, only to have his patient die under his care before the operation had even begun. Guilt-ridden and distraught by his error, the fledgling doctor nearly quit medicine before doubling down on his scholarly efforts while simultaneously developing an addiction to cigarettes.

Cushing went on to study surgery at Johns Hopkins Medical School under the legendary chief of surgery William Stewart Halsted, who revolutionized general surgery with the introduction of general anesthesia, antiseptic technique, and fastidious tissue dissection. Cushing's interest in the nervous system was first piqued after he successfully treated a patient with intractable facial pain by carefully dissecting and then severing the trigeminal ganglion, a bundle of nerves that sits just below the brain. Weighing the pros and cons of restricting his focus to neurosurgery alone, which was unheard-of at the time, Cushing took the advice of another of his teachers, Sir William Osler, the physician-in-chief at Hopkins, and set out for Europe to absorb whatever wisdom he could glean from the few world experts in the field.

Cushing's trip abroad started a tradition among many subsequent neurosurgeons of embarking on international travel to observe trailblazers pioneering new operations not yet taught or widely accepted in the United States. In Switzerland, he observed the Swiss surgeon Emil Theodor Kocher and researched the brain's circulation in the lab of Hugo Kronecker. In England, Cushing watched Sir Victor Horsley, the father of British neurosurgery, and studied under the neurophysiologist Sir Charles Sherrington. When Cushing returned to Hopkins in 1901, Halsted was initially not supportive of Cushing's notion of focusing his practice uniquely on neurosurgery, as so few established brain operations ended in success. But Cushing persisted and Halstead relented. Only a few years later, in 1905, Cushing published his seminal article *The Special Field of Neurological Surgery*, the first monograph on the subject and the field's unofficial birth certificate.

Surgeons in Cushing's day had access to neither MRIs nor CAT scans, so surgeries on the brain were, for the most part, exploratory. The only clues they had were the patients' self-reported symptoms and whatever could be gleaned from physical examinations. Surgeons were then forced to correlate those symptoms with their still-limited knowledge of the organization of the nervous system and forge ahead.

Imagine the combination of ego, sangfroid, and monomaniacal fortitude it must have taken for a young physician like Cushing to put his patients' lives at risk time after time in pursuit of accomplishing what most preeminent surgeons of that era had deemed hopeless. It's nearly impossible for the modern neurosurgeon to conceive of this audacity, since so many of the operations we now perform have been codified, validated, rehearsed, and deemed, for the most part, to have a good chance of success. Cushing faced enormous and understandable criticism from colleagues, but he countered their condemnation of his recklessness with his remarkable results.

Cushing's commitment to uncompromising precision marked both his career and his character. As a result of the death he had witnessed as a medical student while administering the primitive ether rag anesthesia, he pioneered the structured recordkeeping and blood pressure measurements used by anesthesiologists to this day. At the age of thirty-two he was put in charge of neurosurgery at Johns Hopkins Hospital. Only a few years later he was recruited to Harvard's Peter Bent Brigham Hospital in Boston, where he worked for most of the remainder of his career.

Cushing's impact on brain surgery was nothing short of transformative. In his hands, operative mortality went from 50 percent to under 10 percent. In the words of one of his biographers, Michael Bliss, "Harvey Cushing became the father of effective neurosurgery. Ineffective neurosurgery had many fathers." He was also a remarkable artist and documented the details of his operations with Da Vinci–like precision.

Cushing not only annotated each patient's history and illustrated the disease process; he also preserved his patients' brains after death. In studying postmortem specimens, Cushing was forcing himself to confront his own failures and pushing himself to improve. The collection of disembodied brains, each preserved in its own jar, remains on display in the Harvey Cushing/John Hay Whitney Medical Library at Yale University.

Cushing logged fourteen-to-sixteen-hour days, six days a week, taking few holidays. His leisure activities included tennis and collecting rare medical books. He was known to spend hours scouring back-alley shops during his frequent trips abroad. He was also, not surprisingly, an absentee husband and father, leaving his wife, Kate, to raise their five children. After spending two years in Europe at the tail end of the First World War, from 1917 to 1919, Cushing returned home and, rather than take time off to get reacquainted with his wife and children, jumped right back into his work. In a

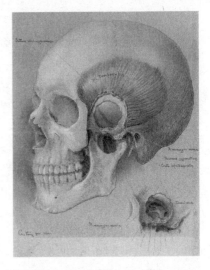

A Cushing sketch from one of his operations.

Medical Historical Library, Harvey Cushing/John Jay Whitney Medical Library, Yale University

letter to her husband, Kate pleaded with him, "Something in me was hurt to the core—perhaps it was my heart." In another letter, she poured out her soul, lamenting the fragility of their marriage, and then closed with the words: "I can't say these things to you. You are always too busy or too tired."

Cushing was known for his repressed, puritanical character, on full display the day he learned of the death of his twenty-three-year-old son, Bill. After completing his third year at Yale, barely passing his classes, Bill spent the night celebrating. On the way home, he crashed his car into a tree and was instantly killed. When Cushing got the news, he was in the hospital on a Saturday, ready to start his first case of the day. Instead of collapsing in grief in a pool of tears or rescheduling his case for another day, he stepped into the operating theater and completed his surgery. Only then did he depart for New Haven to claim his son's body.

Cushing's other son, Henry, dropped out of Yale after failing several classes and never returned, suffering some sort of nervous breakdown,

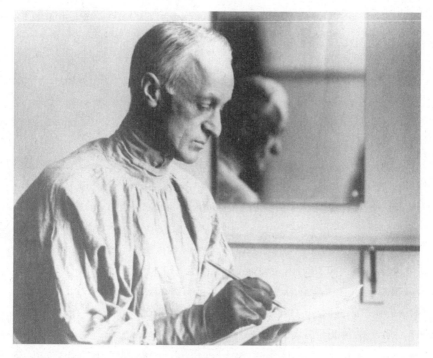

Cushing documenting the results of one of his operations.
The Chesney Archives of Johns Hopkins Medicine, Nursing, and Public Health

although he eventually recovered and went on to a successful business career. Cushing's three daughters, on the other hand, fared much better. Known as the "fabulous Cushing sisters," they married into enormous wealth, the six husbands between the three of them including an Astor, a Whitney, a Roosevelt, a Mortimer, and William S. Paley, the founder of CBS. One might imagine that their mother raised them to seek out men with enough money and time to focus attention on their marriages. When the relationships became loveless, the girls, unlike their mother, moved on.

Cushing's uncompromising personality traits also made him quite unpopular with his staff. In Bliss's words, Cushing "reduced nurses to tears and residents to nervous breakdown with his scorn and sarcasm." One of his famous students, Percival Bailey, who went on to become the head of neurosurgery and neurology at the University of Chicago, euphemistically described Cushing as having a "tart tongue."*

Today, Cushing's behavior with his staff would not be tolerated by hospital administrators; he would no doubt be sent directly to a mandatory anger management class. Somewhat surprisingly, while he could be cold and clinical with colleagues, Cushing was beloved by his patients for his warm bedside manner.

Cushing was not without other faults as well and was subject to the prevailing anti-Semitic prejudices of his times. "I have no objection to Hebrews," he wrote, "but I do not like too many of them all at once." That said, his feelings did not prevent him from training one particularly brilliant Jewish neurosurgeon, Leo Davidoff, who would go on to place his stamp on literally every Jewish medical institution in New York City. Despite his humble beginnings as the son of a Latvian shoemaker, Davidoff attended Harvard College and Harvard Medical School, followed by a residency at the Peter Bent Brigham Hospital in Boston, where he studied under Cushing. During a long and distinguished career, Davidoff led the departments of neurosurgery at the Jewish Hospital of Brooklyn, Montefiore Hospital in the Bronx, and Mount Sinai Hospital and Beth Israel in Manhattan before founding the Albert Einstein College of Medicine in the Bronx. Cushing, in a letter of recommendation, described Davidoff as "a very un-Hebraic Hebrew"—by which he presumably meant high praise.

On the other hand, in response to Hitler's atrocities, Cushing secured positions for Jewish physicians escaping Nazi persecution. He even placed his name on the letterhead of the Emergency Committee in Aid of Foreign

---

*Bailey was quite critical of Cushing's personality, which he documented in his essay "Pepper Pot," delivered in a lecture to the Chicago Literary Club but never published. Bailey tried to publish this essay in his autobiography, *Up from Little Egypt.* He elected not to include it after a copy was sent to Cushing's daughters, who threatened to sue Bailey if it were ever published. Supposedly, a copy of the text can be found in the club's archives at the Newberry Library, Chicago. Paul C. Bucy, "Percival Bailey," in the *National Academy of Sciences of the United States, Biographical Memoirs: Volume 58* (Washington, DC: National Academy Press, 1989).

Displaced Physicians, whose mission was to relocate Jewish refugee physicians and scientists—proof yet again of the complexity of the human psyche, our divided selves, and, yes, even the brain's mysteries. We are all capable of being both Dr. Jekyll and Mr. Hyde, depending upon the context, Cushing no less than anyone else.

Any contemporary neurosurgeon would jump at the chance to travel back in time to witness a Cushing operation. "Watching Cushing operate," one of his biographers wrote, "was like watching Freud analyze a patient . . . or the Pope saying mass." Fortunately, several of his students were able to document the experience, leaving behind a video of his 2,000th brain tumor operation, done on April 15, 1931. The patient was Ida Herskowitz, a thirty-one-year-old woman from New York whom he cured of a pituitary tumor. The gift bestowed upon him by his staff to commemorate this momentous occasion was a silver cigarette case, supposedly containing 2,000 cigarettes, one for each tumor he had removed.

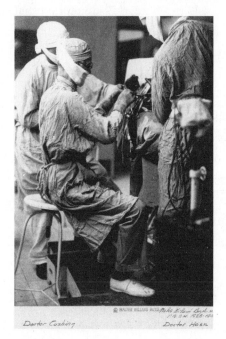

Cushing removing his two thousandth brain tumor on April 15, 1931.

Medical Historical Library, Harvey Cushing/ John Jay Whitney Medical Library, Yale University

Cushing worked in an operating theater with an assistant resident, surrounded by a crowd of observers seated on a mobile balcony, which could be pivoted from one spot to another to provide the best view. One of his residents recalled the experience:

Cushing's operating room was a silent place. He used a set of hand signals to indicate the instrument he wanted, the thumb and forefinger pinched for a scalpel, an open palm with a twist of the wrist for the needle holder, rapid motion of two fingers for scissors, and so forth. . . . A Cushing operation was exasperatingly slow. . . . Through all of these long hours, Cushing seemed impervious to fatigue, the athlete showing his trim.

Another student, who began to nod off while holding a retractor during one of Cushing's long operations, recalls receiving the admonition that Cushing often delivered: "Eyes on the ball!"

In addition to founding the field of neurosurgery, Cushing identified what is now known as the Cushing reflex, when blood pressure rises and heart rate lowers in the face of mounting intracranial pressure, as well as Cushing's disease, a disorder of the pituitary gland in which a small tumor secretes high quantities of steroids. Cushing's name has graced a U.S. warship, a postage stamp, and a neurosurgical society: the Harvey Cushing Society, the largest American neurosurgical professional society today, later renamed the American Association of Neurological Surgeons. In his spare time he penned the definitive biography of his teacher Sir William Osler, for which he won a Pulitzer Prize. Ironically, and perhaps unfairly, the father of modern neurosurgery never won a Nobel Prize in Physiology or Medicine, although he was nominated a startling thirty-eight times.

Cushing's impact on neurosurgery has been so profound that any U.S.-trained neurosurgeon working today can trace their educational lineage straight back to Harvey Cushing with fewer than six degrees of separation.* While Cushing's legacy of excellence weighs heavily on the shoulders of modern neurosurgeons, as it must have weighed on his sons, we also

---

*You can see this diagrammed by going to either neurotree.org and searching "Harvey Williams Cushing" or neurosurgeon.com and searching "Harvey W. Cushing."

benefit from a climate of trust that Cushing did not enjoy. The public today assumes that contemporary neurosurgeons know what they're doing, even when we fail. And unlike Cushing, we are, for the most part, no longer required to be intrepid risk-takers. While neurosurgical training and practice are still time-consuming and emotionally draining, patient outcomes are so dramatically better than they were in Cushing's day that it's now possible to maintain a modicum of work-life balance without risking the depression and drug addiction that was so prevalent during the early days of the field. That said, many of the most difficult brain operations remain fraught with danger. If not performed with expert precision, complications and poor outcomes can become commonplace. Cushing's dedication to his craft and his meticulous operative technique not only formed the cornerstone of our profession but still drives us brain surgeons in the relentless pursuit of perfection.

NO . . . BUT I PLAY ONE ON TV

If you were to stop a random person on the street and ask for the names of the most influential neurosurgeons in the world, my guess is that you would be faced with blank stares. Ask them to name *any* neurosurgeon and you'd probably still hear crickets. Yet Hollywood has created an image of the neurosurgeon that has captured the public's imagination. In typical Hollywood fashion, these fictional caricatures often bear little resemblance to real neurosurgeons. One exception was the Netflix documentary series *Lenox Hill*, which featured two actual neurosurgeons, but these accurate portrayals are rare. Screenwriters mostly latch on to one of the two stereotypes: either brilliant but egotistical renaissance men—White men, more specifically—or sociopathic mad scientists (still mostly White men). Simply put, we are either Harvey Cushing or Victor Frankenstein.

The best examples of the former are Buckaroo Banzai, who, in the film *The Adventures of Buckaroo Banzai Across the 8th Dimension* (1984), was also a test pilot, particle physicist, and rock star. Another is Dr. Steven Strange, who becomes a superhero with mystical powers in Marvel Studio's *Doctor Strange*. But the mad scientist–sociopath stereotype is, unfortunately, the more common of the two. This stereotype includes the racist neurosurgeon in *Get Out* (2017) who keeps his community of White supremacists alive by transplanting their brains into healthy young Black bodies; Dr. Michael Hfuhruhurr in the film *The Man with Two Brains* (1983), another unhinged neurosurgeon obsessed with brain transplantation; and Dr. Hannibal Lecter, who, in the movie *Hannibal* (2001) performs brain surgery on his conscious pursuer and forces him to consume a piece of his own frontal lobe as an hors d'oeuvre.

For the record, although a neurosurgeon named Robert J. White did successfully transplant the head of one animal, a monkey, onto the body of another in 1970 and even managed to keep the head alive for a few hours, this experiment has never been repeated and certainly not tried on humans. As for Lecter's foray into brain surgery, successfully exposing the entire top of the brain and removing the dura, the brain's skin-like covering, would be next to impossible without years of training and an array of fine surgical instruments at hand—particularly for a psychiatrist, which was Lecter's field of expertise. Although some brain surgeries *are* performed on patients who are wide-awake, we use plenty of local anesthesia to make sure they are both numb and comfortable.

The closest Hollywood has come thus far to portraying a neurosurgeon with some semblance of realism was the character of Derek Christopher Shepherd, better known as McDreamy, on the long-running television series *Grey's Anatomy*. In fact, McDreamy (played by Patrick Dempsey) may be the most widely recognized neurosurgeon in America. Moreover, many of the surgeries performed by him, while somewhat sensationalized, were also fairly accurate, due to the script consulting by Dr. Steve Gianotta, the chair of neurosurgery at the University of Southern California (USC).

McDreamy follows the Harvey Cushing model of a neurosurgeon: smart, compassionate, and tirelessly devoted to his patients, but also tough and completely uncompromising. Yet, in contrast to Cushing's cold Puritan demeanor, he's also sensitive and considerate. We can also thank

McDreamy for adding "sex symbol" to the image of neurosurgeons. (One of my young female patients, upon emerging from anesthesia, once asked if McDreamy was still in the room. Sure, she was drugged and had no idea what she was saying, but, hey, I'll take it.)

The public's fascination with brain surgeons reflects the ongoing mystery about what it is we really do. Another show about neurosurgeons, *3 lbs.*, aired in 2006. It featured Stanley Tucci playing the brilliant but arrogant neurosurgeon Dr. Douglas Hanson, who was forced to work for the younger, more sensitive neurosurgeon Dr. Jonathan Seger, played by Mark Feuerstein. Feuerstein and I went to the same high school, so he called me up and asked if he could follow me around for a day to prepare for the role. I'm not sure what it says about my future career as a movie consultant, but the show was canceled after only three weeks.

STILL MOSTLY WHITE MEN

Screen and television writers usually show neurosurgeons as White men, and unfortunately they are not incorrect. As of this writing, only 9 percent of U.S. neurosurgeons are women and a mere 3.8 percent are Black. The number of women entering the field today, while far less than the 53.5 percent of medical school graduates who are female, is, thankfully, rising. Women now represent almost 20 percent of neurosurgery residents currently in training, a rapid upward trajectory that is expected to reach 30 percent by the year 2030. Black trainees still constitute less than 5 percent of the neurosurgery resident pool.

The first female neurosurgeon in the United States, Dr. Dorothy Klenke Nash, finished her training at Columbia's Neurological Institute of New York in 1928. She remained the only female neurosurgeon for the next thirty-two years! It wasn't until 1961 that the first woman received board certification in neurosurgery. Her name was Ruth Kerr Jakoby. It would take another twenty years for the United States to certify its first African American female neurosurgeon, Dr. Alexa Canady. In fact, the numbers are so far from where they should be that Johns Hopkins did not admit its first female Black neurosurgery resident into its training program until 2017.

Neurosurgery also has its own Rosalind Franklin, who, as you may recall, played a critical but unappreciated role in the discovery of DNA alongside James Watson and Francis Crick. In 1915, Harvey Cushing hired an editorial assistant named Louise Eisenhardt to help him write his papers. When Cushing went off to Europe during the First World War, Eisenhardt first put the finishing touches on Cushing's landmark acoustic neuroma monograph, and then enrolled in Tufts Medical School. After graduating with the highest grades in the school's history, she studied pathology and then returned to work at Cushing's side.

Over the remainder of Cushing's career, he and Eisenhardt were inseparable. She kept meticulous records of all his cases, coauthored his papers, and became the curator of his Brain Tumor Registry, including all 2,000 specimens currently housed at Yale. She was elected the first woman president of the Harvey Cushing Society in 1938 and a few years later became first editor of the *Journal of Neurosurgery*. Emblematic of the time, in 1965, when she gave the first Cushing Oration, the president of the Harvey Cushing Society, Dr. Frank Mayfield, bestowed upon her a paternal kiss on the cheek along with her medal.

In all fairness, Eisenhardt's contributions were never swept under the rug, and she has been appropriately lionized in the annals of neurosurgery for her contributions. That said, within the four walls of the operating room she was still not a surgeon and so not a full card-carrying member of the fraternity. Back then, neurosurgery was still more comfortable keeping women behind the scenes. Indeed, in recognition of her role, Dr. Leo Davidoff, Cushing's Jewish disciple, described Eisenhardt as "the midwife for modern scientific neurosurgery." In his eyes, while she may have stood on the field, she was more a cheerleader than a player.

As for Black men, they entered the field slightly earlier than White women, but their path was by no means easier. For the most part, Blacks were forced to acquire their training outside the United States. Three of the first four male African American neurosurgeons received their education in Canada at the Montreal Neurological Institute, since opportunities for minorities in the United States were scant. In 1953, Dr. Clarence Sumner Greene Sr., neurosurgery's Jackie Robinson, became the first African American neurosurgeon in the United States. After receiving his dental degree from the University of Pennsylvania, Greene practiced for a short time before realizing he would prefer to become a physician. He completed the necessary coursework at Harvard and U Penn and then obtained his MD from Howard University. After finishing his residency in general surgery, Greene was accepted to study under Wilder Penfield, the director of the Montreal Neurological Institute. When he returned to the United States, he became the head of surgery at Howard University, a job he held for only two years before his untimely death from a heart attack.

Although Hollywood has not yet embraced the idea of a minority member or female neurosurgeon as a lead character in a drama, most biographical movies depicting the life stories of real neurosurgeons almost always feature members of underrepresented groups. The storylines generally focus on their remarkable and unlikely paths to success, always highlighting the obstacles these individuals had to overcome to establish themselves in neurosurgery. In a sense, it is precisely *because* they do not fit the stereotype created by the media that their stories are worth telling.

The best known of these rags-to-riches heroes is Dr. Benjamin S. Carson Sr. Born in Detroit in 1951, Carson was raised in poverty by a single, nearly illiterate mother, Sonya, who struggled with mental illness. Despite her limitations, she was a strong-willed disciplinarian who instilled a strict work ethic in her children. Carson went to Yale for college and the University of Michigan for medical school, then trained and worked at Johns Hopkins, rising to become the youngest chief of pediatric neurosurgery in the United States at the time. Carson was recognized for his reinvigoration of two complex neurosurgical procedures: the hemispherectomy, in which half the brain is removed to treat epilepsy, and the separation of conjoined twins linked at the head, a condition known as craniopagus.

Carson's inspiring life story—chronicled in his autobiography, *Gifted Hands*—provides compelling evidence for the possibility of overcoming socioeconomic constraints, systemic racism, and opportunity gaps that plague class fluidity in the United States. Emphasizing the stabilizing role of religion in his life and championing a conservative social platform, Carson went on to write several books, work the lecture circuit, and receive numerous achievement awards. He ran for president in 2016 before serving as the secretary of Housing and Urban Development under President Donald Trump.

Carson fits the mold of the neurosurgeon who has something to prove, who sees neurosurgery as the crowning achievement in a life of perseverance and accomplishment, and whose success against all odds is a testament to the enduring promise of the American Dream. At the same time, whether Carson's story is an example of the possibility for social mobility in the United States or a rare exception to its inherent constraints remains unclear.

Perhaps even more astounding than Ben Carson's ascent is the story of Alfredo Quiñones-Hinojosa. Dr. Q, as he is better known, was born in Mexicali, Mexico. At nineteen, he crossed the border illegally into the United States, where he worked as a migrant laborer picking tomatoes and sleeping in his car. Teaching himself English and attending night classes, he managed to obtain a scholarship to UC Berkeley, where he graduated with honors. Dr. Q went on to Harvard Medical School and then neurosurgery training at UC San Francisco. After spending a decade as a professor of neurosurgery at Johns Hopkins, where he overlapped with Carson, he was named the chief of neurosurgery at the Mayo Clinic in Jacksonville, Florida. Using the platform of his memoir, *Becoming Dr. Q: My Journey from Migrant Farm Worker to Brain Surgeon*, he, like Carson, has leveraged his life story to become an inspirational speaker and has received numerous awards for his achievements.

Dr. Q's story, also featured in the Netflix documentary *The Surgeon's* ᵃᵃ3ᵃ

Cut, is exhibit A in the undocumented immigrant debate—namely, their often unjustly thwarted potential to contribute to American society if given an opportunity to take advantage of our educational system. Both Carson and Quiñones-Hinojosa see neurosurgery as the ultimate achievement in a hard-knocks life story of self-reliance and enterprise.

As long as we're on the topic of neurosurgeons who've overcome obstacles, I would be remiss not to mention Dr. Karin Muraszko. Muraszko was born with a form of spina bifida, Latin for "split spine," which left her with limited mobility in her legs, one being a few inches shorter than the other. At age five she spent a year in a body cast, after which she endured several surgeries to correct her uneven legs. Nevertheless, she was able to graduate from Yale University and then Columbia Medical School.

When she walked into the office of the chief of neurosurgery at the Neurological Institute of New York in 1981 for her interview, she stood four feet nine inches tall and was wearing a leg brace and a built-up shoe. Dr. Bennett M. Stein, the chief at the time, while somewhat skeptical about her ability to complete the training, saw something in this woman's will to succeed that compelled him to give her a chance. Not only was she disabled, but she was the first woman ever accepted into the program. She completed the residency and in 2005 became the first female chair of the neurosurgery department at an American medical school, the University of Michigan.

Muraszko sees her disability as a challenge, not a barrier. Her accomplishments have inspired generations of woman, not to mention those with disabilities, to consider neurosurgery as a career despite its reputation for being a physically grueling, male-dominated field. Eventually requiring a wheelchair, in 2022 she stepped down from the leadership position she had held in Michigan for seventeen years. One of her primary goals as chief had been to create a culture of mentorship, and one of her most prominent trainees was none other than CNN's Dr. Sanjay Gupta. He was so inspired by her that he profiled her in 2016 on CNN. When he asked her which has been more difficult, being a woman neurosurgeon or having a disability as a surgeon, she didn't hesitate: "Being a woman was more difficult."

Gupta faced fewer challenges during his career but has become arguably the most widely recognized neurosurgeon of our era. He was born into
an Indian family and attended college and medical school at the University
of Michigan. During his neurosurgery training, Gupta nurtured his interest in politics by working as a White House fellow under Hillary Clinton
when she was first lady. Although he still practices at Grady Memorial Hospital in Atlanta, he is best known as the chief medical correspondent
for CNN.

Ironically, Gupta is well-known precisely because he does *not* focus on
neurosurgery; rather, he reports on broad medical issues with wide public
appeal. (Named one of the sexiest men alive by *People* magazine in 2003,
Gupta is the closest one of us neurosurgeons has gotten to becoming a real-
life McDreamy.)

Another real neurosurgeon whose story captured the imagination of the
American public was neither a minority nor a woman. Dr. Christopher
Duntsch, a White male, was featured in the podcast and series *Dr. Death*
and filled the stereotype of the mad scientist prototype. After completing
an MD-PhD at the University of Tennessee, Duntsch managed to finish his
neurosurgical training with the bare minimum amount of required operative experience. While most U.S. residents participate in several thousand
operations over the course of their training, Duntsch scrubbed in to far
fewer.

Duntsch advertised himself as a spinal surgery expert and began working out of a few small hospitals in Texas where there was little to no oversight. Within a few short years he was responsible for the deaths or
permanent paralysis of at least thirty-three patients, crimes for which he
is currently serving a life sentence in prison—the first time a physician has
ever been convicted on criminal charges based on medical treatments.
Duntsch was, by all accounts, a sociopath. His story terrifies us because it
not only challenges the trust that patients place in their physicians but un-
dermines our faith in medical degrees and titles. Clearly, just because a

trained doctor has been dubbed a neurosurgeon does not mean he or she necessarily possesses the healing and empathic qualities we normally attribute to that label.

The good news is that it's almost unheard-of for a patient to die in the operating room under the care of a neurosurgeon. The only exception to this rule is when a patient arrives with a devastating disease or potentially fatal injury for which their chance of survival is already extremely low, regardless of the experience and skill of the surgeon. The reality is that, while most neurosurgeons are not Harvey Cushing, neither are we Christopher Duntsch.

Then, who are we?

TWO

THE TRAINING

B efore we untangle what it's like to be a brain surgeon, it will be important, first, to understand what it takes to become one. What motivates
a medical student to embark on a neurosurgical career, knowing that
the training is grueling, the time commitment intense, and the hours
long, even after all the schooling is complete? While every kid with a dream
of becoming a neurosurgeon has their own story, I've seen a few common
themes emerge.

Many choose neurosurgery because they become fascinated with the
nervous system and want to gain a greater understanding of the inner
workings of the brain. The workload, to this group, is not intimidating.
They've been grinding away for years in their science classes, even dedicat-
ing extra hours working in a laboratory. Some acquire PhDs along the way.
These often combine neurosurgery with research and hope to contribute
to the field by developing new techniques or devices for operating on the
brain. These are the Urkels (à la *Family Matters*) or the Sheldons (à la *Big
Bang Theory*), who probably watched a lot of *Star Trek* along the way.

The second group are more socially adept and outgoing. These are the
athletes or class leaders who are drawn to the difficulty of neurosurgery.
The required manual dexterity is a technical challenge like any athletic

competition on which they thrive. The length of the surgeries, which often extend late into the night, requires a certain degree of physical stamina, which doesn't intimidate them. On the contrary, these type A personalities see neurosurgery as an honorable profession that will provide them with the same kind of ego gratification as winning the big game. This group is often a bit more narcissistic but no less conscientious or competent. A subgroup of these are the musicians, who are used to training for years to attain technical proficiency and see neurosurgery as a way to redirect their dexterity from instrument to body. To them, surgery itself is a type of performance, a concerto that needs to be executed perfectly from start to finish.

Another type are the Boy and Girl Scouts who always did the right thing, made their parents proud, and were told from a young age that they were special and could accomplish anything with hard work and grit. Some strivers—alas, too few—are women claiming their rightful footholds or ethnic minorities or immigrants who might even have been the first in their family to go to college, let alone medical school. They want to plant a flag.

Some have had a family member, either a parent or a sibling, who's been diagnosed with a tumor or an aneurysm and undergone an operation. Perhaps their relative's life was saved, and in their gratitude they want to pay it forward. In some cases the tumor may have won and they're determined to dedicate their lives to improving neurosurgical care for others. In other cases they're the child or grandchild of a neurosurgeon who spent many a weekend following their mother or father on hospital rounds or listened to stories over the dinner table. For these doctors, neurosurgery is a way to connect with a parent who was both an inspiration but also may not have been as present as they wished during their childhood.

My own story is not atypical. I grew up on the Upper West Side of Manhattan in a Jewish household with my older brother, who was more the athlete and rebel to my more cerebral, conformist personality. The son of a Freudian psychoanalyst and a Holocaust survivor, I was very much a product of my environment. From my father, I soon began to realize that there was a lot going on in the brain about which we are unaware, and that these un-conscious processes can have a profound influence on how we think, feel, and behave. My mother's war experiences, rarely discussed, lent an air of gravity to my childhood, a sense that no matter how well things were go-ing, tragedy lurked around every corner. Perhaps her insecurity gave me the sense that I should never be complacent at any point in my training or career.

In high school, I played on the football team, but my real passion was music. After starting out on piano and then saxophone, I settled on bass guitar and spent hours practicing and studying the instrument. Did years of rapidly running my fingers up the bass fretboard help me manipulate instruments deep in the brain? Sure. Maybe. If I were to fit myself into one of the neurosurgery stereotypes, I'd say I'm mostly a musician, with a side of athlete, a dash of striver, and a pinch of nerd sprinkled on top. And, yes, I watched a lot of *Star Trek*.

One morning during high school, while walking to the bus stop after a snowstorm, I saw a woman struggling to extricate her car from its parking spot near the curb. The vehicle had been completely boxed in by a recently plowed wall of snow. Her wheels were spinning hopelessly. The slush was spitting in all directions. A fellow bystander tried to help by pushing the car from behind, so I ran over to do the same. After a few concerted and coordinated heaves, we managed to free her car, and she went on her merry way with a quick wave and shout of thanks.

I remember the feeling afterward, the emotional high of helping a stranger. For the first time I felt useful, purpose-driven, which during the self-involved teen years of high school was a refreshing departure. I knew at that moment that I wanted to pursue a career that would allow me to help others in need. But I never could have imagined at the time that this epiph-any might propel me into a career as a neurosurgeon, a path that would not only test my will but provide me with challenges on almost every level—emotional, physical, mental, and psychological. I also never could have imagined that I would someday be shouldering the burden of taking care of both of my parents, many of my friends, and even my friends' parents, all of whom would fall prey to a variety of different neurological ailments over the ensuing years. But I am getting ahead of myself and this story.

THE SCHOOLING

Despite my grandmother's insistence since I was a child that I was destined to become a doctor, when I arrived at college I declared astrophysics as my major, which was more in line with my own childhood dream of becoming an astronaut. After briefly exploring the solar system via an introductory astronomy seminar, I soon realized that my ability to achieve a high score on the math SAT did not translate into an agility with the convoluted equations of rudimentary theoretical astrophysics. I quickly abandoned my celestial ambitions and changed my major to a dual concentration in philosophy and English literature.

While I enjoyed my sojourn in the humanities, I ultimately fell back on my family trade, completed the premed requirements, and went off to medical school determined to become a doctor of some sort. Neurosurgery—or any kind of surgery, for that matter—was not even remotely on my radar. Then one day, during the neuroanatomy module taught by a female neurosurgery resident—the term "resident" derives from the fact that back in the days of Cushing, they literally lived in the hospital—we were learning about the anatomy of the cranial nerves: which ones move the eyes, which control the pupils, which are for hearing, and which move the face. After reviewing each in detail, she then described a patient scenario to see if we could figure out what was going on, based on what we had just learned.

A young girl is in a car accident. Her head hits the dashboard. She has a contusion on her scalp to prove it. She rolls into the ER unconscious. You shine a light in her eyes and see that her right pupil is bigger than the left.

"Quick!" she urged. "What do you do? She'll die unless you act!"

What could make the pupil dilate like that? The answer was that there must be a blood clot enlarging somewhere in her skull that was pushing on her brain, which, in turn, must be affecting the nerve that controls the pupil. The solution was to rapidly drill a hole in the girl's skull to release the clot. But where was the clot? And where do you put the hole? There was no time to get a CAT scan, and the patient's fate would be determined in the next few minutes if you didn't do anything. So we had to figure it all out based on the anatomy we'd just learned.

If you'd been paying attention in class, you could save her life. If you'd dozed off when the instructor was reviewing the location of the presumably torn middle meningeal artery and the nerve that regulates the size of the pupil, she was gone. This experience was an adrenaline rush for someone like me, who had spent the last four years squirreled away in a library, studying esoteric theories of philosophy. I remember thinking, *So neurosurgeons can save people's lives in an instant, based on knowledge they acquired from books and skills they develop through practice?* I had no idea such a field existed.

I was immediately intrigued but not yet sold. I needed more information before committing to a specialty with a reputation for having the most brutal training, never-ending work hours, and a sky-high divorce rate. I put this thought on the back burner.

My first two years of medical school were mostly spent in a classroom. The next two years we rotated through teaching hospitals, spending time in each of the different medical and surgical specialties for a month or two, shadowing and assisting the residents, and helping them get through their daily mountain of tasks. At this stage, medical students possess little skill and only a superficial knowledge of a smattering of topics. Occasionally, the residents would ask for your help entering orders, transporting patients, placing IVs, and holding retractors in the operating room. You were mostly just in the way. You spent 30 percent of your time trying to absorb new information and the remaining 70 percent trying to impress everyone enough to get a decent grade, which might boost your chances of landing a residency spot of your own. And we had only sixteen months to figure out what field we wanted to enter before making a lifetime commitment.

I decided to spend a month working on the neurosurgery service at

Massachusetts General Hospital, or MGH. By that time I had read a bit about neurosurgery, but I had never actually worked alongside a neurosurgeon to see if the myths in magazines and books matched the reality. I was not disappointed. The neurosurgery residents there were brilliant, confident, and enthusiastic. They functioned at what seemed like a superhuman pace. Their fingertips and brains were equally nimble, storing not only the requisite muscle memory to perform intricate delicate operations but an encyclopedic knowledge of the vast published literature on neurosurgery. Would it take me three lifetimes to learn what they already knew and could recall at will? I didn't care. I wanted in.

More impressive than the residents were the attendings, the fully trained neurosurgeons, who were the ones primarily responsible for tackling the grueling operations. I spent hours standing—or sitting, if I was lucky enough to find a stool in the corner of the operating room—watching them as they stood hunched forward over the spotlighted operative field, working on the human brain with both intense concentration and finger movements so subtle, it looked as if their hands were barely moving. The anatomy was so fine that the critical portions of the surgeries were performed under an operating microscope. Perched atop motorized chairs specifically designed for microsurgery, their arms resting on cushioned extensions to reduce tremors, these neurosurgeons reminded me of the astronaut heroes of my childhood, cradled in the cockpits of their starships. Only they were venturing into the remote microcosm of the human brain.

I was so enthralled with the experience that I brought my camera into the operating room to capture these first moments of discovery.

I was terrified that I didn't have the right stuff: the stamina, the precision, the cool-under-pressure intelligence, and nerve. Perhaps even a bigger problem was that standing in the operating room was brutal on my back. I could hardly last for twenty minutes standing still. How was I supposed to train myself to stand for five or six hours at a stretch? I tried eating with chopsticks in my left hand to hone my dexterity. I began noticing

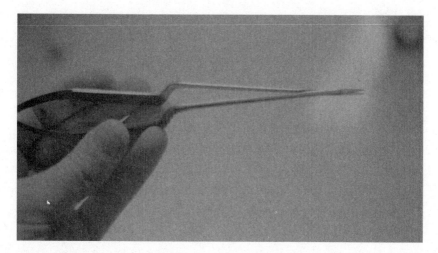

As a medical student, I took a photograph of the first time I held a neurosurgical micro-scissors.

Courtesy of the author

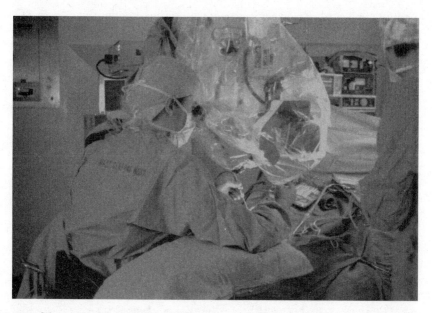

One of the Massachusetts General Hospital neurosurgery residents sitting in the oper-ating chair with his arms supported, working under the microscope.

Courtesy of the author

small tremors in my fingers and questioned if I would have to forgo coffee for the rest of my life: a nonstarter.

But despite these misgivings, by the conclusion of my monthlong rotation, I had made my decision. I was going to become a neurosurgeon. It was the whole gestalt that convinced me: the extraordinary challenge, the intensity of the work, the life-and-death stakes, my interest in the brain and how it worked, the commitment, the respect I would command, and the impact I could have. At this point, I couldn't imagine doing anything else.

"We thought you were going to be a pediatrician!" my mother lamented in disappointment.

During my first surgery rotation, I spoke with Dr. Paul S. Russell, a legendary transplant surgeon at MGH. He was the chief of surgery from 1962 to 1968 and director of the transplantation unit from 1968 to 1990. We were in a small group, just a few medical students with Dr. Russell, and we were expected to ask questions. Facing my own fork in the road, I asked him how he had dealt with the sacrifices required of his demanding career. His calm, direct answer was so perfect, it stuck with me to this day. "Ted," he said, "it's simple. If you want people to depend on you, you have to be dependable."

That was it. I repeated it in my head for good measure. *If you want people to depend on you, you have to be dependable.* Would it be inconvenient? Probably. Would it interrupt other aspects of my life? I imagined so. But would it be worth it in the end? I had to believe it would. I wanted people to depend on me. So I would have to become dependable.

LET THE GAMES BEGIN

Once a medical student has overcome the psychological hurdle of selecting neurosurgery as their career choice, the chance of earning a spot is surprisingly not so difficult. Every year, roughly 35,000 medical students apply for 5,000 medical and surgical residency positions. In neurosurgery, there are only 400 applicants applying for 230 spots. In other words, neurosurgery, while clearly competitive, given the small number of open positions, is also self-selecting, given the remarkably small number of applicants. The biggest challenge is to find a position in the program, or even the geographic area, where you want to live. Each of the approximately 100 training programs offers only two or maybe three positions, so if you have your heart set on one hospital in a specific city, you are competing with 400 highly qualified people for only a few spots. The training then lasts six to seven years after the requisite four years of medical school.

Positions in medical and surgical training programs are allocated yearly based on an antiquated, *Hunger Games*–type system called "the Match." Each applicant parades from program to program for a nerve-wracking day of mandatory in-person interviews with the neurosurgery attendings.* Given the limited number of available spots, the average candidate applies to multiple programs; ten to fifteen is the norm. I remember, not very fondly, my own residency interviews. At one program the interviewer handed me a needle and thread, counting the number of failed attempts as I tried to pass it through.

At another interview, the surgeon looked down at my résumé, then up at me, and said, "You went to Harvard College and Harvard Medical School, so you're probably a wimp.† How do we know you can handle the work?" The truth is, neurosurgery is, at its core, a very blue-collar occupation. Don't get me wrong: there's nothing blue-collar about the average salaries, but neurosurgery is *not* a desk job; if you are not willing to get your hands dirty—and I mean *really* dirty—it's not the career for you. It's not a coincidence we change into scrubs to do our work. Like a mechanic, whose blue coveralls get covered in grease and grime, we often leave the OR covered in blood, Betadine, and bits of brain.

---

*Since the COVID-19 pandemic, virtual interviews replaced in-person ones, but this is slowly shifting back.

†The interviewer didn't actually use the word "wimp." He chose a more vulgar word that I altered to avoid offending anyone. You can use your imagination.

At the end of the interview process, applicants rank each training program in order of preference, and the programs do the same with the applicants; then a computer algorithm matches applicants with spots. As we say to our kids: you get what you get, and you don't get upset. It was disconcerting that the next seven years of my life would be spent in a city not directly of my choosing. Thus began the process of giving up control. No longer would I decide where I lived, when I ate my meals, what I wore, when I slept, or with whom I would spend my waking hours.

While the lifestyle of a neurosurgeon is demanding, it's the reputation of the residency training that strikes fear into the hearts of most medical students and probably winnows the neurosurgery applicant pool as much as any other factor. One tale, possibly apocryphal, described an esteemed member of the Harvard Medical School faculty who, as a resident, spent one hundred consecutive days in the hospital before returning home. His wife, a few weeks into her hundred days of solitude, apparently grew so frustrated that she left him but then, feeling guilty, returned a few weeks later. When the resident finally arrived home, he was completely unaware of his near divorce, thinking his wife had simply been there the whole time.

I placed the Neurological Institute of New York, the program affiliated with Columbia University, at the top of my rank list because I figured at least if I ended up in New York, I could spend what little free time I would have with my family and friends. My parents were also getting older, and who knew what the future held for them? It was, in my opinion, the best training program in the city at the time, and I had already spent a month there as a medical student, so they knew I was interested.

Established in 1909 and originally located on New York's Upper East Side, before moving to its current location on 168th Street and Fort Washington Avenue, the Neurological Institute of New York held a storied place in the history of neurosurgery. The first freestanding building and institute in the United States devoted entirely to treating disease of the nervous system, its founding neurosurgeon, Dr. Charles Elsberg, was one of the first surgeons after Harvey Cushing to dedicate their surgical practice uniquely to neurosurgery. I was thrilled when the letter arrived in the mail stating that I had matched at Columbia, and I spent the summer mentally preparing for what was to come.

SKULL'S ANGELS

In the March 1989 issue of *Rolling Stone*, Steve Fishman published an article entitled "Skull's Angels," in which he described the brutality of the NYU neurosurgery training program and the grit and determination required to succeed. Spending nearly every waking hour in the hospital, the residents were completely isolated from the outside world and often became angry and depressed, receiving little positive feedback from their instructors. Although in some sense a perfect example of why the traditional abusive neurosurgery training system needed to change, for some odd reason I found the piece inspiring.

The number of hours a resident worked in the U.S. hospital system when I trained, prior to regulations imposed in 2003, was unrestricted. I was on call every third night and every other weekend, which meant one thirty-six-hour shift, followed by two twelve-hour shifts, and then back to another thirty-six-hour shift. This three-day rotation repeated itself *ad exhausteam*. Like Bill Murray in *Groundhog Day*, I felt stuck in an endless loop: the scream of my alarm clock at 4:30 every morning would jerk me back into the same unremitting predicament from which only sleep provided a brief respite. Every other weekend was spent in the hospital. The on-call room consisted of a single bed, a phone, and bathroom. If you were lucky, housekeeping had cleaned the sheets from the night before.

My first year as a neurosurgery resident was spent rotating through the various surgery services as an intern. I remember my first night on call. I was at dinner in the cafeteria when my beeper emitted its first chirp. I called the number: a new trauma had just rolled into the ER. They needed me right away! I slammed down the phone, leapt out of my chair, and prepared to sprint down to the ER to save my first life before realizing . . . I had no idea how to get to the ER.

I stopped in my tracks and turned sheepishly to a nearby nurse to ask for directions.

I quickly realized that I was about as helpful in emergency situations as I was knowledgeable about the layout of the hospital. In fact, I was dangerous. One afternoon I was paged to a code, which is called when a patient has a sudden change in condition and may require placement of a breathing tube—called intubation—or even chest compressions and a shock to restart the heart. The senior resident in charge, who ran the code, needed to inject a medication into the patient's IV as quickly as possible, and she asked me to retrieve a vial of saline from the pharmacy closet to help flush the drug through. I grabbed what I thought was a small vial of saline, or sodium chloride—salt water to you and me. The resident drew up the solution I handed her and injected it into our patient. Suddenly the patient, who was already pale and weakened but still conscious, looked up and said two words I'll never forget: "Oh my."

Her head dropped and her body slumped forward. Alarm bells rang out, alerting the room to the fact that her heart was no longer beating. I felt as if my heart had stopped as well. I looked down at the vial in my hand and read the words "potassium chloride," an identical-looking fluid in a vial indistinguishable from sodium chloride, except that it had a pink-colored top, not green. When injected in high enough doses, potassium chloride causes instant cardiac arrest. Its reliable deadliness has made it one of the three drugs in the lethal injection used for capital punishment.

Two thoughts immediately crossed my mind. First, I knew I needed to do everything in my power to fix the situation or I could never live with myself. That was priority number one. But I also wasn't sure of the legal ramifications of my medical error or my own personal liability. The push-pull morality play contained in that microsecond was thankfully that—only a microsecond.

I ran over to the senior resident and pulled her aside. I showed her the vial and told her what I had done in the vague hope that this knowledge would allow her to rectify the situation. She looked me directly in the eye, took the vial out of my hands, and said, "Don't tell anyone what you just told me." She then ran back over to the patient and saved her life.

It was a defining moment, one I will never forget and one which I have never shared until now. I also learned a valuable lesson: When in doubt, always put the patient's health and safety first in your mind and the rest will sort itself out. Whether hiding my error was appropriate or unethical was not my main concern at that moment, since I had been given a direct order by the senior resident who had just prevented me from suffering the psychological burden of committing an unpardonable sin—a result of my own incompetence.

Live and learn. Hopefully without inadvertently killing anyone.

In 2001, Britain's National Health Service created their own National Patient Safety Agency to guard against inadvertent medical errors like the one I had made. Their first directive? An alert on the handling and storage of potassium chloride, due to the frequency of medical errors committed from accidental administration. I guess I wasn't the first person to make that mistake.

Was it possible that lack of sleep was the cause of my medication error? Or was it my inexperience? Or something else? Back in the early '80s, there was a strong push to limit resident work hours based on the tragic death of Libby Zion in the Cornell emergency room. Zion, the daughter of a lawyer and a *New York Times* correspondent, had been administered two medications that when given together can lead to a fatal reaction. Sidney Zion, her father, sued the hospital and the residents taking care of her, claiming that they were too tired after thirty-six hours on call to make coherent decisions. They were eventually exonerated when, in court, six prominent medical doctors all testified that they, too, were unaware of the rare interaction. Not letting the truth get in the way of a good story, the case led to the passage of national resident work hour restrictions called the Libby Zion Law.

In my opinion, neither of these two errors—mine or the death of Libby Zion—were due to sleep deprivation, and to make that claim is pure revisionist history. Yes, more sleep for residents is a positive thing, but in both my error and the Libby Zion case, the root causes were system-wide errors. In the latter, residents were expected to recognize a rare drug interaction unknown to six prominent chairs of medical departments. Today, hospital computer systems raise alerts if anyone tries to give these two drugs in combination. As for my error, I had fallen into a common trap unintentionally set for me by the hospital: storing a deadly fluid next to and in a similar container as salt water. Now potassium chloride has its own unique label and sits in a locked cabinet, requiring two signatures for removal.

Once my internship was completed, I became a junior resident in neurosurgery, and my primary responsibility was caring for patients before and after surgery. Rather than clipping aneurysms, removing tumors, and reconstructing the spine, we spent most of our time drawing blood, replacing dislodged IVs, and refilling orders for stool softeners. Maybe Luke had to clean Yoda's toilets at the beginning of his Jedi training, but they never showed that part in the movies. Moreover, the sound of my beeper was beginning to feel less like the Bat-Signal and more like a car alarm.

On occasion the senior residents would regale us with stories from the operating room, about the amazing cases they had witnessed and were beginning to learn how to perform. These tales of adventure sustained us and provided just enough hope that life would get better so we wouldn't quit. Although drug abuse is reportedly higher in doctors, I witnessed none of that in our program. Divorces, sadly, yes, and one unfortunate and deeply unhappy resident eventually took his own life many years later. (The suicide rate for male physicians is 40 percent greater than the general population, and for women it's 130 percent greater!)

Looking back, the work we did at the time that seemed menial and tedious and below our pay grade was, in fact, the essence of what it means to serve others and care for the sick. In my exhaustion, I had undoubtedly missed out on chances to truly connect with the patients under my care, human beings who were probably scared, lonely, facing their own mortality and the prospect of several weeks of recovery after surgery. In retrospect, I was too busy feeling sorry for myself—my lack of time, connection with loved ones, sleep, food, showers, etc.—and more concerned with checking the clinical boxes on my to-do list than checking to make sure my patients were emotionally cared for and comforted. To this day, I feel bad about my own youthful neglect of some of those patients. Placing an IV in their arms at 3:00 in the morning was clearly more miserable for them than for me. Perhaps I was experiencing the requisite anguish associated with my transformation into a physician, resentful of the fact that my life was no longer my own, but now devoted to serving the greater good. This seems so obvious to me now. Then, not so much.

But times have changed. Resident work hours are now legally limited to eighty (or a maximum of eighty-eight hours for surgeons) per week. Although it *is* critically important to have the mental and physical wherewithal to perform under pressure at any hour of the night, our brain's ability to consolidate new information and our body's capacity to master mechanical skills require sleep, nutrition, and exercise, at least as much as endless repetition. But still, I don't think that exhaustion leads as much to *medical* errors as it does to *humanistic* ones. It's not a challenge to remember the correct name of a medication or order a CAT scan when you're woken up from a deep sleep. What *is* challenging is to have the patience to sit at someone's bedside, ask them how they are feeling, and grapple with their fears and anxieties when all you want to do is get back in bed for a few hours before the onslaught of the next day begins anew.

Once my first two years of training were complete, my life improved. At long last, it was time to begin learning how to operate.

FEAR OF FLYING

Neurosurgeons learn their trade by operating on living human patients through an iterative process with a gradual increase in responsibility, starting with the simplest, least risky tasks and progressing in complexity. At first, residents work on "the opening" and "the closing," as in opening and closing the skin, muscle, and skull on the way in and out of the brain. Once the brain is exposed, the attending usually takes over and the resident is relegated to watching and assisting. While this might sound terrifying, both to the patient and to the resident, constant oversight and supervision are most definitely part of the package. This goes on for years.

Only near the end of their training will residents be granted permission to work on the brain by themselves, and even then they may not be allowed to perform the more complex or dangerous parts of the operation. Some moves carry such a high risk of calamity if not done perfectly that a resident may never be allowed to attempt them during their training. These riskier moves include peeling a tumor away from the nerve that controls facial movement—which if not done perfectly can lead to facial paralysis— or putting a clip on an aneurysm sitting deep in the brain, whose rupture would result in irreversible paralysis or even death.

In fact, some neurosurgeons may never perform a few of the most vitally delicate maneuvers by themselves until the patient on the table is their responsibility and theirs alone. This makes the first few years of neurosurgical practice—after residency is complete and the training wheels come off—extraordinarily stressful, sometimes even more so than residency itself. While the public doesn't want neurosurgery residents "practicing" on them, they also want surgeons to emerge as fully trained experts—but you can't have it both ways.

What makes neurosurgery different from other skilled professions, such as sports and music, in which prodigies emerge young and careers often peak in one's twenties, is that experience and judgment are far more important than youth and dexterity. Skill certainly plays a role, and there are neurosurgeons whose technical gifts allow them to work faster and more smoothly than others. However, sometimes knowing *what* to do and *when* to do it is more important than being able to do it quickly. Neurosurgery is not a race. The surgeries can routinely take between four and six hours. The ability to anticipate surgery's land mines—to see and understand the anatomy of the brain so well that you know, without having to think, which structures lie hidden around every corner—is key.

You also must know when to slow down and take your time to avoid damaging those nerves and arteries that can sometimes never be repaired once injured.

While there is no proven ideal age for a brain surgeon, let's just say that during the first five years after residency, we are still getting our sea legs. Over time, as with any learned skill, a subtle transition occurs. Suddenly, surgeries seem to take less effort. Movements become second nature as we enter what psychologist Mihaly Csikszentmihalyi called a "flow state," where pursuit of a singular goal creates a transcendental state of purposeful concentration on the task.

On days when I am operating, I may first look at the clock around 10:00 in the morning. The next time I look up, it is already late in the afternoon. I am completely present. The instruments feel indistinguishable from my fingers. The microscope becomes an extension of my eyes. Together, we pivot, zoom, and focus in a smooth and seamless dance. As with yoga, where positions are assumed and held for extended periods of time, neurosurgery requires that we stand or sit for hours on end, hardly moving a muscle. The key is to be both relaxed and alert. This explains how we can operate all day without food or a bathroom break. When my patients ask me how long an operation will take, I give them a very rough idea, but in the end I tell them I don't really know. It will take as long as is required to get the job done right.

But achieving neurosurgical nirvana takes years of practice. Residency is the time when you train your muscles and brain through endless repetition. It takes effort, like rehearsing your scales and arpeggios before improvising a solo. The average neurosurgery resident will assist in 2,000 cases during their seven-year training. In each case they will tie, on average, some 50 knots for a total of 100,000 knots. That's a lot of knots.

Neurosurgeons perform most operations with only two instruments: a suction and a bipolar cautery. One instrument goes in each hand: generally the suction in the left (or nondominant) hand, and the bipolar with the right (or dominant) one. The bipolar is a long, tweezer-like instrument that allows surgeons to pass an electrical current between its tips by stepping on a pedal, instantly charring and cauterizing small vessels or softening hard tumors so they can be removed with the suction. The bipolar was invented in 1940 by neurosurgeon Dr. James Greenwood while he was working at Houston Methodist Hospital. Before this time, the only method of cautery available was the Bovie, the electric scalpel developed with the help of Harvey Cushing. Another neurosurgeon, Dr. Leonard Malis, further refined the bipolar at Mount Sinai Hospital in New York into the device we use today.

The suction, a metal straw with a gentle bend, is grasped in a very specific manner, as a drummer holds a drumstick in the traditional grip between the fingers of their left hand—palm and forearm facing the ceiling, with the working end controlled between the third and fourth fingers. This arrangement puts the thumb over a teardrop-shaped inlet on the top of the suction, which gets closed off to varying degrees to regulate the strength of the vacuum. After years of practice, neurosurgeons become so skilled at rolling their thumbs over this teardrop opening that it becomes second nature.

Although we have other instruments at our disposal, to deploy as needed, these two instruments stay in our hands and essentially become an extension of them for most operations. It may seem surprising that technically complex surgeries can be performed with such simple instruments, but the tools are less critical than the mind and muscles controlling them. Although few neurosurgeons are as talented or visionary as transformative artists, think of what Michelangelo could do with just a hammer and a chisel, or Pablo Picasso with a simple brush and some oil paints.

The other key part of training is learning from failure, a path that is obviously problematic in the context of neurosurgery. One well-known neurosurgeon was once asked how he became so good at his craft. His answer? "There's a graveyard full of my mistakes behind the hospital."

One of my own slipups during residency occurred during the removal of an arteriovenous malformation, a tangle of blood vessels in the brain. Once the mass was removed, a rare view of a remote region of the brain's anatomy suddenly came into view, a sight I can only describe as startlingly beautiful. Though it may seem odd to describe brain anatomy this way, no other words suffice. Operations are like voyages into unknown parts of the natural world, exposing sights rarely seen by other human beings, even other neurosurgeons. There are some anatomical structures in the brain that even an experienced neurosurgeon may have encountered only in textbook illustrations before seeing them for the first time during one of their operations.

Because of this, we often preserve these aurora borealis moments through pictures and videos, which we share with our colleagues as if they were slides from our last family vacation. We do this partly to educate but also partly to show off where we've been and what we've seen. And that's what got me into trouble, as I decided to take a photograph of the image to keep for my records. Back when I was a resident, we didn't have the technology to take digital pictures directly through the microscope the way we can now. We used old-fashioned handheld SLR cameras. I asked the nurse for a new pair of gloves—a third pair—to place over the other two that I normally wear. (We put on two pairs in case one gets torn). My plan was to pick up the camera with this third pair of gloves, shoot the picture, and then discard the camera-contaminated gloves before closing the patient back up again, finishing the case with the remaining two pairs of sterile gloves.

Once I had finished closing the skin, I began to wrap the patient's head in a bandage. At this point I usually take off the outer pair of gloves, which are often smudged with blood, to prevent any staining of the clean white gauze. (I've learned that splotches of blood on a bandage can alarm the family when they first see the patient in the recovery room: they may think there is ongoing bleeding from the head.) I removed my first layer of gloves and then realized, to my horror, that I was still wearing two more pairs. In other words, I had just performed the final closure of the operation wearing a contaminated set of gloves!

The possibility that this patient's wound might get infected and require prolonged antibiotics or even a another operation—and that my inattention might have been the cause—was sickening. At this point the attending surgeon had already left the room and was not aware of my error. Rather than try to hide my mistake, I immediately called him on the phone. Although I knew he'd be frustrated by my oversight, I also knew I had to face up to what had happened and deal with the consequences. My suspicion was correct: he was none too pleased. But, to my surprise, he told me not to do anything about it, hoping that the antibiotics we'd given her before and during the surgery would prevent any future infections.

I thought about it for a moment, and in an act of disobedience decided that if I didn't do everything in my power to prevent an infection, I might look back in regret. If this patient did, in fact, get an infection, it would have weighed heavily on my conscience. I told the nurses we were going to reopen the wound, irrigate it for a few minutes with antibiotic solution, and then re-close it. I was a senior-level resident at that point and was technically capable of doing this safely on my own.

After the fact, I let the attending know what I had done, and he was fine with my decision. Most important, the patient never got an infection, and I learned a valuable lesson, which prevented me from ever making that mistake again.

By the end of my seven years of training, I was more adept and less prone to rookie mistakes. One day, an uninsured immigrant came into the emergency room complaining of a stuffed nose and trouble breathing. He'd been diagnosed with a brain tumor in his home country of El Salvador and told he needed surgery. Rather than having the procedure done there, he got on a plane, flew to New York, and walked into our emergency room. He was in his mid-thirties, with long, straight black hair and a round, trusting face. He spoke no English. His tumor was enormous, filling his entire nasal cavity and extending up into his brain, which was quite swollen from the pressure. Something needed to be done fast. Although he had no insurance, patients were never turned away. Free care is provided this way at hospitals throughout the country. He was scheduled for surgery the next day. I was the chief resident at the time, and I presented the case to the attending on call who specialized in brain tumor operations.

Given the location of the tumor, which sat between the top of the patient's nasal cavity and the bottom of his brain, we elected to take the tumor out using a craniotomy: creating a large opening at the top of his skull. After making an ear-to-ear incision over his head like a tiara, we pulled the skin down, excised the large piece of the bone that makes up the forehead—which would be replaced at the end of the operation—and exposed the brain and the tumor below. Over the course of the next eighteen hours, we extracted the tumor in its entirety.

To this day, it remains the longest operation I've ever done. I think we started at around 1:00 in the afternoon and finished at 7:00 the next morning—just in time to start the next day's work. (As an aside, I can now do this same operation in a fraction of the time without making a single incision, using long, thin endoscopes passed through the patient's nostrils.)

What was also significant about this surgery, beside its length, was that the attending neurosurgeon took me through the operation and sat by my side for the entire eighteen hours. He let me perform what I could of the operation and helped me when I needed assistance. We stayed up all night together, providing this undocumented immigrant with the best we had to offer. The attending who did the case with me gave the gift of his time generously and willingly, not only to help this needy patient, but also to educate me and, in turn, benefit my future patients.

I remain forever grateful to the surgeons who trained me. They ceremoniously handed down the collective wisdom of a hundred years of trial and error that comprise the ever-expanding neurosurgical canon.

Eventually my residency training ended and I was at long last ready to begin my career. I was thirty-three years old.

THREE

PENETRATING HEAD TRAUMA

ead trauma, both blunt and penetrating, remains neurosurgery's bread and butter, in the same way that skateboards and trampolines keep our orthopedic colleagues in business. Traumatic brain injury, or TBI, not only makes up a significant portion of any modern neurosurgeon's on-call responsibilities, but it is the predicament we've historically treated most frequently. The field of neurosurgery owes both its origins and the inspiration for many of its earliest innovations to the management of head trauma.

Early cranial surgery—which generally consisted of making holes in the skull called trephinations—was performed almost solely for the treatment of whacks to the head, whether in the hands of the Incas, the Egyptians, or the Greek founders of modern medicine. Given the generally hostile nature of humankind, the frequency of combat-related injuries throughout history is hardly a surprise. As a result, nearly every neurosurgical pioneer, almost without fail, learned his craft while attending to fallen soldiers on the battlefield.

During neurosurgery training, the few cases in which the junior residents—trainees in the first two years of residency after the internship year—are allowed to participate are mostly head traumas. This is where we start to log the first of our 10,000 hours. Because these surgeries are almost always done on an emergency basis, the attendings—the surgeons in charge—have not met the patients or their families prior to surgery, meaning they have not promised to perform every aspect of the surgery, as we are so often asked to do. More important, the procedures themselves are not that technically complex. For these reasons, the attendings generally let the residents do a bit more than they might during an elective (i.e., scheduled) surgery.

Because these head traumas are often where the junior trainees start to get their hands dirty, this is where we, too, shall begin.

Head trauma can broadly be divided into two categories: penetrating and blunt. Examples of penetrating trauma are arrow injuries, nail gun accidents, and gunshot wounds. Blunt trauma, on the other hand, occurs when your head hits something—the windshield, a wall, pavement—or is bludgeoned by something—a hammer, a rock, or any other object that doesn't pierce the skull, such as a baseball or another helmeted head. In 2021, there were 69,000 TBI-related deaths in the United States. That's 190 a day.

I once operated on a young man who arrived at the emergency room with the handle of a Swiss Army knife sticking out of his head. Swiss Army knives are not that thick or long, yet when jabbed in precisely the right location they can be surprisingly dangerous. The blade had passed through the thinnest part of his skull, just behind the temple, where the bone is only one or two millimeters thick. The knife had gone all the way through, into the left hemisphere of his brain, the tip coming to rest just next to his carotid artery: the blood vessel that supplies oxygen to most of the critical parts of that hemisphere.

Treating this precarious situation was not so straightforward. Simply pulling the knife out would have risked injuring the artery, causing massive fatal bleeding. Instead, we elected to bring him to the OR, put him under anesthesia, and open his skull to expose the tip of the knife so we could remove it under direct observation. How the assailant knew that the bone was so thin in this area, I will never know. It was probably just a fluke.

A few hours later, we had successfully removed the knife without causing any additional brain damage and saved the victim's life. He spent the next few days in the hospital recovering while handcuffed to a gurney with a police officer at his side. I wanted to ask him what had happened. How had the knife ended up in his skull? Whatever the true story was, I was never going to hear it with the officer present. Not surprisingly, once the staples holding his incision together were removed, I never heard from him again.

But despite the occasional misplaced Swiss Army knife, the most common penetrating brain injuries, by far, are those caused by firearms.

CAMELOT LOST

For a brain surgeon, repairing a bullet wound to the head is both messy and inconvenient.

Messy because the skull has been opened haphazardly by the explosive force of the bullet, rather than elegantly, in the refined manner of a fastidious neurosurgeon. This more volatile method for breaching the cranium is also unpredictable, embedding fragments of bone and metal in the soft, spongy brain, which begins to swell, squeezing its way out of the skull in a slimy purple ooze. Very messy.

Inconvenient because people with gunshot wounds to the head invariably crash on the shoals of our emergency rooms in the middle of the night: the witching hours when people with guns often go about their business. When these emergency cases arrive at the hospital, the on-call neurosurgeon will be awakened from a deep sleep with an alert. If the assault occurs during daylight hours, as might be the case for a suicide attempt or an assassination, it's equally inconvenient: a diversion of resources that often interrupts another scheduled operation or a clinic full of patients.

Obviously, the true mess and inconvenience falls upon the victim, who rarely makes it out alive.

THE CASE OF
PRESIDENT JOHN F. KENNEDY

We all know the sad story. On November 22, 1963, John F. Kennedy, the thirty-fifth president of the United States, was traveling with his wife, Jackie, in the back seat of a Lincoln Continental limo with the top down. Three bullets were fired that day and Kennedy's skull was struck by the third. Within five minutes he was rushed to Parkland Memorial Hospital. Despite multiple attempts at resuscitation, he was pronounced dead within seventeen minutes of arrival.

With the possible exception of the assassination of Archduke Ferdinand, which kicked off World War I, JFK's assassination might be the most highly publicized gunshot wound in history, if not the most controversial. It haunts our collective memory, having been captured in Technicolor by bystander Abraham Zapruder on his 8mm home movie camera. We can't forget the look of terror in Jackie's eyes when we first watched her climb out of the back of the car, enveloped in pink, and witnessed as she first caught sight of her husband, Jack, in a jarring juxtaposition of colors, suddenly covered in red.

The event also haunts historians, who must deal with the enormous controversy surrounding the details of the shooting—not only the motivations of the assassin, Lee Harvey Oswald, but also the trajectory of each bullet.

While there are conflicting reports of the damage wrought by the bullet that pierced Kennedy's skull, we will first consider the words of his neurosurgeon, Dr. William Kemp Clark. Kemp, as he was better known, was raised in Dallas. After a surgical internship in Indiana, he served two years in the U.S. Air Force and then completed his neurosurgical training at the Neurological Institute in New York. Dr. Clark returned to Dallas, where he rose to become the chief of the division of neurosurgery at UT Southwestern and chief of neurosurgery at Parkland Memorial Hospital. After briefly assisting with attempts to resuscitate Kennedy, Dr. Clark turned his attention to examining the head wounds. He noted that the wound was in the "right posterior part" of the head and it appeared to be "tangential," meaning it had glanced off the skull rather than penetrating it. He also clearly recalled having seen some cerebellum, the smaller hindbrain that sits just below and behind the cerebrum, protruding from the wound. And this is where the ensuing controversy began.

Dr. Clark's statements that day—(1) no entrance site; (2) protruding cerebellum—contradicted both the autopsy report and the official government-sponsored Warren Commission report, which stated that there was most certainly an entrance wound in the back of the head, in direct line of sight of Oswald's location, and that the damage had occurred to the right occipital, parietal, and temporal bones. There was no mention in the Warren report of damage to the cerebellum, as Clark had claimed, and which lies below the occipital lobe.

The fact that Clark did not find an entrance wound raised suspicion that perhaps the bullet may have come from a different angle, implicating a possible second, yet unidentified shooter. Clark later retracted his original version of the injury, saying that, in retrospect, he must have been mistaken. He must have *overlooked* the entrance site. Once the conspiracy theorists learned of his correction after the fact, they did what conspiracy theorists do: they looked for holes in the story of the holes in the president's head.

To better understand Dr. Clark's confusion regarding the bullet's path, and whether this supports a second-shooter hypothesis, we'll first need to review some basic anatomy of the brain and the skull.

NEUROSURGERY 101

Although we tend to imagine the brain as one homogeneous organ, it is really made up of several different components. The largest part of the brain, which is what we usually think of when using the term, is really the cerebrum, which, in turn, is divided into four lobes, each of which controls different functions. These lobes are the frontal lobe, the parietal lobe, the occipital lobe, and the temporal lobe. Directly below the cerebrum, specifically just below the occipital lobe, lies a smaller sub-brain called the cerebellum. They both have Latin roots: *cerebrum* means "brain"; *cerebellum* means "little brain."

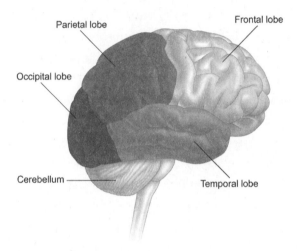

While the smaller cerebellum primarily controls coordination, the four lobes of the cerebrum together are responsible for everything else: movement, touch, hearing, vision, speech, memory, and awareness. The frontal lobe, for example, controls movement and is responsible for short-term memory. On the left side only, the frontal lobe also controls language production. The parietal lobe is critical for sensation, calculation, and, on the right side, visuospatial processing. The temporal lobes process hearing and help store memories. The left temporal lobe also processes language comprehension. Last is the occipital lobe, which has only one function: vision.

Another key concept to grasp—perhaps you remember this from high school biology—is the crossed control by the brain, meaning that the right side of the brain controls the left side of the body and vice versa. For example, the right frontal lobe controls movement of the left side of the body, while the left frontal lobe controls the right side. Equally, the right occipital lobe processes the left field of vision, and the left occipital lobe processes the right side. You get the picture. Or, rather, your occipital lobes are sending neural signals to your right parietal lobe to help you create an image of this phenomenon. Got it?

Now, the skull encasing and protecting the brain, also called the cranium, is not just one solid piece of bone. Rather, it's made up of several bones, each of which is named after the underlying lobe of the brain. So the frontal bone protects the frontal lobe, the parietal bone encases the parietal lobe, the temporal bone overlies the temporal lobe, and—this is important—the occipital bone shelters *both* the occipital lobe *and* the nearby underlying cerebellum.

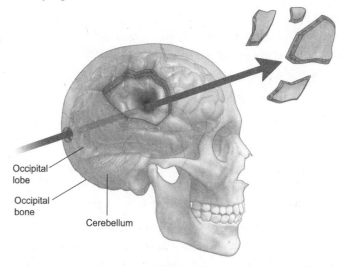

Occipital lobe

Occipital bone

Cerebellum

Artist's rendition of trajectory and damage caused by the bullet as it passed through JFK's skull with the occipital bone and relevant brain lobes designated.

With only this basic anatomical understanding of the largest components of the brain and skull, we already have enough information to make sense of Clark's retracted observations. Since the occipital bone encases both the occipital lobe *and* the cerebellum, which sit right next to each other, it's possible that when Clark saw brain material oozing out of a crack in the occipital bone, he mistakenly thought he was looking at the cerebellum, when in fact it was the occipital lobe. Clark's error, made in the heat of the moment in a crowded trauma room, doesn't necessarily prove there was a conspiracy. More likely it reflects the fact that bruised and bloody brain tissue, whether coming from the cerebellum or the occipital lobe, looks pretty much the same: like purple mush. Bottom line? Clark never saw oozing cerebellum, since the bullet passed just above this part of the brain, through the adjacent occipital lobe.

But what about the missing entrance site in the occipital bone? How do we reconcile that oversight? As it turns out, Clark was not the only neurosurgeon present on that fateful day as JFK rolled into trauma room 1 at Parkland Memorial Hospital. Dr. Robert Grossman, a second neurosurgeon, six months out from his residency also at the Neurological Institute in New York, was in attendance. He was standing right next to Dr. Clark, a well-trained eyewitness, yet his testimony was never taken, his expert account never considered—neither by the Warren Commission nor by any of the subsequent government investigations.

In 2003, exactly forty years after the assassination, Grossman published an article in *The Journal of Neurosurgery,* documenting exactly what he saw.

According to Grossman, both he and Clark clearly identified a small wound in the occipital region consistent with an entry site. He wrote, "Kemp and I lifted [JFK's] head to inspect the occiput. There was a laceration approximately 1 inch in diameter located close to the midline of the cranium, approximately 1 inch above the external occipital protuberance." Not only did Grossman confirm the existence of an entry site; he also described its location *above* the occipital protuberance, which is important because the cerebellum lies well below this landmark.

Grossman was puzzled why Clark would leave this critical piece of information out of his testimony. Clark's hypothesis had been that the bullet had hit the head tangentially, essentially grazing it, since he couldn't locate an entrance wound. Grossman, on the other hand, was positive that there'd been an entrance site in the occipital region, which confirms that the bullet passed *through* the head from a posterior trajectory, and that Oswald acted alone. His recall of the facts not only supports the findings of the Warren Commission but also eliminates any whiff of controversy. As for whether they saw cerebellum or not, Grossman confirmed that Clark "must have mistaken macerated brain for cerebellum."

So all the facts line up. As far as I'm concerned: case closed.

SIC SEMPER TYRANNIS

In the same way we can reexamine JFK's assassination through the lens of neurosurgery and learn a few facts about the brain along the way, it's helpful to revisit Abraham Lincoln's as well. But first, the story:

THE CASE OF
ABRAHAM LINCOLN

On April 14, 1865, John Wilkes Booth entered Ford's Theatre in Washington, DC, and shot Abraham Lincoln, the sixteenth president of the United States, in the back of the head. Booth then jumped down onto the stage, held up a dagger and yelled, *"Sic semper tyrannis!"*—"Thus always to tyrants!" Although he broke his leg during his leap, Booth managed to escape the theater. A few minutes later, Dr. Charles A. Leale, a twenty-three-year-old surgeon, attended to Lincoln, who was still alive at the time although the right side of his body was already paralyzed. He was later cared for by Dr. Charles S. Taft, a physician who happened to be attending the performance that evening, but little could be done, given the limited abilities of surgeons at the time. He passed away several hours later, at 7:22 the next morning, roughly nine hours after the shooting.

These are the known facts. They are part of history and the public record. But as a neurosurgeon, I'm interested in the path the bullet took through Lincoln's skull and brain, and the many hours he managed to stay alive.

The bullet entered on the left side, passing through and shattering the occipital bone. It then traversed the occipital and parietal lobes, moving through the long axis of the brain, ultimately lodging itself in the frontal bone, where it caused a fracture. As with Kennedy's assassination, debate erupted and to this day there remains disagreement regarding the exact trajectory of the bullet, with some historians believing it eventually crossed over to the right side of the brain.

Both Lincoln and Kennedy were shot from behind, as is often the case with surprise assassinations. Lincoln was attended to by an inexperienced general surgeon before the field of neurosurgery even existed. Kennedy, by contrast, was cared for by two Columbia-trained neurosurgeons nearly one hundred years later. So why did Lincoln live so much longer than Kennedy?

To answer that question, we first need to understand why someone dies of a gunshot wound to the head. One of the most critical factors that determines the outcome of such an injury is the velocity of the bullet when it hits the target. The Philadelphia Deringer that shot Lincoln propelled its bullet at around 400 feet per second. Compare this with the 6.5mm Carcano rifle used to kill President Kennedy, which shot its bullet at 2,500 feet per second, or about six times as fast. There's a simple equation for measuring the damage that a gunshot wound does to the head. It's a product of the weight of the projectile and the *square* of the velocity. This means that the biggest determinant of damage is velocity.

Although the two bullets were shaped quite differently, each weighed roughly the same amount: between 10 and 12 grams. The bullet used to kill Lincoln was spherical with a diameter of 44 millimeters. Kennedy's bullet was 6.5 by 52 millimeters and shaped like a torpedo. Based on the laws of physics and the speed of each bullet, a far greater force was delivered to Kennedy's brain than Lincoln's, which likely led to JFK's speedier demise, despite the century of neurosurgical progress between the two shots. In fact, if we plug the data from each assassination into our equation and square the relative speed difference, we can estimate that Kennedy's brain received *forty times as much force.*

So, what can a neurosurgeon do, in the face of such devastating injuries, to save a gunshot victim's life? Well, if the impact of the projectile is not direct, or if the brain damage is limited, sometimes an intervention can be performed rapidly, and neurosurgeons can change the course of history.

———

THE SURVIVORS

THE CASES OF
JAMES BRADY, GABBY GIFFORDS, AND MALALA YOUSAFZAI

James Brady was the White House press secretary when he was shot in the head on March 30, 1981, by a stray bullet meant for Ronald Reagan, sixty-nine days into his presidency. The gunman? John Hinckley Jr., who, in a deluded effort to impress the actress Jodie Foster, decided he needed to assassinate the president.

Reagan was shot in the chest and lungs—injuries that are generally easier to repair. He made a full recovery. Brady, on the other hand, was in critical condition. The bullet had entered his head through the left frontal bone, which was completely shattered. It then passed through the left frontal lobe and crossed over into the right frontal and temporal lobes, where most of the damage was done.

Within minutes of his injury, Brady was rushed to George Washington University Hospital, where neurosurgeon Dr. Arthur Kobrine immediately performed a bifrontal craniotomy—meaning he removed both the frontal bones that make up the forehead—to clean out the bullet fragments, damaged brain, and blood clots. Brady's injuries were so severe that, even as he was still undergoing surgery, several news anchors, including Dan Rather of CBS, reported that he'd already died. When informed of this, Dr. Kobrine replied, in a Chuck Yeager–meets–Mark Twain deadpan style, "Well, no one has yet told that to me or the patient."

Brady surprised everyone and lived, but he was never the same. After a long recovery, he was left in a wheelchair with severe weakness on the left side of his body and slurred speech. Since the injury was to the right hemisphere, and language is localized on the left side of the brain, he didn't lose his ability to speak altogether. However, the damage to his frontal lobes left him with subtle alterations in personality, almost as if he'd undergone a frontal lobotomy. The most frontal parts of the frontal lobes—unlike previously mentioned areas of the brain, each of which controls a specific bodily function—connect to every other part of the brain. They control short-term memory, long-term planning, emotions, mood, and behavior.

In the words of Dr. Richard Cytowic, one of Brady's physicians, "Though he is technically a different person from the one he was before the shooting, he has retained enough of his characteristically 'personal' repertory that most people recognize him as Jim Brady." Nevertheless, he was clearly more emotionally labile and easily distracted, and had lost some degree of his memory and higher-level cognitive faculties.

Once Brady recovered from his injuries, he became a staunch advocate for gun control. Not only was he a Republican, *he took a bullet* for one of the most popular Republican presidents, so he was able to gain enough public and Capitol Hill support to move the political needle. The Brady Bill, requiring background checks through the National Instant Criminal Background Check System and a mandatory five-business-day wait period to purchase a gun, passed in 1993. From 1998 to 2014, more than 202 million background checks were conducted, resulting in the prevention of *1.2 million* attempted purchases of deadly weapons.

Almost thirty years after Brady was shot in the line of government duty, on January 8, 2011, Gabrielle "Gabby" Giffords was shot in the head outside a Safeway supermarket in a failed assassination attempt. Giffords, a Democrat representing Arizona's Eighth Congressional District in the U.S. House of Representatives from 2007 to 2012, was only the third woman from Arizona to be elected to Congress.

The bullet entered the back of her head on the left side and exited an inch above her left eye, passing through the left side of her brain. She was immediately evacuated to University Medical Center in Tucson, still conscious and responsive.

Within thirty-eight minutes, neurosurgeon G. Michael Lemole Jr. (who happens to be Mehmet Oz's brother-in-law) was in the operating theater, performing a procedure on Giffords called a hemicraniectomy. In a hemicraniectomy, half of the skull—hence "hemi-"—is removed. This lifesaving surgery allowed her brain tissue to swell without raising her intracranial pressure, so the remaining healthy brain could recover. Lemole also placed a drain called a ventriculostomy into the ventricles of her brain to remove some of the cerebrospinal fluid, which is another trick neurosurgeons have in their arsenal to keep the pressure low inside the head.

Four months later, on May 19, 2011, Giffords's missing skull bone, which had been fractured by the bullet and discarded by her surgeon, was replaced by a prosthetic one. She then underwent intensive rehabilitation and has since made an astonishing recovery. Although she was left with some weakness on the right side of her body and has some speech difficulty—also called aphasia—she continues her valuable political work. (Brady's slurred speech was a result of damage to the motor aspects of speech production, such as moving the lips and tongue, rather than a deficit in language processing, as occurred with Giffords.) In 2013, shortly after the Sandy Hook Elementary School shooting, Giffords and her husband founded the nonprofit super PAC Americans for Responsible Solutions (ARS), now called Giffords, to support pro–gun control candidates. Since its formation, Giffords has played a key role in passing more than 200 new gun laws.

Another important voice that extremists failed to silence with a bullet was that of Malala Yousafzai, now an author and winner of the Nobel Peace Prize—the youngest person ever to receive this honor. Malala was an outspoken activist when she was shot in the head on October 9, 2012, on her bus to school. Her sin, according to the Taliban? Speaking out against their misogyny, including forbidding girls and young women from the basic human right to a formal education.

The assassin boarded Yousafzai's school bus, then shot her in the left side of the head in full view of all the other children. The bullet didn't penetrate Yousafzai's skull but rather grazed it, causing multiple bone fractures. Nevertheless, the shock wave created by its force led to both brain swelling and internal bleeding. She was immediately airlifted to a military hospital in Peshawar, where neurosurgeon Colonel Junaid Khan performed a hemicraniectomy—the same procedure Giffords had received—to reduce the pressure inside her skull. The removed piece of bone was then placed inside her abdomen for safekeeping, as a kangaroo might store a joey in its pouch. The intention was to replace the bone later once her brain swelling had subsided.

Four months after the assassination attempt, Yousafzai's skull was replaced using a prosthetic, rather than her own skull, which was removed from its temporary resting place inside her abdomen and discarded. Since undergoing extensive rehabilitation, Malala has made a remarkable recovery. She started her own foundation, the Malala Fund, which continues to advocate for the education of children, particularly young girls, and women around the globe. In fact, her influence and position as a human rights advocate arguably increased after the failed assasination attempt.

———

So why did Brady, Giffords, and Yousafzai live while Kennedy and Lincoln did not? Was it the force of the shot, the trajectory of the bullet, or the speed and scope of the neurosurgical care that made the biggest difference in their outcomes?

With respect to force, although it's difficult to make a direct comparison, we can assume relative parity in the cases of those who lived. The bullet that shot Giffords weighed 8 grams and was shot from a Glock 9mm at 1,250 feet per second, carrying more force than Lincoln's bullet but less than Kennedy's. Brady was shot with a Röhm RG-14, a Saturday night special, a poor-quality handgun that can be purchased for under $50. The ammunition was a .22-caliber "Devastator" bullet, and devastate it did: weighing only 2 grams, it was designed to explode on contact, so the damage to Brady's brain was far greater than it would have been by just the force of the bullet alone. The projectile in Malala's case was shot from a Colt .45 weighing 15 grams. It was discharged at 915 feet per second, which was similar in force to the one that hit Giffords.

But it's not all about force and the path of the bullet. Arguably the most important factor that leads to injury or death after head trauma is our ability to control brain swelling.

Swelling in the brain occurs in direct response to the shearing of tissue and damage to blood vessels, which leak a serum made of fluid, proteins, and white blood cells. Serum is the fluid within which the red blood cells travel. This vessel permeability allows the elements of the serum to temporarily exit their normal paths of circulation and rush, like first responders, to the site of the tissue damage.

The brain, like any injured tissue in the body, soon becomes engorged. But unlike in your ankle or wrist after a twist or a fall, which has room to swell outward under elastic skin, brain tissue is confined in a rigid container. Picture a coconut shell that cannot expand if there is an increase in the fluid or soft flesh inside. The swelling has nowhere to go. Therefore, as the brain swells, the pressure rapidly rises.

But a bullet doesn't just cause swelling; it also tears through blood vessels, which rupture, allowing the blood contained within to jet into the brain, leading to a blood clot, also known as a hematoma. The combination of brain swelling and bleeding is a dire emergency. That's when the neurosurgeon is called in to open the skull and remove the clot to bring down the pressure. The goal is to save whatever remaining brain remains unharmed. This generally entails opening the skull through a craniotomy ("crani-" refers to the skull, or cranium, and "-otomy" comes from the Greek -tomos, meaning "that cuts").

The brain does not rest directly against the skull like coconut flesh against its shell. Rather, it floats in a pool of liquid with the consistency of water. This liquid is called cerebrospinal fluid, or CSF. If you picture an egg yolk suspended inside the shell of an egg, the yolk would be the brain, and the white would be the CSF. Unlike a yolk, however, the brain also has

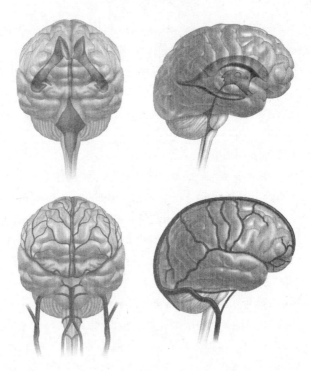

The ventricles within the brain (top left and top right) contain and circulate CSF and help keep the brain from collapsing on itself. The arteries (bottom left) bring oxygenated blood to the brain, and the veins (bottom right) bring deoxygenated blood back to the heart and lungs, where it's reoxygenated.

internal compartments that hold CSF. These are called ventricles. The hard protective shell of the skull therefore shields the brain, the CSF, and its blood vessels, all of which take up some of the intracranial space. A delicate balance of these three substances must be maintained to keep the pressure inside the head constant.

LETTING THE MUFFIN OUT OF THE CAN

Since the skull is a closed container, the fastest way to lower pressure is simply to open the lid.

The hemicraniectomy, the operation in which half the skull is removed, does just that: it allows the neurosurgeon to safely remove the lid, so to speak, and leave it that way for several days or even months until the brain's swelling has subsided. Unlike the snake in the can party trick, however, the brain does not shoot out of the skull. Instead, the swollen brain slowly mushrooms outward like the top of a muffin, a condition called fungus cerebri, *fungus* literally meaning "mushroom" in Latin.

The first scientific description of the hemicraniectomy was published in 1896 by the French doctor Charles Adrien Marcotte, and the first hemicraniectomy to lower intracranial pressure after brain trauma was performed that same year by Swiss physician Emil Theodor Kocher. Kocher was the chief of surgery at the University of Bern and in 1909 became the first Swiss to win the Nobel Prize. Given the simplicity of the concept, the procedure has not changed much since then, although the tools used to perform it are now vastly improved.

Throughout most of the twentieth century, the hemicraniectomy was hardly ever offered to patients with severe head trauma because the

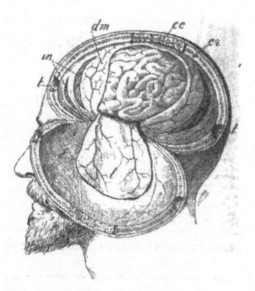

Illustration from the first scientific description
of the hemicraniectomy procedure in 1896.

procedure was usually prescribed too late, after all other medical therapies had failed. By that time the damage was irreversible. It took until the late 1990s for neurosurgeons to realize that a hemicraniectomy could control intracranial pressure long enough for the remaining healthy brain to survive, but only if the procedure was performed quickly—more specifically, within five hours of the injury.

Let's take a closer look at how neurosurgeons crack open the skull without damaging the underlying brain.

The skull is designed for one purpose and one purpose alone: to protect the brain. It doesn't want to be cut into or removed. It wants to stay there, intact, doing its important brain-sheltering work. And it has a design that enhances its ability to do just that.

The skull is not a single solid piece of bone but rather comprises three different layers. Between two hard shells—also called the outer and inner tables—lies an intermediate layer called the diploe, which looks like a honeycomb with small struts and buttresses. Biomechanical studies have shown that this three-layered design confers greater strength to the cranium. So to remove a 1-centimeter-thick piece of skull slightly bigger than a hockey puck—and to do so without damaging the fragile brain beneath it—is no simple task. The surgeon must use tools powerful enough to penetrate all three layers while also having the skill to know exactly when to stop before the drill plunges into the brain.

One of the earliest neurosurgical drills, called the Hudson brace, was a hand-powered twist drill shaped like a crank with a rounded handle on one end and a metallic bit jutting downward on the other. First described in 1518 and still in use until only a few decades ago, the drill was designed so the neurosurgeon could lean with one hand on the handle to push or brace it against the skull while the other hand manually rotated the vertical connecting bar, which would turn the drill bit. The motion is akin to stirring a bowl of thick batter with a long wooden spoon. With each turn, a worm-shaped fragment of bone wriggles up through the drill's grooves and is irrigated away by an assistant. The trick to this maneuver was to learn to recognize the sensation that occurs when the very tip of the drill penetrates the innermost part of the bone. It's a subtle catch that lets you know when you've reached the right depth and need to stop before the drill penetrates through that last remaining thin layer of bone. Should you fail to appreciate the tactile feedback and continue drilling, the results would be catastrophic.

When I started my training back in 1993, these drills were still standard equipment, although they were soon replaced with the power tools we use

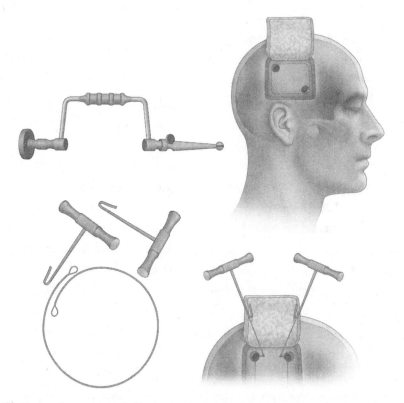

The Hudson brace (upper left) was used to make the initial burr holes (upper right). Then a Gigli saw (bottom left) was passed from one hole to the next and handles were attached to connect the burr holes and remove the bone flap (bottom right).

today. To muster enough force to puncture the skull, you really had to lean quite hard against the drill. While a skilled surgeon learned to recognize the precise moment to let up on the pressure, the beginner had to acquire this feel through trial and error. *Talk about scary!* I'd always imagine the drill plunging straight through. Luckily, this never occurred in my hands, but I did hear about cases where it had. The natural reaction was to stop every few turns to check and be sure, which could drag the process on for so long that a single burr hole could sometimes take five or ten minutes to complete. While this may not seem like such a long time, remember that sometimes craniotomies are done in emergencies where minutes of delay can mean the difference between life and death.

A similar type of handheld drill would have been used back in 1981 to perform James Brady's surgery. Ironically, the electric drill was introduced more than seventy years earlier by two French surgeons, Eugène-Louis Doyen and Thierry de Martel, but these primitive power tools never caught on in the United States. Cushing preferred the Hudson brace, which he considered a much safer technique. Like good soldiers, all his disciples followed in lockstep.

After creating several equidistant burr holes strategically placed at what would become the corners of the eventual bone flap, Brady's team then had to link them together so the appropriate wedge of frontal bone could be detached and lifted away from the skull. This connection between the burr holes would have been performed with a Gigli saw, essentially barbed wire, which would pass under the bone from one burr hole to the next via a thin metal rod pushed just above the dura. Think of a needle and thread going down into one hole, under the skull bone through the thin metal rod, then up and through the next hole. Only instead of a needle and thread, it's a wire with saw teeth. Handles were then attached to the ends of the wires, and the neurosurgeon would pull back and forth to saw through the bone from the inside out like an aggressive dentist with a thick piece of floss. The safety of this "inside-out" cutting was the reason Cushing favored the manual Hudson brace and Gigli saw over the French mechanical devices that penetrated the bone from the outside in.*

Today, craniotomies are performed with power tools driven by compressed air or electricity. A single burr hole is created in a matter of seconds with a high-speed drill, and then a device called a craniotome, a thin, side-cutting drill with a footplate, is used to disconnect the bone flap from the rest of the skull while protecting the underlying brain. The electric drill and the craniotome are two of the many devices that have made modern

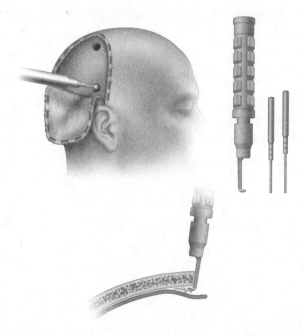

A pneumatic drill (top left) is used to drill a burr hole, which is then used as an access point to place a craniotome (top right). The footplate (bottom) of the craniotome sits beneath the skull and protects the dura from injury.

---

*As an aside, the Gigli saw was named after the Italian obstetrician Leonardo Gigli, who designed it in 1893 to unhinge the bones of the pelvis during difficult childbirths, a surgery he dubbed the "lateral pubiotomy." Yes, it was as horrific as it sounds. Gigli's saw was later adapted to cut down trees, which eventually morphed into the modern-day chain saw.

neurosurgical operations safer and speedier than surgeries performed just thirty years ago, when I started my training.

B ut let's get back to our hemicraniectomy.

After the bone is removed, what does the neurosurgeon do with it? If the patient survives the surgery, the bone will need to be replaced after the brain swelling has subsided. For this, we have three options: The bone can be stored in a sterile location such as a freezer in the hospital. It can be implanted in what is essentially a storage pocket made just under the skin in the patient's abdomen, as was done with Malala Yousafzai. Or, thanks to recent technological advances, we can 3D print a new prosthetic plate to replace the missing bone and simply discard the piece removed during the hemicraniectomy.

The first option, freezer storage, is the one traditionally used in most hospitals outfitted with a bone bank. The second option is commonly used on the battlefield or in places where resources such as freezers, let alone fully equipped modern hospitals, are scarce. For example, abdominal storage of cranial bone was frequently used in the Iraq War, from 2003 to 2008. The initial surgeries were performed at forward combat hospitals, and the bone flaps of the young soldiers were stored inside their bodies, traveling back with them to larger hospitals in the States, such as Walter Reed.

The third option, which is made possible by 3D printing, enables neurosurgeons to fabricate a prosthetic plate designed to fit the exact dimensions and shape of the opening created by the hemicraniectomy.

Both Giffords and Yousafzai received prosthetic plates. In Gabby's case, her bone had been shattered and could not be reconstituted. It's not clear why Malala's British neurosurgeon chose not to use her own bone, but sometimes bones stored in a freezer or the abdomen have a tendency to shrink in size without the proper nutrient environment. Eventually, they can shrivel down to the point where they may no longer be large enough to cover the gap in the skull.

So, based on the cases we've reviewed so far—JFK and Lincoln, on the one hand, and Brady, Giffords, and Yousafszi on the other—we can draw a few general conclusions. First, without immediate neurosurgical intervention, the latter three would certainly have perished. James Brady, Gabby Giffords, and Malala Yousafszi survived because they were transported immediately to a hospital; because those hospitals were staffed with well-trained neurosurgeons with access to fully equipped operating rooms; and because they then underwent early, aggressive, and appropriate neurosurgical interventions—namely, the removal of enough cranial bone and macerated brain to keep the pressure down inside their heads (pressure being the real killer in severe cases of TBI). Another critical piece of each of their stories is that the brain damage they suffered was not *so* severe that their situations were hopeless. One of the best predictors of the success of a hemicranitectomy is the level of alertness of the trauma victim prior to surgery. If they are already too far gone, little can be gained from an operation, regardless of how quickly it's performed.

Given the velocity and trajectory of Booth's bullet, along with the duration of Lincoln's survival with essentially no care whatsoever, had his injury occurred in the present, it's likely that he would have survived. During the Civil War, mortality from a penetrating injury to the head was nearly 71 percent. If you count deaths from ensuing infections, the rate approached 95 percent. Between World War I, when Harvey Cushing was alive, and World War II, the mortality from similar injuries decreased from roughly 40 percent to 14 percent. By the Vietnam War, it dropped again to 10 percent. By the time Operation Iraqi Freedom was in full swing, it was down to 6.8 percent.

Had Lincoln been saved, however, it doesn't mean he could have delivered another speech to rival the one he gave at Gettysburg. Given his injuries, Lincoln would have been paralyzed on the right side and aphasic—unable to talk. The left hemisphere of the brain processes speech in 99 percent of right-handed individuals. Although it's hard to know for sure that Lincoln was a righty, it turns out that the left hemisphere controls speech in most lefties as well. JFK, on the other hand, was doomed from the moment the assassin's bullet entered his skull. No amount of surgical skill no matter how rapidly administered could have saved him.

THE CASE OF
ROBERT F. KENNEDY

In a cruel twist of fate, five years after JFK's assassination, his brother Robert was also shot in the head as he was campaigning in the Democratic primary. The bullet, fired at close range from a .22-caliber Iver Johnson "Cadet" revolver, entered just behind the right ear, passing through the right cerebellum, occipital lobe, and temporal lobe. The shooting occurred at 12:17 a.m. Due to both an error in communication and the dispatcher's ignorance of the severity of the injury, RFK was first rushed to a small local hospital where there were no neurosurgeons on staff. There he was stabilized before being transferred to Good Samaritan Hospital in downtown Los Angeles. He arrived there at 1:00 a.m., roughly forty-five minutes after the accident.

At this point RFK was completely unresponsive and unable to move. This was back in 1968, before the CAT scan. The damage to his brain was not as bad as had occurred with his brother, roughly on par with Lincoln, Brady, and Giffords, but more severe than Yousafzai. Without the benefit of any imaging or knowledge of the extent of the injury, neurosurgeon Dr. Henry Cuneo wheeled RFK into the operating room, but not until 2:45 a.m., a solid two and a half hours after his injury. That's a long time in injured brain hours. Too long. He drilled five separate burr holes with a Hudson brace around the bullet entry side. Then, using the Gigli saw, Cuneo extracted a 5-centimeter piece of bone. Over the course of almost four hours, the surgeon removed the bullet fragments as well as RFK's severely bruised cerebellum and occipital lobe.

After the operation, RFK was able to move his right side a bit. Cuneo reached out to neurosurgeon J. Lawrence Pool for advice. Dr. Pool was the chair at the Neurological Institute of New York, who, after hearing all the details, concluded that the prognosis was grim and nothing could be done.

Pierre Salinger, RFK's campaign manager, telephoned another neurosurgeon, Dr. James L. Poppen, a friend of the Kennedys' who worked at the Lahey Clinic in Boston. Poppen was flown over on Air Force One and assisted with the postoperative care, but to no avail. I mention both Pool and Poppen here because we will learn more about them later. Both were not only two of the most well-respected neurosurgeons of their era but also at one time practitioners of the frontal lobotomy.

The next day RFK eventually succumbed to his injuries. The autopsy revealed that the bullet had not only damaged his cerebellum and occipital lobes but it sheared several arteries and veins in his brain. The resulting swelling, which was massive, killed him.

A few neurosurgeons from Duke reexamined RFK's case and concluded that, had RFK been treated more quickly and with modern neurosurgical know-how, he, like Lincoln, might very well have survived. Today, if RFK rolled into our hospitals with the same injury to the head, we would immediately obtain a CAT scan, which we can now do at the patient's bedside with portable units. A ventriculostomy would be placed in the depths of his brain to lower intracranial pressure, and he would receive a hemicraniectomy. Also, today his arterial and venous injuries might be reparable using the operating microscope, a device not widely available at the time of his injury. He would be cared for in a modern ICU staffed with critical-care specialists monitoring his respiratory settings, intracranial pressure, and even the temperature of his brain to maximize his recovery.

The subsequent historical events are well-known. Hubert Humphrey won the Democratic primary, then lost to Richard Nixon in the general election. While it is fanciful to imagine that history might have been changed and the United States spared the embarassment of the Watergate scandal had RFK's life been preserved, the truth is that RFK's recovery would have taken years. He would have been severely impaired and not even remotely the same robust candidate he had been before Sirhan Sirhan's bullet pierced his brain. Saving the life of a head trauma victim is one thing. Restoring function to a devastated brain is quite another.

FOUR

HEAD-ON COLLISIONS

very so often a neurosurgeon will intervene in a case that leaves such an indelible mark that the memory remains as vivid as the day it occurred. This happened to me early in my career, only a few months into my first job as an assistant professor at the University of Medicine and Dentistry of New Jersey, which at the time was more commonly known as UMDNJ. Fresh out of training, I was eager to test my mettle operating independently, without the safety net of a more expert surgeon backing me up.

UMDNJ—which has since been absorbed into the RWJBarnabas Health conglomerate of hospitals and become a part of the Rutgers University School of Graduate Studies—is the primary academic university-based medical center serving the state of New Jersey. While UMDNJ is composed of a network of hospitals, its busiest trauma center, University Hospital, is in Newark, which is where I was stationed primarily. Because University Hospital is one of only three trauma centers providing level 1 emergency care to the entire state, the volume of cases that funnels into that hospital on a busy night can be overwhelming. Its roof supports a helipad that acts like a turnstile for the most critically injured patients. It was not uncommon for me to get little to no sleep when I was on call there, managing the wide assortment of head trauma cases that came barreling through its doors.

On this one evening, I had been at home, enjoying a rare moment of rest and relaxation, when my beeper went off. A girl ten years old, maybe, had been thrown from a horse. She was riding with an instructor and even wearing a helmet when a motorcycle roared past on a nearby road and spooked the animal. It reared and off she flew. When she hit the ground, her head collided with a rock, which landed squarely on her left temple just below the helmet, the thinnest part of the skull through which courses the middle meningeal artery. She was airlifted to my hospital and whisked down from the helipad for a CAT scan, which revealed a large epidural hematoma, a collection of blood between the skull and the dura, the thick membrane that covers the brain. The blood clot was pushing inward, exerting tremendous pressure, and scalloping the normally spherical organ. Her torn meningeal artery was undoubtedly the cause of the bleeding.

By the time I arrived at the hospital, the patient was already in the operating room. I checked her pupils as the anesthesiologist began putting her to sleep and saw that the left one was already dilated, or "blown," as we call it. A blown pupil is an ominous sign of catastrophically high intracranial pressure. It was unclear if it was already past the point where we could turn things around, but if we didn't at least try, she surely wouldn't have survived more than a few more minutes. Moving as rapidly as safety allowed, we shaved her head almost completely on the side of the injury, cut into her scalp to create a large U-shaped flap of skin, drilled a single burr hole, and from there cut a wide ellipse with the craniotome to unroof a large portion of her skull.

The moment we lifted the wedge of bone away, an enormous blood clot expressed itself under such high pressure that it literally exploded out of her head, sliding down the surgical drapes and onto the floor in one slimy solid lump. The snake had most certainly been released from the can. But now the middle meningeal artery, pulsing with fresh arterial blood, still had to be dealt with. We immediately cauterized it with the bipolar. Once the skull bone was replaced and the skin sewn back together, our little patient was brought to the intensive care unit for monitoring. She was kept under heavy sedation at first, which was gradually reduced on an hourly basis to see if she would regain consciousness. Although her life had been saved, we could only hope that we had moved quickly enough to remove the clot and relieve the pressure inside her head before irreparable brain damage had occurred.

When I left the OR, I walked out into the hallway and began searching for the child's family. I didn't know who they were, since we hadn't had time to meet before the surgery. I spotted a woman pacing back and forth, her face a mask of worry and fear. I knew instantly that this was the girl's mother. When our eyes met, no introductions were necessary. I told her that we had acted as fast as we could, that we'd given her daughter the best chance possible for survival, but, still, the prognosis remained uncertain. The good news was that the blood clot had not been *in* the brain but rather outside it, so the clot itself had not caused any obvious damage. There was still hope that the brain might recover, but it was too soon to know.

Every day I'd visit this child's room on my morning rounds and spend a few moments with her mom, who was there 24/7, often curled up in bed next to her daughter when I arrived. The routine was the same. I'd ask if she'd seen any movement and then I'd perform a quick examination, stimulating the girl's hands and feet in the hope of eliciting a response. For ten days I got nothing. My little patient, breathing tube still in place, filling her small lungs with air, just wouldn't move. She wouldn't respond to voices, wouldn't flinch when pinched. Her pupils were normal in size—a good sign—but after this long, I would have expected at least *something* if she were going to recover.

On day eleven I stopped by and found my patient's mother in tears. I asked what had happened, and she told me that one of the doctors in the pediatric ICU had just broken the news: given the amount of time since surgery, he had said consolingly, recovery at this point was unlikely. It had, plain and simple, just been too long. I was frustrated, to say the least, with this doctor's insensitivity. Hope is a terrible thing to steal, especially from a parent. I've always believed that it's irresponsible to douse optimism until the prospect for improvement has completely vanished. Which in this case it hadn't.

A brain MRI had been obtained a few days earlier, and propitiously it showed no obvious damage to the girl's brain. Recalling a useful bit of teaching impressed upon me during my training—*eventually, all patients end up looking like their MRI scan*—I was still sanguine. In other words, if the MRI scan appears normal, then there's still hope. (Conversely, if the MRI reveals severe damage, the patient probably won't recover.)

I told the mother in no uncertain terms that I still thought her daughter had a good chance. I saw the thick, tense creases relaxing in her face just a bit, and I knew that I'd given her a gift. I just hoped it wasn't a temporary relief from the inevitable reckoning we both feared might be coming.

For the next few days my patient remained comatose, not moving a muscle, not responding. Every day I made sure to connect with her mom and to repeat my message: "I think she's going to improve. Just give it a little more time."

Then one day it happened. I saw a slight flicker in the little girl's finger. Then her arm. Then her eyelids. Slowly, as if she were purposefully taking her time, not eager to arouse from her slumber, she began to wake up. Over the next few weeks she made a full recovery, left the hospital, and eventually returned to school. Within a year she was back in the same grade with her friends. Every year since then, without fail, I've received a Christmas card from her mother along with a photograph of her daughter. The girl's picture is always accompanied by a short account of her accomplishments— the normal milestones most parents take for granted, nearly lost to a horseback riding lesson.

WHEN THE BOUGH BREAKS

When a child comes into an emergency room with head trauma—and if they haven't clearly fallen off a horse or been hit in the head with a baseball in front of dozens of witnesses—the ER staff are trained to suspect child abuse. A more common situation involves a very young child, either an infant or a toddler, who's brought in by a caregiver who allegedly found them in bed, difficult to arouse after a nap. If the ER doctor's examination confirms that something's not right, a CAT scan of the head may be performed, which might reveal a shocking amount of internal trauma, including swelling in the brain and a subdural hematoma—blood that has collected between the brain and the dura, in a compartment one layer deeper than would occur in an epidural hematoma.

At this point, a call will go out to the pediatric neurosurgeon covering the emergency room, since the infant's life is in imminent danger. In the meantime, the ER doctor might examine the baby's eyes. The presence of small hemorrhages in the retinas provides further evidence that the baby may have been the victim of abuse, perhaps at the hands of their parent or caretaker, who may not be just an innocent bystander in this saga.

Of the 3 million cases of child abuse reported every year in the United States, only 700,000 are confirmed. That's one in five. The disparity between these two numbers is obviously chilling, but proving the heinous crime of child abuse, like all crimes, depends on evidence. If only the abuser and the child are in the room together, there are no witnesses to the crime other than the victim, who may be both prelingual and possibly in a coma, and the perpetrator, who may not be so inclined to incriminate themselves.

But what if the signs of child abuse were so clear-cut and objective that the infant's own body and the results of their medical tests could provide incontrovertible evidence of misconduct? Such was thought to be the case with the phenomenon called shaken baby syndrome, or SBS.

The mechanism of SBS seems simple enough. When a caregiver becomes frustrated with a baby's incessant crying, they shake the baby, often quite violently, to stop the irritating noise. Because babies' necks are weak, the head whips back and forth, and this to-and-fro motion supposedly causes the damage. The jerking motion injures not only the infant's brain but also small blood vessels in the retina—a telltale sign of abuse—which an astute physician can spot by looking through the infant's pupils into the back of the eye with a handheld ophthalmoscope.

When the head moves rapidly in one direction, the brain moves along with it. But since the brain floats in a sea of cerebrospinal fluid, it lags slightly behind. This delay causes it to bang up against the side of the skull. Eventually, the brain accelerates to catch up. When the skull stops moving, the brain's momentum propels it into the other side of the skull, causing a second blow. This type of injury is called a coup contrecoup, from the French *coup,* which means "blow." More simply, a single bang to the head results in two separate bruises, also called contusions, one on each side of the brain. (Imagine taking Jell-O out of a mold and moving it into a new, slightly larger mold of a similar shape, then rapidly jerking the mold from side to side.)

Shaken baby syndrome was first described in 1971 by British neurosurgeon Arthur Norman Guthkelch. Guthkelch, who began his career during World War II and was Britain's first dedicated pediatric neurosurgeon. While working at the Royal Manchester Children's Hospital, he observed a few cases in which babies had been shaken for disciplinary purposes, a practice that was apparently common in northern England at the time. In Guthkelch's own words, "One has the impression that a 'good shaking' is felt to be socially more acceptable and physically less dangerous than a blow on the head or elsewhere."

The parents were not *trying* to harm their babies; they were just letting them know that this sort of tantrum would not be tolerated going forward. Unfortunately, harm was done—significant harm—but given the mechanism of injury, there were no external marks, such as bruises about the head, that might provide a clue to the cause of the injury. After witnessing this devastating event repeatedly, Guthkelch issued a warning to his colleagues recommending that should they come across cases of infantile subdural hematoma, they must "keep in mind the possibility of assault." Guthkelch hypothesized—with no biomechanical evidence to support his claim, mind you—that "the relatively large head and puny neck muscles of the infant must render it particularly vulnerable."

In a follow-up article, published a few years later, Dr. John Caffey, a pediatric radiologist, defined the term "whiplash shaken infant syndrome," in which he described a triad of symptoms caused by shaking that included subdural hematoma, retinal hemorrhages, and brain swelling. Caffey's goal in describing this syndrome was to educate caregivers about the risks of shaking their babies. He never imagined that his description of these three findings would be relied upon as unassailable clues to identify abuse cases, which might then trigger protective intervention.

Once defined, SBS was quickly adopted by the medical community as a means of establishing proof of child abuse, even if there were no external signs of trauma. All that was needed to trigger a criminal investigation was for the doctor to document the classic triad of symptoms: subdural hematoma, hemorrhages in the retina, and severe brain swelling. Armed with this supposedly ironclad definition, a physician could act as a forensic detective, providing irrefutable evidence to implicate the perpetrator as an abuser and, in so doing, defend the most vulnerable and voiceless members of society.

In 1974 the U.S. Congress passed the Child Abuse Prevention and Treatment Act (CAPTA). This act reinforced the mandatory reporting laws that already existed in most states, requiring designated professionals to report cases of suspected child abuse to the state. Once the law passed, nurses and physicians were not merely recommended but *required* to report parents and caregivers to the authorities. While statistics are not precisely known, the CDC estimates that roughly 1,000 cases of SBS are reported every year in the United States. As many as 25 percent of these infants will ultimately die of their injuries, and 80 percent of the survivors will go on to suffer permanent brain damage. The devastation is unequivocal, but the conundrum remains: How to separate the accidental from the intentional?

Because SBS is a form of traumatic brain injury, pediatric neurosurgeons are often called upon to perform emergency surgeries, such as hemicraniectomies and ventriculostomies, on its victims. Once the SBS diagnosis is made, litigation often follows, so these same neurosurgeons then become expert witnesses in trials where their testimonies can determine the outcome. Neurosurgeons have also been instrumental in studying SBS, desperately trying to understand how shaking a child can cause so much injury. In these cases, Sherlock Holmes and Dr. Watson are one and the same, drawing upon deductive and inductive reasoning as well as medical research to solve the case.

GUILTY UNTIL PROVEN INNOCENT

THE CASE OF
MATTHEW EAPPEN

Louise Woodward was a nineteen-year-old British au pair working in the United States. In 1997 she was hired by two physicians, Sunil and Deborah Eappen, to take care of their eight-month-old son Matthew. On February 4, Woodward called an ambulance to report that Matthew had stopped breathing. Once in the pediatric emergency room, Matthew was found to have a fractured skull, a subdural hematoma, retinal hemorrhages, brain swelling, and an old wrist fracture.

Matthew's injuries were so severe that, despite emergency brain surgery, he died a few days later. Louise was charged with abuse in a case of shaken baby syndrome. During the police interview, Louise admitted she had "tossed Matthew onto the bed." The official report went on to say that Louise had admitted she had been "a little rough" and that she "might have dropped him on the bathroom floor." When questioned, Louise acknowledged that she was frustrated. However, she later testified that she had *never* been rough with the child and clarified that she said "popped" the child on the floor, not "dropped."

Woodward was defended in her trial by a team of lawyers that included Barry Scheck, the founder of the Innocence Project. This organization reexamines cases in which people are imprisoned based on the illegitimate testimonies of inept forensic pathologists relying on antiquated and inaccurate techniques like bite mark analysis. Using new and more reliable DNA technology, the Innocence Project has been able to exonerate several formerly convicted criminals. Scheck argued that this couldn't be a case of shaken baby syndrome based on two claims. The first was that there were no neck injuries. The second was his suggestion that the bleeding in Eappen's brain may have been a "re-bleed," an exacerbation of an earlier injury that occurred before Woodward began caring for Eappen. The prosecution, on the other hand, called as a witness the treating pediatric neurosurgeon, Dr. Joseph Madsen, who disagreed with Scheck. The injuries to Matthew were much too acute and severe to have been from a distant trauma.

On October 30, 1997, after twenty-six hours of deliberations, the jury found Louise Woodward guilty of second-degree murder. The following day, Judge Hiller Zobel sentenced her to life in prison with a minimum of fifteen years. At a post-conviction relief hearing, Woodward's lawyers managed to reduce her sentence to time served and she was freed.

To understand the arguments raised by each side in the Eappen case, we must first review some of the research on shaken baby syndrome. Remember, when Guthkelch and Caffey first introduced the concept, they lacked any scientific evidence that shaking a baby can indeed cause trauma to the brain. The first such evidence emerged from the work of a neurosurgeon by the name of Dr. Ayub Ommaya, once the chief of neurosurgery with the National Institute of Neurological Disorders and Stroke in Washington, DC.

Ommaya was trying to understand the mechanism behind the whiplash injuries that resulted from rear-end collisions during automobile accidents. His experiments, on adult rhesus monkeys, were designed to tease out the degree of rotational forces required to cause brain injury when one car smashes into another, absent any direct impact to the head. In a paper published in 1968, he showed that it was possible to cause brain injury purely from whiplash, but he also noted that, in over half the animals he studied, such an injury was often accompanied by neck injuries, which is why Scheck used the *absence* of such injury as a crucial argument in Woodward's defense. Whether these findings were relevant to human infants and whether it might be possible to generate sufficient rotational forces merely by shaking a baby were never discussed by Ommaya. Nevertheless, this mostly unrelated data was appropriated by paid expert witnesses, lawyers, and the courts as the scientific basis for SBS.

The first biomechanical studies that directly examined whether a whiplash injury to an infant could truly cause brain trauma (and SBS) were carried out by pediatric neurosurgeon Ann-Christine Duhaime during her training at the University of Pennsylvania. (At the time of this writing, she is the director of pediatric neurosurgery at Massachusetts General Hospital.) Duhaime examined a few infants who had been diagnosed with SBS and discovered that every one of them had at least some evidence of blunt head trauma. Basically, she showed that Guthkelch was wrong. Shaking alone was *not* sufficient to cause head trauma unless the baby's head also hit something, in which case one should also find bruises on the scalp or other such evidence.

Using a mechanical model of an infant embedded with an accelerometer to measure energy, Duhaime compared the forces created from violent shaking with those created from direct impact—namely, striking the baby's head against an object. She found that direct impact caused 50 times more force than violent shaking. In fact, she was never able to reproduce the required injury by shaking the model without smacking the head against something. Impact was such a critical prerequisite that she argued the name of the syndrome should be changed to shaken impact syndrome to emphasize her point.

Two years later, in response to Duhaime's study, another group of neurosurgeons at the Barrow Neurological Institute in Phoenix, led by neurosurgeons Mark Hadley and Harold Rekate, identified a few cases in which shaking a baby alone, absent any impact to the head, caused brain injury. However, these authors also noted that to achieve the requisite amount of torque, the shaking must be so intense that neck injuries *had* to occur, just as Ommaya had found in his car crashes involving monkeys.

So, while impact is the most common and likely cause of injury to a baby's brain, shaking an infant *can* cause brain damage, but the force required to cause this damage would also lead to a neck injury. Bottom line, for SBS to occur, you must have either scalp bruises or a neck injury.

As it turns out, most infant abuse cases are also accompanied by signs of direct head trauma. They rarely involve just shaking. The treating physician often finds such evidence in the form of a skull fracture or scalp swelling. Accordingly, the term "shaken baby syndrome" has been replaced by a more inclusive description: "abusive head trauma." The new label renders the mechanism of injury irrelevant. The resulting trauma becomes the crux of the case.

In the case of Matthew Eappen, the fact that no signs of neck injury were found—one of the main lines of the caregiver's defense—becomes irrelevant so long as the prosecution proved there was direct head trauma, which it did.

I had the opportunity to speak with Dr. Joseph Madsen, the neurosurgeon who operated on Matthew Eappen and testified at the trial. I've known Joe for over thirty years. In fact, he was the first neurosurgeon I ever met, back when I was a medical student.

Madsen is now a professor of pediatric neurosurgery at Harvard Medical School and the director of epilepsy surgery at Boston Children's Hospital. I asked about Eappen. He reiterated what he'd stated in court. "This was a clear case of a traumatic acute subdural hematoma," he said. "The scalp was swollen, and Matthew's head showed signs of a recent injury. There is no way this could have been an old hemorrhage or due to anything else other than severe recent head trauma."

As the treating neurosurgeon in the case, Madsen also testified at the trial. On the defense side, Scheck called two expert witnesses. One was Dr. Ommaya, the neurosurgeon who had published the original article on vehicular whiplash injuries in monkeys. The other was Dr. Ronald Uscinski, another pediatric neurosurgeon, who was recently featured in the documentary *The Syndrome*, which raised doubts about the scientific basis of

SBS. They both testified that when a baby shows up in the ER and is found to have subdural hematomas, brain swelling, and retinal hemorrhages, violent shaking is not necessarily the cause, thereby supporting Scheck's claim that Woodward was possibly innocent.

But who really cares if the cause was shaking or just plain old abusive head trauma? So what if Woodward didn't shake Matthew? She dropped and possibly hit him. Whether Woodward *intended* to harm Eappen, or whether she was just impatient and careless, can never be known without a confession. The only thing we know for sure is this: a child was unquestionably harmed while in her protective care.

Today, it's generally agreed that cases of infant abuse should not hinge solely on the SBS triad of signs but rather on a careful weighing of the sum of all the evidence on a case-by-case basis. Several courts in England, Australia, and Canada have tried to go back and review their SBS abuse cases to see if a false conviction might have hinged solely upon the presence of the original three symptoms. Only a small handful have been overturned, the original evidence pointing to abuse being so convincing.

It may sound harsh, but if a baby comes into an ER with swollen hemorrhagic brain, retinal hemorrhages, external signs of trauma, evidence of older healed fractures to other bones, or any combination thereof, it's abuse until proven otherwise, *even without the three signs of a clinical syndrome defined in a cursory fashion decades ago.* In this situation, the caregivers are guilty until proven innocent.

THE LUCID INTERVAL

The two situations we just described—falling from a horse and child abuse—are both forms of *blunt* head trauma, which differs from what we described earlier, namely *penetrating* head trauma, as when the brain is pierced by a bullet or a Swiss Army knife. Other common forms of blunt head trauma include motor vehicle accidents and violent assaults, followed by falls and sports injuries. When sufficiently severe, these injuries can be devastating and often warrant neurosurgical intervention. Performed quickly enough, such surgeries can be lifesaving. But as we have already seen, if surgery is delayed, the result can be fatal.

THE CASE OF
NATASHA RICHARDSON

A blunt head trauma felled Britain's Natasha Richardson, daughter of legendary star Vanessa Redgrave and director Tony Richardson. She was a Tony Award–winning actor in her own right, with a highly successful international television and film career, where she met her second husband, the actor Liam Neeson.

On March 16, 2009, Richardson, then forty-five, was on a ski vacation with one of her sons at Mont-Tremblant, outside Montreal. According to reports, she was standing on a bunny slope, taking a lesson, when she slipped and fell, hitting her head. She was not wearing a helmet. She was evaluated by the ski patrol, deemed fine, and even overheard joking about the fall.

Nevertheless, protocol is protocol. At 12:43 p.m. the paramedics were called, and at 1:00 p.m. she was transported by sleigh to the infirmary. Some accounts of that day claim that she was told she should go to a hospital for further evaluation but refused. Regardless, she felt okay and was signed out at 1:10 p.m.

By 1:30 p.m. she was back in her room. Reports of what happened next are murky, but some say she developed a headache and started feeling unwell. At 2:59 p.m. she began to deteriorate. Richardson was put in an ambulance at 3:47 p.m. and brought to a small hospital, where she was stabilized. She was then transferred to a larger hospital at 7:00 p.m., where she remained overnight. The next day, at 12:30 p.m., she was flown to yet another hospital, this one in New York City, where she was declared braindead and removed from life support. The cause of death was "epidural hematoma due to a blunt impact to the head." Did she have a CAT scan during her first two hospital admissions? Was the hemorrhage identified that was enlarging and compressing her brain? (A hemorrhage is an ongoing bleed and a hematoma is one that is no longer enlarging). Was she offered surgery? These questions remain unanswered.

The sad truth is that, had Richardson's hemorrhage been diagnosed in a timely fashion and operated upon, she very likely would have survived. The evacuation of an epidural hematoma is one of the most common and simplest operations in the neurosurgeon's arsenal, performed thousands of times per year in the United States alone. As far as brain surgeries go, it's even more straightforward than the hemicraniectomy. The surgeon performs a craniotomy, removing a piece of bone and exposing the blood clot that sits right below the skull. The clot is then evacuated with a suction or a forceps. The middle meningeal artery is often bleeding from where it was torn and needs to be cauterized. But that's it. The dura is never opened and the brain is never exposed. It's the same surgery I performed on the girl who was knocked off her horse.

Richardson's story resonated so intensely with the public because the mechanism of her fall seemed so mild and commonplace. Most of us have fallen and hit our heads in a similar fashion. Even more terrifying was the fact that Richardson appeared perfectly fine after the injury. How is one to know, after a similar bump to the head, that there isn't a life-threatening blood clot enlarging inside their skull?

To understand exactly what happened to Richardson and the reason she seemed fine for several hours before she deteriorated, we first need to review a bit more anatomy.

Between the skull and the brain lie several layers of tissue where blood can pool and expand. The first layer, just beneath the skull, is called the dura mater, or "tough mother" in Latin. Often just called the dura, this membrane looks like a thick piece of skin. When blood collects outside this layer, between the skull and the dura, it's called an *epidural* hematoma. When blood collects below this layer, between the dura and the brain, it's called a *subdural* hematoma, which is what occurs in shaken baby syndrome.

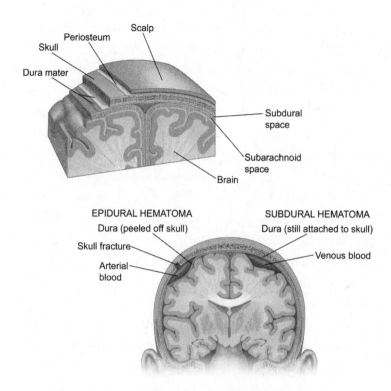

Layers between the skin and bone of the brain include the dura mater and the arachnoid membrane, which is adherent to the brain. An epidural hematoma occurs when blood collects between the bone and the dura. A subdural hematoma occurs when blood collects between the dura and the arachnoid.

The period of time after Richardson bumped her head but before the onset of her symptoms has a name; it's called the lucid interval. That you or your loved one could have a traumatic brain injury, appear completely normal, and then collapse a few hours later from a fatal brain bleed is a terrifying prospect. That fear runs through the mind of any parent, neurosurgeon or not, watching on the sidelines as their child experiences a blow to the head while playing a contact sport. Concerns over missing a growing blood clot have led many a parent to the misguided notion that they should keep their child awake throughout the night. Given the rarity of this event during contact sports, which we will soon explore in more detail, suffice to say that these fears are unwarranted.

The lucid interval was first identified by John Abernethy, a surgeon working in London in the early 1800s. He described the case of a man who got hit in the head by the hook of a crane. Briefly stunned, the man got up, walked home, and went to bed. Later that day he could not be aroused. His family transported him to Abernethy, who took the man straight into surgery, where a large epidural hematoma was discovered and evacuated. Abernethy speculated that the source of the bleeding, in this case, was the middle meningeal artery, which runs along the dura just under the thinnest part of the skull near the temple.

Abernethy, we now know, was correct—though his patient died anyway because the surgery was not done promptly enough. The most common cause of an epidural hematoma is, indeed, bleeding from a severed middle meningeal artery, which can be torn when the adjacent bone fractures. In adults, most of the skull is thick and strong. But in one location—just next to the eye around the temple—the bone is quite thin, to make room for the

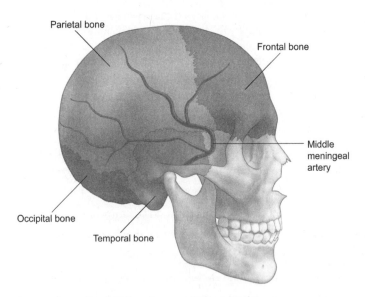

The middle meningeal artery runs just under the bone in its thinnest location, i.e., the temple.

thick temporalis muscle, which allows us to chew. This region is quite prone to fracturing, as happened when my young patient fell off her horse. It's even thin enough for a Swiss Army knife to penetrate if thrust just right.

———————

The man Abernethy treated had been able to walk home after his injury before falling asleep. But if his patient had indeed ruptured his middle meningeal artery, which was spurting blood into the epidural space, how was it possible that he remained alert for so long? It didn't make sense. If arterial blood was pumping into the narrow space between the skull and dura, it should have filled up rather quickly.

The answer to this last piece of the puzzle wouldn't be clear until the 1980s when a group of researchers in Norway figured out that blunt force head trauma not only tears the middle meningeal artery but also tears the nearby veins. Since the pressure in the artery is much higher than in the vein, the pressure gradient forces the blood back into the veins, which slows its accumulation. It's like turning on a faucet to fill the bathtub but forgetting to plug the drain. Eventually the tub fills up, but it takes twice as long.

So how long can a lucid interval last? To answer this question, it's first important to note that not all epidural hematomas have a lucid interval. Depending on the intensity of the blow, some patients may never wake up. Likewise, not all lucid intervals after trauma are caused by epidural hematomas. Sometimes the cause is a blood clot *within* the brain or a bruise to the brain, so the victim stays awake for a while until the brain starts to swell, at which point they lose consciousness in a delayed fashion.

But when a lucid interval is caused by an epidural hematoma, as is true of nearly half of all cases, it can last anywhere from fifteen minutes to four days. On average, however, patients with an epidural hematoma will deteriorate within six hours of their injury.

Richardson, tragically, fit right into the expected time frame.

———————

THE OLD MAN IS SNORING

THE CASE OF
BOB SAGET

In 2022, sixty-five-year-old Bob Saget, who'd hosted *America's Funniest Home Videos* and played Danny Tanner in *Full House*, was found dead in his hotel room. The previous night, he'd performed a two-hour stand-up set in Orlando, Florida. Security cameras caught him very much alive and entering his room at the Ritz-Carlton Orlando just after 2:00 a.m. His dead body was found at 4:00 p.m. the next day.

Rumors swirled of drug abuse, foul play, and even murder until the coroner's report emerged, which concluded that Saget had died from head trauma. The only drugs in his system were clonazepam, a prescription antianxiety medication he'd been taking for years, and trazodone, an antidepressant. No alcohol was found. Saget was Covid positive but asymptomatic. The official story, released by the medical examiner and endorsed by the family, was that he had fallen in his hotel room, bumped his head, thought nothing of it, crawled into bed, and died that night.

The timeline of events reported by the press alleviated fears of foul play, but careful scrutiny of the coroner's report, once it was released, confused the matter. It read like exhibit A in the case of *Saget et al. v. Unnamed Intruder*. The autopsy showed that Saget's skull was fractured in several places and his brain was severely damaged by internal bleeding. Major news outlets interviewed experts, most of whom opined that a simple fall in the bathroom should not result in such severe injuries. In fact, the injuries were so extensive that it would have been highly unlikely that Saget could have so easily climbed back into bed—and even if he could have managed it, he would have realized that he was in trouble and called either 911 or his family for help.

The question is this: Do all the pieces fit together? Is it possible that a fall in the bathroom, as seemingly harmless as Richardson's fall on the bunny slope, can lead to such extensive injuries?

To get to the bottom of this mystery, we need to do a bit of research and run the stats on what we neurosurgeons call "fall from standing." (Yes, this injury is so common it has its own name.) As many as 30 percent of people over sixty-five—Saget's age at the time of his accident—will at some point fall and hurt themselves. Some 10 percent of all head trauma patients admitted to the hospital will have sustained their injuries just by falling from a standing position. Of those, as many as 8 percent will die.

Several factors dictate the extent of the injuries from such a fall. The first is the impact velocity, which depends on the subject's height and weight and whether the fall is broken, either by their outstretched hand or by their rear end hitting the ground first. The second is the impact surface: Is it flat, like a sidewalk, or sharp, like a curb? The third is the angle of impact: Sideways or straight on? The fourth and last is the thickness of the bone where it's struck. Although all these factors contribute to the likelihood of a skull fracture, the most important one is the contour of the impacted surface. When a skull hits a curb or any other non-flat surface, a skull fracture often results. Why? It's a matter of pounds per square inch hitting the non-flat, pointed surface and the concentration of the force on the skull when it does.

In one 2014 study of people who died after such a fall, skull fractures were found in 94 percent of cases, contrecoup contusions in 90 percent, subdural hematomas in 84 percent, orbital roof fractures in 44 percent, and periorbital hematomas in 28 percent. These were Saget's exact injuries. Not only are such falls common and occasionally lethal, but if Saget fell in the bathroom and his head hit something before striking the floor—the edge of the bathtub or toilet or an open drawer—his injuries were completely consistent with the mechanism of injury. To definitively confirm the fall-in-the-bathroom hypothesis would require evidence like a piece of skin or hair identified on the object his head might have hit. Alas, the full results of the CSI investigation have been blocked by Saget's family.

I admit that I, too, was initially skeptical when the circumstances surrounding Saget's death emerged. It just didn't *feel* right that someone could fall in the bathroom and die so quickly.

But then, two weeks after the story broke, I received a call from the wife of one of my patients. He'd collapsed in the bathroom of their home. I'd operated on him a few weeks earlier, and his surgery had gone smoothly. His tumor, which was a malignant cancer, had been removed completely. The surgery was a success. He'd left the hospital a few days later in perfect condition.

That morning his wife had heard a loud clunking sound coming from the bathroom and the sound of drawers being knocked about. She ran through the door only to find her husband on the floor, with blood seeping from his ear. He was rushed to a local emergency room, where a CAT scan revealed massive bleeding throughout his brain. He died a few days later.

I was devastated, not only because he and his wife were my friends, but because he'd fallen so soon after I had performed his surgery. Even though, logically and medically, I knew I was not to blame, I couldn't help but feel that in some way I was responsible.

He'd probably had a seizure, which can occur after a brain tumor operation, even if you're taking the appropriate anti-seizure medications. When I spoke to his wife, I expressed my deep sadness at her loss and my apologies if the surgery had, in any way, contributed. I asked if her husband was taking any aspirin or anticoagulation medication that might explain the severity of the injury. He was not. To my surprise and appreciation, rather than try to pin her anguish on me, she proceeded to thank me for all that I had done and express their gratitude for my help. Even in her time of deepest sorrow, she found the strength to ease my heartache, as trivial as it was in comparison with her own.

When I hung up the phone, two thoughts ran through my mind. One was the coincidental timing of this event, so soon after Bob Saget's death, and its confirmation of the plausibility of the coroner's story. The second was a feeling of sympathy for Saget's family—not only for their loss but because they had been forced to suffer both it *and* the public's scrutiny and suspicion of foul play.

It's so much easier to assume improper behavior to explain the unimaginable. None of us wants to believe that our loved ones, or we ourselves, could simply slip or fall in the bathroom—or on a bunny slope, for that matter—and die from a traumatic brain injury. But such is life's tightrope and the fragility of the human brain. Our skulls are excellent protectors, no doubt, but they cannot protect against everything.

THE DEAD-BALL ERA

THE CASE OF
RAY CHAPMAN

The 1920s were considered a turning point in the game of baseball, wedged between an earlier period, the "dead-ball" era, during which home runs were rare, and the modern steroid-fueled, high-scoring, home run derby of a game. Prior to 1920, not only were the fields larger but balls were poorly made and rarely replaced. This led to an accumulation of grime and scuff marks, which made them fly erratically, rendering them tremendously difficult to hit. Pitchers would purposely cover the balls in mud, debris, and even saliva, creating "spitballs." Although Babe Ruth's free-swinging slugger style has often been credited for transforming the game into its current version, another, lesser-known player, Ray Chapman, may have had an even bigger impact.

On August 16, 1920, Chapman, the shortstop for the Cleveland Indians, came to bat in the fifth inning against Ruth's Yankees. Both teams were in a close race for the American League pennant. Chapman was one of the most well-liked players of his day, and he was near the end of his career, having recently married Kathleen Daly, the daughter of a prominent

Cleveland businessman. Their first child was on the way. The pitcher Chapman faced that day was Carl Mays, one of the most loathed players in the league. Mays, an introvert, was known for his submarine pitches, which are thrown in a side-arm low-to-high trajectory, which he often delivered a bit inside to threaten batters who crowded the plate.

It was late in the afternoon, the sun was setting, and a fog was drifting in, making visibility poor. Mays hurled a high fastball that walloped Chapman squarely in the temple. Players at that time didn't wear helmets, so the crack of the ball against Chapman's skull was loud—so loud, in fact, that everyone thought the ball had been struck by a bat. Hearing the sound, Mays picked up the ball, which had ricocheted off Chapman's skull and dribbled back toward the pitcher's mound, and threw it to first base, where it met the glove of Wally Pipp. (Pipp, as some baseball fans may recall, would permanently lose his starting position five years later to the "Iron Horse," Lou Gehrig.)*

Chapman collapsed, was helped to his feet, walked a few steps, and then fell over again. He was rushed to St. Lawrence Hospital, where a skull X-ray revealed a depressed skull fracture. He was admitted for observation. A few hours later Chapman began to deteriorate and was taken to surgery just after midnight by T. M. Merrigan, a general surgeon.

At the time, the specialty of neurosurgery was still in its infancy, so there were very few brain surgeons around. Most emergency work on the brain was handled by general surgeons. The operation lasted just over an hour. A three-inch piece of fractured bone was removed from the left side of Chapman's head and a few blood clots were evacuated. Chapman died a few hours later, at 4:40 in the morning.

More than 2,000 people turned out for his funeral, held at St. John's Cathedral in Cleveland. Another 3,000 had to be turned away for lack of space, but they lined the nearby streets to catch a glimpse of the procession.

---

*After Pipp called in sick with a headache, Gehrig was brought off the bench to fill in for him. Pipp never stepped on the bag as a starter again. His story has since become a cautionary tale for the risk of missing a day of work.

Although other baseball players have perished from a similar injury, Chapman remains to this day the only Major League player to die from injuries sustained during a game. His death precipitated several changes to the rules of Major League Baseball, such as outlawing the purposeful scuffing of balls, mandating frequent ball changes, and eventually wearing protective batting helmets—policies that have saved countless lives.*

The batting helmet has its own story that also overlaps with neurosurgical history. The first batting helmet was designed in 1905 by the A. J. Reach Company in a desperate attempt to reduce the mounting number of fatalities resulting from "beanballs," particularly among amateur players. Billed as the Reach Pneumatic Head Protector for Batters, it looked more like an inflatable catcher's mitt attached to the side of the head than a helmet. Not surprisingly, this unsightly and cumbersome device didn't catch on, nor did a series of other equally clunky subsequent prototypes. In 1940, after the beaning of Brooklyn Dodgers superstar shortstop Pee Wee Reese, followed by a second beaning of another player on the team, Joe Medwick, general manager Larry MacPhail recruited two surgeons from Johns Hopkins to design a new protective cap. One of these doctors was neurosurgeon Walter E. Dandy.

Walter Dandy, second only to Harvey Cushing, was the best-known neurosurgeon of his era. He was Cushing's most famous and influential pupil, as well as his foremost rival. In 1940, the year after Cushing's death, Dandy replaced his mentor as the preeminent North American neurosurgeon. He was also a huge fan of the game of baseball. Between operations at Johns Hopkins, he was known to sneak out of the hospital to catch a few innings watching his home team, the Baltimore Orioles.

Dandy was acutely knowledgeable of the anatomy of the skull and its

---

*Chapman tragically missed out on the Cleveland Indians' World Series victory that same year, spurred on by Bill Wambsganss's miraculous one-man, unassisted triple play, the only time such a feat has ever been achieved in a World Series game.

areas of vulnerability, so he designed a rigid plastic insert that could be fitted into the linings of existing baseball caps to protect not only the rounded sides of the head but also the temporal bone at its thinnest point overlying the middle meningeal artery. He designed his first prototype while working out of his living room; it was sewn together by his wife and daughters.

In 1943, after a prolonged patent dispute with MacPhail, on November 8, 1943, Walter E. Dandy was issued patent no. 2,333,987 for a Protective Cap, a version of which now resides in the Baseball Hall of Fame in Cooperstown, New York. The cap was used by most teams until 1952, after which the Pittsburgh Pirates introduced a fiberglass batter's helmet, a precursor to the modern version in use today. It took until 1956, thirty-six years after Chapman's death, for the National and American Baseball Leagues to make protective helmets mandatory.

We will never know exactly what felled Ray Chapman in the CAT scanless 1920s, but we can surmise, given the mechanism of the injury, the location of the impact, and the delay until he deteriorated, that it was most

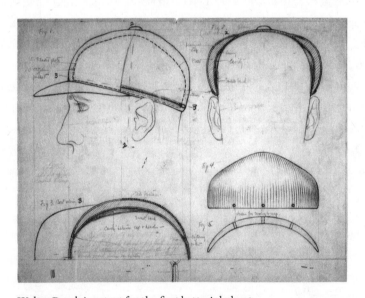

Walter Dandy's patent for the first batter's helmet.
The Chesney Archives of Johns Hopkins Medicine, Nursing, and Public Health

likely an epidural hematoma. Like Richardson's, Chapman's life also could have been saved—and easily at that—had the correct diagnosis been made and the proper operation been performed in a timely fashion. Even better, the whole incident might have been prevented had he been wearing Dandy's helmet.

THE NUTCRACKER SUITE

The neurosurgeon's role as an advocate for better skull protection has not been limited to defense against baseballs. Having to deal with much more serious injuries coming from motorcycle accidents, not to mention bullets and mortar shells, provided neurosurgeons with the motivation to design more effective protective helmets in these other arenas as well.

The most famous of all the dome defenders was undoubtedly Sir Hugh Cairns. Cairns was born in Australia but then spent time studying in England as a Rhodes scholar and went on to Oxford University to obtain his medical degree. In 1926 he obtained funds from the Rockefeller Foundation and set sail for the United States, where he trained with Harvey Cushing.

Cairns served with the Australian and New Zealand Army Corps in the Gallipoli Campaign against Turkey. (He was overheard saying, in jest, that the year he spent as Cushing's resident was more stressful than his time on the front lines.) Cairns's interest in trauma was piqued when he was called to attend to World War I hero T. E. Lawrence, better known as Lawrence of Arabia, who had been injured while riding a motorcycle without a helmet. Lawrence had swerved to avoid two boys on their bicycles and was thrown over his handlebars, smashing his head against the ground. He died a few days later.

Cairns soon began tracking the astonishingly high rate of head trauma in British motorcycle messengers. Working with a physicist, he improved the design of motorcycle helmets and was instrumental in making them mandatory, thereby dramatically reducing the incidence of head and neck injuries. By 1941, motorcycle helmets were compulsory for military personnel, a law that was extended to civilians in 1973. Cairns's helmets reduced the risk of motorcycle-related brain trauma by 70 percent and the risk of mortality by 40 percent.

Cairns eventually moved back to Oxford, becoming one of the earliest surgeons in England to devote his practice uniquely to neurosurgery, carrying on the tradition of the first British neurosurgeons, Sir William Macewen in Scotland and Sir Victor Horsley in England. Starting out his career at the National Hospital, Queen's Square, in London, Cairns faced strong opposition when he tried to implement Cushing's deliberate, meticulous techniques because the more senior general surgeons favored rapid, often more clumsy interventions, hurried as they were by the erratic and unpredictable effects of early anesthesia. Cairns, like the other neurosurgeons of his day, also battled with the neurologists—medical doctors who care for the nervous system using nonsurgical methods—who felt that neurosurgery was a mostly unsafe therapy of last resort that should be regulated and under their control.

His career was once again sidelined by the onset of the Second World War. Since Oxford was spared the relentless bombings suffered in London, Cairns's unit, fondly nicknamed the "Nutcracker Suite," became the primary center for the management of all head trauma. Recognizing the value of rapid surgical treatment, Cairns came up with the idea of creating mobile neurosurgical units that could deliver quality care up near the front line. (Again we see the importance of timing and access in treating head trauma.) The units were so effective that the idea was adopted by the U.S. Army, which expanded it into what are now called mobile army surgical hospitals, or MASH units (as in the '70s and '80s TV show). For his many contributions, Cairns was knighted by King George VI.

Even more prevalent at the time than motorcycle injuries were those caused by cars. Following the end of World War II, dramatic growth in the automobile industry led to a corresponding rise in the incidence of car crashes. Neurosurgeons found themselves at the front lines in a new war, this time against dashboard and steering wheel collisions. In 1955, one in ten cars on the road was involved in an accident; of those, one-third of the accident victims were severely injured. Cars were designed purely for comfort, not for safety. In response to mounting casualties, neurosurgeon C. Hunter Shelden published an article in *The Journal of the American Medical Association* warning of the alarming rise in accident statistics and the mounting frustration of his beleaguered colleagues, who were often called in the middle of the night to clean up the mess. Shelden pointed out that more U.S. citizens had been killed in automobile accidents in the last fifty years than in both world wars combined and highlighted several design flaws that made cars of that era particularly unsafe.

Shelden's piece appeared in *JAMA* ten years before Ralph Nader's book *Unsafe at Any Speed*, which was credited with galvanizing the public outcry that led to the passage of the first seat belt laws in 1968. But Shelden didn't just identify the problem; he tried to fix it. Working alongside neurosurgeon Dr. Frank Mayfield, the two created the first seat belt, which was offered by the Ford Motor Company as an optional feature. Named Lifeguard, the seat belt, along with some other safety features, was only installed upon request, at a surcharge. It was initially a complete failure since consumers refused to pay. Only when car manufacturers were forced by the federal government to include these safety features were they routinely placed in every vehicle.

THE ACCESS PROBLEM

Prompt access to competent brain surgery is not a given. In fact, it's very much dependent on circumstances that are out of the victim's and sometimes even the neurosurgeon's control. Successful management of severe brain trauma has two components. First is an understanding of exactly what needs to be done. Second, and perhaps more important, is the ability to get the patient into the neurosurgeon's hands in time.

In 1993, recognizing that the treatment of traumatic brain injury, or TBI, varied greatly from one medical center to another, three neurosurgeon experts—Drs. Jamshid Ghajar, Randall M. Chestnut, and Donald W. Marion—teamed up to compose a clear set of recommendations. They recruited nine other neurosurgeons to review the existing published studies and created a set of recommendations that they made available to any hospital in the world. First published by the Brain Trauma Foundation in 1996, these guidelines outline when to place a ventriculostomy (the catheters that drain cerebrospinal fluid from the brain to lower pressure), when to perform a hemicraniectomy, and when to evacuate epidural and subdural hematomas. They also provide a cookbook-style recipe for how to regulate blood pressure and intracranial pressure to optimize outcomes.

Implemented correctly, these guidelines have been shown to reduce mortality after TBI by as much as 50 percent. Brain injury accounts for up to one-third of all trauma-related deaths, with a currently estimated annual cost to the United States of upward of $75 billion. This simple set of guidelines has saved literally millions of lives, not to mention trillions of dollars worldwide.

But here's the thing: if a patient can't reach a level 1 trauma center quickly enough, it doesn't matter how smart the Brain Trauma Foundation's protocols are or how skilled the surgeon. The patient won't make it. Mont-Tremblant is only seventy-five miles from the nearest hospital capable of performing basic brain surgery: a lifesaving distance. But Natasha Richardson was first taken by land to a local hospital that wasn't equipped to handle her condition and then transferred in another land vehicle, a process that took over six hours from the time of her fall. Had a helicopter picked Richardson up from her hotel, she could have been in the hands of a neurosurgeon within an hour and her life easily saved. Alas, no such helicopter was forthcoming, which is an infrastructure problem not unique to Canada.

RFK's care, too, we saw, was also delayed by circuitous and inefficient transport.

In an ideal world, surgery to remove a traumatic hematoma should happen within four hours of injury. Earlier is even better. If a mechanism is in place to deliver a patient directly to an equipped trauma center, without stopping at a local community hospital first, this four-hour goal is attainable in most higher-income countries. However, if patients are first brought to a local hospital, where they're assessed, stabilized, and then transferred— all of which takes time, as anyone who has ever visited an emergency room can attest—treatment delays go up considerably.

Several studies have clearly demonstrated that the availability of a transport helicopter increases survival rates after severe TBI. What's less clear, for those counting beans, is whether the incremental cost can be justified. Once readily available, helicopters can be overused, dispatched overzealously to retrieve cases of moderate or even mild TBI—situations where rapid delivery provides no benefit.

One 2010 study closely examined the cost-benefit ratio for helicopter transport. Of the 70,000 flights sent to retrieve trauma victims, at a cost of $240 million, over half were for minor or non-life-threatening accidents. Worse, in a single year, twenty-eight patients *died* from accidental helicopter crashes! Justifying the cost of medical helicopters requires that they decrease mortality by 17 percent, a threshold that has not yet been met. So the cost of the helicopters doesn't justify the few lives that might be saved. Although we don't like to put a value on human life, this is how healthcare dollars are allocated in the face of limited resources. I find the bean counting infuriating. In my opinion, the government's lack of willingness to create appropriate infrastructure to serve the public's needs, such as ensuring rapid transportation of trauma victims to well-staffed trauma centers, is shortsighted.

In low- and middle-income countries the situation is more dire, attributable not only to the lack of transportation and resources but to the paucity of neurosurgeons. There are some 50,000 neurosurgeons working worldwide, which translates to one neurosurgeon for every 230,000 people. High-income countries have one neurosurgeon for every 100,000 people. In sub-Saharan Africa, there is one neurosurgeon for every 5 million, or 0.02 neurosurgeons for every 100,000 people. This is equivalent to a fiftyfold neurosurgery gap between high- and low-income countries.

Lower-income countries also have a more scattered population, with fewer inhabitants living in proximity to trauma centers. In 2018, eleven countries had no practicing neurosurgeons whatsoever, seven of which were in sub-Saharan Africa and four in East Asia. Compare this with Japan, where they have one neurosurgeon for every 17,000 people. Why so many neurosurgeons in Japan? Japan doesn't limit the number of residents who train in neurosurgery and accepts all that apply. Given the oversupply, many neurosurgeons in Japan find work in the emergency rooms and ICUs or in research or radiology.

Access to neurosurgical care is just another example of the unequal distribution of resources on our planet without an easy solution. We neurosurgeons stand at the end of a long line of circumstances regulated by geopolitical and socioeconomic factors out of our control. Until our governments decide to devote more resources to bolster and prioritize medical infrastructure, missed opportunities with tragic outcomes like Natasha Richardson's will continue to break our hearts.

FIVE

SPORTS NEUROSURGERY

As one of the few neurosurgeons in my town, Scarsdale, New York, hardly a week goes by that I don't field a concussion-related phone call from a concerned parent. I usually ask for the student athlete to be brought over to my home after the game for a quick neurological exam. Then I recommend a step-by-step incremental increase in their activities: return to school; light exercise; attending practices; and only then, absent any symptoms, return to play. Most children who sustain a concussion will be fine, and their symptoms will resolve after a few days.

Although we don't have a neurosurgical treatment to shorten the duration of concussion symptoms per se, neurosurgeons often care for patients with concussions in their medical practices, meaning we are the first line of defense after a kid falls or butts heads with another. While football is the most likely sport to lead to a concussion, girls' soccer is a close second, followed by girls' basketball, leading experts to hypothesize that the adolescent female brain may be more susceptible to concussion than the adolescent male brain.

Despite all the attention they've received, concussions in football are relatively rare. Less than one in ten thousand helmet impacts result in a concussion. While "concussion" used to be defined as a loss of consciousness after a head injury, this is no longer the case. With most concussions, there is no loss of consciousness. The damage to the brain caused by a concussion occurs on a microscopic level, well below the resolution of a CAT scan or an MRI. The diagnosis is usually made based on symptoms: headache, sensitivity to light, dizziness, nausea, vomiting, and amnesia that can last anywhere from mere seconds all the way up to weeks or even months.

"Concussion" is another word for mild TBI. Any rapid acceleration-deceleration of the head can transmit a wave of pressure through the brain that can temporarily stun the neurons. If the impact is hard enough, long-lasting damage may result. The parts of the brain that are most susceptible to this type of injury are the wires—also called axons—that connect the neurons with each other. Traumatic damage to axons is also called diffuse axonal injury, or DAI. Imagine the axons in your brain as a handful of well-cooked spaghetti. Head injury does to them what whipping your hand above your head does to the soggy pasta.

Blows to the head can also damage blood vessels, which regulate blood flow, disrupt cell metabolism (the amount of energy consumed), create inflammation (the white blood cell response to injury), and cause scarring, or gliosis, named after the glial cells, which nourish and clean up the excess waste and chemicals produced by neurons.

Luckily, most sports-related concussions in high school athletes don't result in a significant or long-lasting brain injury. Even the trouble focusing, headache, drowsiness, and irritability of post-concussive syndrome mostly resolve on their own. Don't get me wrong: I'm not minimizing the potentially life-altering long-term psychological and cognitive effects that a concussion can have on some children. It's just that these situations are rare and there is nothing a neurosurgeon can do to help. Our services aren't needed. We get involved only if a blow to the head leads to a life-threatening injury such as a brain hemorrhage or swelling.

A brain hemorrhage from a sports collision, such as an epidural hematoma with its concomitant lucid interval, is very rare. That's why you *should* let your child sleep if they are concussed so their brain can heal. A recent fifty-year review of the medical literature on all youth sports-related injuries, published by Vanderbilt's neurosurgery department, found reports of only a handful of epidural hematomas. Moreover, these cases were almost always related to golf and transpired when a child was hit in the head *while watching someone else swing the club.* Of the cases in which the child was participating in a sport, only six cases—three related to skiing and one each related to skateboarding, soccer, and basketball—resulted in an epidural hematoma. That's it! Six cases in fifty years. The real danger to our children, then, is not a concussion, which often resolves, or an epidural hematoma, which is extremely rare; it's a phenomenon called second impact syndrome, and in this situation the symptoms are immediate and severe.

SECOND IMPACT SYNDROME

THE CASES OF
MATTHEW GFELLER, JAQUAN WALLER, NATHAN STILES,
AND ZACKERY LYSTEDT

Matthew Gfeller was a fifteen-year-old boy who played inside linebacker for his high school in North Carolina. In 2008, during his first varsity football game, Gfeller took a hard helmet-to-helmet hit. He struggled to get back up on his feet. He was taken to the nearest hospital, where doctors found an acute subdural hematoma. Despite rapid surgery to remove the blood, he slipped into a coma and died the next day.

Less than a month after Gfeller's injury, a similar situation occurred to Jaquan Waller, a sixteen-year-old running back. Waller suffered a concussion in practice and was taken off the field by the school's injury management specialist. When his symptoms resolved two days later, he was cleared to play. He got hit again while carrying the ball near the line of scrimmage, hard enough that it caused him to fumble. Stunned, he made it to the sideline, where he collapsed. By the time he got to the hospital, he was already brain-dead.

Nathan Stiles was a seventeen-year-old senior from Kansas. In 2010, following one of his games, he told his mom that he had a headache, which quickly got better. Later that week, at practice, the headache returned. He went to a doctor, who ordered a CAT scan. It was normal. The doctor suggested that Nathan take a week off. His headaches resolved and he was cleared to play. The following week he competed for an entire game without a problem. A week later, after scoring his second touchdown of the game, Nathan stumbled off the field, screaming that his head hurt. A moment later he collapsed and couldn't be aroused. An ambulance was called that whisked him from the field to the hospital. There, a CAT scan revealed a subdural hematoma and massive brain swelling. Nathan required an emergency hemicraniectomy and the subdural hematoma was evacuated. Despite these heroic efforts, the next day—four days before his eighteenth birthday—he, too, was declared brain-dead.

As if these three tragic cases were not enough, we cannot forget the case of Zackery Lystedt. Zackery was a thirteen-year-old middle school football player at Tacoma Junior High School in Washington State. In 2011, after getting hit near the end of the first half of the game, he began rolling on the ground, clutching his head in his hands as if it were going to explode. Zackery was kept out for the next few plays but returned to the field for the second half. After another, similar hit, he collapsed to the ground. He was heard saying that he could no longer see anything. Zackery was rushed to the hospital, where a CAT showed hemorrhages on both sides of his brain: subdural hematomas. Neurosurgeons evacuated the blood clots and removed the skull on the left side to give his brain room to swell. Zackery survived but was left with severe brain damage that weakened his right side and garbled his speech.

These four middle and high school football players were considered victims of a condition called second impact syndrome. SIS, as it is more commonly known, was first described in 1973 by neurosurgeon Richard C. Schneider, the chair of neurosurgery at the University of Michigan. Schneider was a huge Michigan football fan and the first neurosurgeon to take an active interest in football-related head and neck injuries. He was also involved in designing the modern football helmet, for which he was nick-named the Father of Sports Neurosurgery.

SIS is diagnosed when a blow to the head leads to massive brain swelling out of proportion to the seriousness of the injury. In the original definition, the head strike must be preceded by a prior head injury that caused a concussion within a certain time frame. The fear of second impact syndrome has been such a successful catalyst for concussion-related legislation that it may come as a surprise to know that there is still debate about whether it really exists.

So how common is SIS? According to a report put out by the CDC in 2017, injuries to the brain and spinal cord caused 2.8 deaths per year in high school and college football athletes. Of these, only 18 percent were preceded by an earlier concussion, which translated to roughly one SIS-related death every two years. Not such a high number. But these statistics probably underestimate the problem, since they don't include devastating but nonfatal brain injuries.

What's more important, though, is how often *any* sports-related head trauma leads to a fatality or other catastrophic brain injury. Whether it meets the criteria to be considered a case of SIS is somewhat irrelevant. One of the main sticking points is the use of the word "second," which may be more misleading than it is helpful, as it implies that one hit is not sufficient to trigger the syndrome. Zackery Lystedt, for example, didn't first have an obvious concussion, so his case didn't fit into the classic definition of SIS. Likewise, Nathan Stiles was asymptomatic for two weeks before his fatal head trauma, and he'd played in a full game without an injury the week prior. He most certainly got hit at some point during that game. Why didn't one of those earlier hits trigger SIS? Perhaps it takes only one of the right *type* of hit to cause severe brain swelling in a susceptible brain?

Another unanswered question is, how much time is permissible between hits? While in some cases the hits can be hours apart, in other cases they are separated by several weeks, with multiple harmless hits in between. Experts also debate whether the presence of a subdural hematoma, rather than just brain swelling, nullifies the diagnosis of SIS. Finally, why is the incidence so high in the United States, and why doesn't SIS occur elsewhere in the world?

————

We now know that most catastrophic brain injuries from football are *not* caused by SIS but rather by severe brain swelling or acute subdural hematomas following a single impact event. So, in the interest of protecting our young athletes, let's stop focusing on whether the athlete had a prior concussion. If we want to reduce the incidence of catastrophic sports-related head injuries, we need to focus on preventing *all* high-velocity head-jarring impacts, not just those that occur immediately after a prior concussion. As with shaken baby syndrome, trying to create a disease by lumping together a hodgepodge of symptoms and imaging findings can sometimes do more harm than good. Although the intent is to protect patients and make the doctors' jobs easier, until the real cause of the problem is understood, it may be best to just describe the findings and treat them individually rather than concern ourselves with whether a case is manifestation of a syndrome such as SIS.

SIS is indeed real, but it's not a comprehensive description of all catastrophic sports-related head-on collisions. So the definition of SIS has now expanded to include the presence of a subdural hematoma in addition to massive brain swelling, and the impact doesn't have to follow a prior concussion. It can be a onetime event. Still, the name remains second impact syndrome, even though there doesn't have to be anything "second" about it. Moreover, with increasing awareness, reports are finally coming in from around the world of SIS, or whatever you want to call it, happening in other sports, such as rugby, hockey, and soccer.

But what's the mechanism? How does a blow to the head lead to uncontrollable brain swelling and why is it more common in youth athletes?

The culprit is believed to be a problem in what neuroscientists call "cerebrovascular autoregulation," which is the brain's ability to adjust the amount of blood perfusing it. SIS causes this mechanism to go haywire, so that too much blood floods the brain, which leads to a breakdown in the filtration system that keeps fluid and toxic chemicals from seeping in. As a result, the brain swells, intracranial pressure rises, and then not enough oxygen gets into the brain. Without oxygen, the neurons slowly starve and die, which leads to further swelling and inflammation as well as to the release of more toxic chemicals, which cause even more swelling, and so on in a vicious circle.

There's just something unique about the teenage brain that impairs its ability to regulate blood flow in the face of repeated brain injuries, or even one significant hit. In contrast to the older brain, which starts to atrophy after age twenty-five, the brain of a young adult is as voluminous as it will ever get, so there is less room in the skull to accommodate any swelling.

Since SIS is so dramatic and devastating, it has provided the wake-up call that was needed to raise political awareness of the dangers of mild and moderate TBI in youth sports so that concussion safety laws could be enacted. After the deaths of the four student athletes listed above, the Zackery Lystedt Law was passed in 2009 and the Gfeller-Waller Concussion Awareness Act and Kansas's School Sports Head Injury Prevention Act were passed in 2011. Now all fifty states have similar rules requiring students with suspected concussions be removed from games, examined, and then cleared by a physician before returning to play.

After the new laws were enacted, ironically, the rate of concussions and ER visits from high school or college sports *increased* by at least 50 percent. Why? Once made aware of the risks, doctors suddenly began identifying and treating more concussions. But the laws weren't intended merely to prevent concussions as much as to reduce the incidence of severe brain injuries and deaths. Whether the laws have been successful in this regard will take more time to unravel, since deaths on the field are so infrequent, roughly one for every million athletes. (In high school players, the rate is slightly higher, but still only one for every three hundred thousand participants.) On the bright side, the most recent data from the National Center for Catastrophic Sport Injury Research led by neurosurgeon Dr. Robert C. Cantu has already shown that fatalities from sports-related head injuries seem to have declined by almost 50 percent in the last five years.

This report also revealed another surprising statistic: the most common cause of death during high school and college football was not impact related at all but rather indirect injuries such as heatstroke or heart attacks. These causes, which occurred more during practices, outnumbered direct injuries by more than 3 to 1. In fact, from 2018 to 2022, when there were only thirteen deaths related to tackling or hitting, there were forty-five indirect fatalities. Clearly, safety in youth sports will require additional efforts at many different levels, including medical screening and education regarding safe practice and hydration policies, but we have every reason to believe that efforts in these areas will be as successful as the laws that have helped identify and treat concussions.

CTE OR NOT CTE?

The National Football League, originally called the American Professional Football Association, was founded in 1920. Initially made up of only eleven teams, the NFL now consists of thirty-two teams, with an annual revenue of nearly $16 billion. If you look up the most-watched television events of all time, in the United States the Super Bowl takes twenty-nine of the top thirty slots. Number nine was the *M*A*S*H* farewell episode.

Maintaining a vise grip on both the industry itself and its entertainment value is a high priority of the league. Football is a violent sport. The combination of aggression and finesse are what make it popular. As a result, injuries abound, including a high incidence of concussion, or mild traumatic brain injury (TBI).

For the last twenty years, the NFL has been deeply involved in a controversy over the severity and long-term sequelae not only of concussions but also of what have been called sub-concussive injuries. Mounting evidence has shown that repeated head impacts, even those that don't cause concussions, can result in a disease called chronic traumatic encephalopathy, or CTE, a progressive neurological illness that leads to symptoms of dementia, irritability, forgetfulness, and emotional instability. The risk of developing CTE is unknown, since the diagnosis can be made definitively only by finding structural changes in the brain on autopsy, and players who submit their brains for autopsy already have severe symptoms. Until a reliable, noninvasive, and accurate test for CTE is developed—one that can be administered to athletes while they are still alive—the true incidence remains obscure.

Preliminary evidence leads us to believe that CTE may be occurring more often than we think. Even more frightening, signs of CTE can be identified in teenage players. Imagine the impact on the sport if one day scientists prove that four years of high school football can cause irreversible brain damage in susceptible youth athletes. I'm not saying this is the case—merely that we still don't have all the data to know that it's *not* the case.

What many people may not know is the remarkable role that a small group of neurosurgeons played in the early chapters of this still evolving story. In fact, nearly the entire CTE controversy played itself out on the pages of one of our leading journals, *Neurosurgery*, well before the public or the reporters had a clue. At that early point, the NFL was managing its players' head injuries internally, relying on their own sports medicine doctors. Very few neurosurgeons were involved, and those who were involved held no leadership positions in the NFL. They were merely consultants. The articles that appeared in *Neurosurgery*, and the ensuing disputes they engendered, provide a fascinating window into what can happen when neurosurgical expertise is sidelined.

In its early days, the NFL was always vaguely aware that concussions might be a problem for its players, but they were not thought to be a bigger issue than other health-related troubles, such as knee injuries or the illegal use of anabolic steroids. When questioned, the league was mostly dismissive about the long-term consequences of mild TBI and generally responded that they were "looking into it." Following a series of high-profile concussions in players such as Troy Aikman and Steve Young, league commissioner

Paul Tagliabue created the Mild Traumatic Brain Injury Committee to address and formally study the issue. Tagliabue selected Dr. Elliot Pellman—a rheumatologist and former Jets team doctor with no special training in either neurology or neurosurgery—as its chair.

Pellman and his medical team performed a series of investigations on the incidence and effects of concussions on the league's players. He then published his findings as a collection of articles that appeared in *Neurosurgery*. To introduce them, Tagliabue scripted an editorial in which he praised the NFL's commitment to safety, its support for independent research, and the "groundbreaking" nature of the studies that were going to appear in the journal. The editor of the journal, Michael L. J. Apuzzo, a well-respected Los Angeles neurosurgeon and a team doctor for both the USC Trojans and the New York Giants, introduced the articles with a letter, in which he called the work "highly responsible."

According to Apuzzo, Pellman phoned him up after the articles were submitted, confirming that they would be published as written. But Apuzzo insisted that they undergo the usual rigorous peer review scrutiny required of all published research. What Pellman, Tagliabue, and the rest of the back office and billionaire owners in the NFL couldn't have predicted was how these articles would be received by the neurosurgeon reviewers. They soon learned that controlling the messaging in a scientific journal was not as easy as managing the timing and pageantry of a halftime show. They were ill-prepared for the squabbling and acerbic back-and-forth match that was about to play out on the pages of one of our most prestigious journals.

The first two articles, published in May and August 2003, described the types of hits that caused concussions. They were not particularly controversial and generally well-received. As was the custom in *Neurosurgery*, the articles were followed by commentaries reflecting the opinions of the reviewers, none of which were antagonistic or called into question the reliability of the data. Three reviewers of note, neurosurgeons Robert Cantu, Joseph Maroon, and Julian Bailes, have been leaders in the field of concussion research over the years.

In the October 2003 issue, Pellman published an opinion piece in which he outlined his goals: "This research should be funded to independent scientific researchers; and . . . the NFL's Mild Traumatic Brain Injury Committee should be charged with oversight of the project." But herein was the problem. The members of the NFL's Mild Traumatic Brain Injury Committee were far from independent. One of the key principles of scientific research is that the scientists can't have any (pig)skin in the game. It's as silly as the tobacco companies funding their own scientists to examine the risk of cigarette smoking (which they did, and we all know how that turned out).

In the next article, published in January 2004, Pellman examined three issues: the incidence of concussions, which players in which positions were most at risk, and whether it was safe to allow a player back into the game after a concussion. He found that only one concussion occurred every two games, that quarterbacks were most at risk because they repeatedly got sacked, and that at least half the players with concussions could safely return to play without incident.

In the comments section, the neurosurgeon reviewers started to raise questions about the reliability of the data as well as the league's handling of its concussions. Several of the reviewers pointed out that most concussions were never reported by the players, since their primary concern was not their own brain health but rather their desire to continue playing. In fact, the players with the most severe symptoms were more likely to opt out of participating for fear of being benched. That being the case, the incidence of concussion would be grossly underreported. Even worse, testing was never performed immediately after an injury, when the symptoms were at their most obvious. Rather, assessments were done several days later, after players had had time to recover. The NFL also failed to provide any long-term cognitive data on players who had been in the league for decades, so they never addressed the risk of CTE, which often takes years to manifest. It was also noted that the NFL didn't routinely use neurosurgeons as advisors despite the specialty's obvious experience dealing with head injuries. Moreover, in many circumstances in which a player clearly had sustained a concussion, there was no on-field medical examination to determine the level of injury. Players were generally sent right back into play without having an expert assess their level of incapacity or the risk of further impacts.

As more articles were released and reviewed, it became apparent that the NFL's "sponsored research" and Pellman's data were seriously flawed and biased. The NFL was simply reporting what had been observed and what was done about it—as if their ability to measure concussions were flawless and their management strategy optimal. A better study would have determined how many concussions were *missed* and what *should* have been done to identify them.

For example, every player could have been given objective neuropsychological and eye movement tests before and after each game by a group of independent and unbiased examiners to determine the number of concussions that *actually* occurred. (Eye movement abnormalities are one of the most sensitive ways to pick up on a concussion.) This number could have then been compared to the number of concussions the team doctors *thought* had occurred, based on the players' own reports. But the NFL didn't employ on-field examiners, and the team doctors who made the assessments were not neutral. In fact, as employees of a team to whom they were loyal, they were inclined to overlook concussions because they didn't want to keep their players off the field and risk losing games.

As more of Pellman's articles emerged, the conclusions became increasingly dubious, and the neurosurgeon reviewers became progressively more critical. In his last few articles, Pellman concluded that repeat concussions did not cause long-term brain injury and that returning to the same game after a concussion was not dangerous, even if the player still had a headache. In response, the neurosurgeon reviewers stopped pulling their punches and asserted that the NFL's findings were "flawed with respect to the study design and the interpretation of the findings" and that their conclusions were "very suspect."

THE EVIDENCE MOUNTS

THE CASE OF
MIKE WEBSTER

Mike Webster was a hard-hitting center who played for the Pittsburgh Steelers and then for the Kansas City Chiefs between 1974 and 1990. Nicknamed "Iron Mike," Webster was known as one of the toughest players in the NFL. He won four Super Bowls, was named All-Pro seven times, and played in nine Pro Bowls. Having competed in a total of 245 games, he was inducted into the Hall of Fame in 1997. After his retirement, Webster's behavior grew more erratic. He became increasingly aggressive, forgetful, and disorganized, exhibiting symptoms of early dementia. He ran into financial troubles, and near the end of his life he was homeless, divorced, and depressed. He applied to the NFL for disability, claiming that his cognitive issues were a result of repeated blows to the head, like a boxer who becomes "punch drunk." Neuropsychological evaluations confirmed his mental decline, and in 1999 the retirement board of the NFL approved his request.

In 2002, at the age of fifty, Iron Mike died of a heart attack. His body was brought to the morgue at the Allegheny County, Pennsylvania, coroner's office, where pathologist Dr. Bennet Omalu was assigned to perform the autopsy. Omalu had been trained in emergency medicine in Nigeria but then came to the United States and completed a residency in pathology at Columbia-Presbyterian's Harlem Hospital Center in New York City, followed by a fellowship in neuropathology in Pittsburgh. When Webster's body came across his table, Omalu had just finished his training and knew next to nothing about the game of football.

Even to Omalu's relatively inexperienced eye, what he found in Webster's brain was completely unexpected and, for that reason, also worth reporting. So he submitted for publication an article describing his findings. The journal he chose was, coincidentally, the same one where Pellman had just published his controversial concussion articles. In July 2005, *Neurosurgery* published Omalu's article, in which he documented the pathological changes he had found in Webster's brain, including a buildup of tau proteins and amyloid plaques in the neocortex, the brain's outer surface.* These findings were consistent with chronic traumatic encephalopathy. CTE was not a new disease, having been described in 1973 in a study of retired boxers who developed severe memory loss, aggressive behavior, and mood disorders, a condition called *dementia pugilistica*. Omalu naively assumed the NFL would be interested in the effect the game was having on its players' brains and would appreciate the information.

Omalu's conclusion stopped short of claiming that football *caused* Webster's CTE, since causation had not been definitively proven, but the underlying message was loud and clear. Like the sound of a blitzing middle linebacker snapping the quarterback's femur, the report was a shot heard round the world. The neurosurgeons who reviewed this paper were not at all surprised by the findings, but they also acknowledged that more evidence was needed to establish a definitive relationship between professional football and CTE.

The biggest criticism of the paper that was raised by the reviewers was the lack of proof that Webster had ever been diagnosed with a concussion. If Webster had never been concussed, how could he have CTE? The most likely explanation, of course, was that Webster had indeed suffered multiple concussions but had either failed to recognize them as such or simply hid them from the trainers. Or equally plausible was that the trainers just didn't believe that mild concussions were worth noting. They occurred so frequently that no one thought they were dangerous. Another, more insidious possibility was that CTE could develop, absent any obvious

---

*The neocortex is another name for the gray matter of the brain. It's the outer centimeter which contains all the neurons. The deeper white matter consists mostly of axons, the connecting cables that the neurons use to talk with one another. The reason white matter is white is that these cables are covered with a fatty substance called myelin, which helps them transmit information faster.

concussions, from the normal hits experienced by a player during a career. At the time, such a concept wasn't even entertained, although we now know that CTE is probably caused by a combination of frequent undiagnosed and undisclosed concussions along with thousands of smaller hits, or "sub-concussive" impacts.

The NFL's response to Omalu's article, published in the May 2006 issue of *Neurosurgery*, was swift, harsh, and utterly misguided. Written by several members of the NFL head trauma committee, they first accused Omalu of a "complete misunderstanding of the relevant medical literature," then urged him to "retract the paper or sufficiently revise it and its title after more detailed investigation of this case."

Pellman and colleagues pointed out that the classic tetrad of neuropathologic findings present in the original 1973 description of CTE in boxers—which included scarring in the cerebellum, neurofibrillary tangles, abnormalities in the septum pellucidum (a small membrane that sits in the middle of the brain) and degeneration of the substantia nigra—were not all present in Webster's brain. Since Omalu's findings didn't demonstrate the classic tetrad, Webster couldn't have had CTE. The NFL was essentially using the same disingenuous tactic as Scheck used to defend Woodward in the Eappen case—as in, even though there are clear signs of head trauma, because the classic triad of symptoms is not present, this cannot be shaken baby syndrome and thus cannot be child abuse.

Pellman and his colleagues also had the gall to claim that Webster never had any concussions, since he'd never been removed from any games. Not only does this bogus argument assume that team doctors were appropriately and cautiously preventing players from returning to play after concussion—which we know was not the case—but it ignores the NFL retirement committee's conclusion that Webster's cognitive issues were the result of playing football.

As additional evidence mounted in support of Omalu's hypothesis, another key paper was published in the October 2005 issue of *Neurosurgery* by a group led by neurosurgeons Julian Bailes and Robert Cantu, along with Kevin Guskiewicz at the Center for the Study of Retired Athletes at the University of North Carolina. In this paper, the researchers questioned more than 2,500 retired professional football players, asking them whether they had noticed any symptoms of memory loss, particularly if they had sustained repeated concussions.

The findings were dramatic and demonstrated a higher-than-normal incidence of cognitive decline at the end of a football career. Another piece of the puzzle was now falling into place—namely, evidence for a causative link between football-related head trauma and long-term mental and emotional deterioration.

In the November 2006 issue of *Neurosurgery*, Omalu reported a second case of CTE—found in NFL veteran Terry Long. Long played for eight years in the NFL. According to official records, he'd never suffered a concussion, although interviews with his wife revealed that he clearly had multiple minor but unreported ones. He exhibited many of the same symptoms as Webster and, after several failed attempts at suicide, took his own life by drinking antifreeze at the age of forty-five. Under Omalu's microscope, Long's brain looked different than Webster's. It had no amyloid plaques, and the tau proteins were found in Long's hippocampus, a part of the brain important for memory, not the neocortex, as the case with Webster had been. The authors raised the possibility that CTE might take many different forms and that our understanding of the disease was incomplete, requiring further study.

In that same issue, Pellman published yet another letter, the latest salvo in his back-and-forth exchange with Omalu. In it, Pellman accused Omalu of leaving out the fact that Long had died by consuming antifreeze (although this had been clearly stated in Omalu's report). Pellman went on to propose that the effects of antifreeze on the brain could cloud the pathology results (which, by the way, is not true). Pellman and colleagues then spent several paragraphs discussing Omalu's specific choice of words, questioning his definitions of "sparse" and "widespread," and pointing out how the diagnosis of CTE hinges on the use of these two words. In essence, the NFL's arguments were rhetorical, as if they were arguing a case in the court of public opinion rather than in a scientific journal, indicating their complete unwillingness to even consider the possibility of CTE in their players.

NEUROSURGEONS ENTER THE GAME

In 2008, Boston University School of Medicine established the Center for the Study of Traumatic Encephalopathy. Cofounded by Cantu, neuropsychologist Robert Stern, and neuropathologist Ann McKee, at the time of this writing, the center had examined the brains of over 600 former concussed athletes and diagnosed CTE in more than 350 of them. The NFL eventually "released" Pellman from its concussion committee and, in 2010, brought on two neurosurgeons to be its co-chairs, Drs. Richard Ellenbogen and Hunt Batjer. Under their leadership, the NFL made over twenty-two official rule changes back in 2011 to improve the safety of the game, including penalties for head-to-head contact, and they continue to review and update their policies. The NFL also donated $100 million toward research on the long-term consequences of concussion and, to protect its players, created a game-day concussion protocol.

This protocol includes the placement of athletic trainer spotters in the stands to identify injuries and unaffiliated neurotrauma consultants on the sidelines to examine players. At the first sign of a possible concussion, such as loss of consciousness, ataxia (or stumbling), confusion, or amnesia, players are taken out of the game. If these symptoms are not present, the players must then answer a series of orientation questions named after the Australian neurologist D. L. Maddocks and are examined by an unaffiliated head trauma consultant, often a neurosurgeon or neurologist from a local hospital, who scrutinizes their speech, balance, pupils, and eye movements. Players then must pass a comprehensive sport concussion assessment test called the SCAT5 before returning to play.

A player diagnosed with a concussion is required to abide by the

Madden rule, named after John Madden, the legendary coach of the Oakland Raiders. The rule, which also found its way into the video game *Madden NFL*, mandates that a player diagnosed with a concussion be escorted off the field to the locker room, not to return to play for the rest of the game. They then must pass through a five-step return-to-play protocol, starting with limited activities and graduating up through aerobic activity, heavy lifting, drills, and full practice before being cleared.

In 2013, Cantu's CTE center published an article in the journal *Brain* in which they defined several varieties of CTE and the different stages of the disease that manifest over a broad spectrum of pathologic findings not limited to just the previously identified tetrad. That same year, the NFL finally settled a class action lawsuit filed by thousands of former players that, to date, has paid out over a billion dollars.

The conclusion of this story suggests that, given enough time, science trumps convenient lies. In 2016, the NFL publicly admitted the role the game plays in the development of CTE. Omalu was vindicated, and the NFL has paid out massive reparations to its former players. But the concussion saga is far from over. While the role of repeated head injuries in causing CTE is mostly accepted in the United States, the same is not true internationally. In 2023, consensus statements released by the International Conference on Concussion in Sport still raise doubts about the causative role of head injury in CTE, emphasizing unanswered questions, such as why some athletes get CTE while others do not and the uncertainty regarding the number of collisions needed to trigger the disease. Guess who's supporting the research behind these doubters? The Fédération Internationale de Football Association (FIFA), the International Olympic Committee, as well as the governing bodies of Formula One and World Rugby—the very same leagues that would be faced with massive lawsuits should an association be found. Sound familiar?

In 2017, the NFL created a new position in its organization: chief medical officer. They named neurosurgeon Dr. Allen Sills to the role. Sills is a professor of neurosurgery at Vanderbilt University and the co-director of its concussion center, whose involvement, according to the NFL's website, has already decreased the incidence of concussions by 24 percent at the time of this writing.

Will the new system miss some concussions? Certainly. Football remains an inherently violent sport in which men willingly put their bodies and brains on the line for our entertainment. But they are playing a game they love and being compensated well for taking these risks. The league is obliged to make the game as safe as possible, but if all risk were eliminated, the very nature of the game would be fundamentally altered. The reason sports are so engaging for the spectator is that the struggles and risks inherent in human conflict are amplified and focused into brief, intense moments that result in a clear outcome: victory or defeat. The athletes become our avatars, allowing us the cathartic experience of emotional highs and lows from a safe vantage point.

A part of us may still feel that these athletes are taking undue risk and that contact sports should be further regulated to make them safer. But all jobs carry risk of some sort or another: whether you are an airline pilot or a window washer, your safety is not guaranteed. For example, why is it more acceptable for young men in the military to put their lives on the line to go to battle—sometimes even against their wills if they are drafted—to fight for ideals they may not fully share or to satisfy the ambitions of a leader for whom they may not have voted? Yet, at the same time, we feel obliged to protect football players, who also willingly place their health on the line for their profession. In fact, football, unlike war, empowers its athletes with money, fame, and the opportunity to alter the economic trajectory of their lives and the lives of their families. In some sense, sports, with its inherent meritocracy, clear rules, and referees, may be the fairest of all professional pathways to success. Now, in the post-Omalu era, the risks of football are understood, and the players are choosing to participate despite these known risks.

Having served as a neurosurgeon on the sidelines of a few NFL games myself, I've experienced the complexity and conflicting loyalties of the position. While it might seem obvious on one level that a neurosurgeon should step in and remove players from risk at the first sign of concussion—to protect them—on another level this decision is not as clear-cut as it may seem. As physicians, we have an obligation to ensure that our patients make informed decisions about their health. In the case of a neurosurgical emergency, for example, when a patient's life is on the line, we must step in and act immediately—sometimes without their consent, particularly if they're unconscious. But if a patient walks into my office with a potentially lethal brain tumor, I educate them about their diagnosis. We discuss what their future might look like either with or without treatment. We frankly review the risks of both options, and then I let *them* choose what they want to do. I don't force them into making one decision or another about how to proceed so long as they are competent enough to make their own decisions. We label cigarettes to advertise their risks, but we don't prevent able-minded adults from purchasing them.

Perhaps the role of the concussion expert should reflect a similar logic. In the end, maybe it should be up to the players to decide what they want to do. It's their body, after all. Who are we to say that they shouldn't put themselves at risk to have what may amount to the only fair chance they may ever get to partake in the American dream? If the league wishes to enact rules to protect its players, to avoid the public relations nightmares and lawsuits that might arise from catastrophic injuries, that's their prerogative. But then, for whom are the doctors on the sidelines working: the league or the players? Let's face it, if we were there to represent the players' best interests—to prevent any brain injuries—we wouldn't let them step onto the field in the first place.

Qualified doctors at the ready will no doubt mitigate the risks of the game. Damar Hamlin, who was successfully resuscitated after he suffered a cardiac arrest on the field, is a great example of that. But let's not kid ourselves into thinking that parking a neurosurgeon on the twenty-yard line will prevent or even reduce the incidence of serious or potentially permanent brain injuries when two men hurl themselves at each other running twenty miles per hour and collide head on.

II

HOW DO
BRAIN SURGEONS THINK?

SIX

WEIGHING THE RISKS

Sometimes I try to imagine what it would be like to be one of my patients. One minute you're feeling great, exercising, enjoying time with family and friends, and working a full-time job. The next thing you know, you're on a stretcher, in the back of an ambulance, waking up groggy. You open your eyes and spot the EMT next to you.

"What happened?" you say.

"Not sure," you hear. "Looks like you might have had a seizure."

A . . . *seizure*? Your mind starts racing. What does that even mean? Vague fragments learned or overheard start to come back to you, but you're still not quite sure what a seizure is. You've never had one before. Don't epileptics have seizures? Maybe your blood sugar was low? Maybe you were dehydrated from that workout? Blaming yourself, you think, *I knew I shouldn't have skipped lunch*. You try to sit up, but your head is pounding.

"Just stay down," says the EMT as he gently pushes you back down onto the stretcher.

They roll you into the ER and park you in the corner for what seems like an eternity. It's loud and chaotic. Doctors, nurses, and the family members of patients are walking and running this way and that. Voices and moans erupt from every direction, punctuated on occasion by a scream. Your back is stiff from lying on the stretcher, and your mouth is dry. You see a pitcher of water on the table next to you and reach over to pour yourself a drink, only to realize that your arm is tethered to an IV pole by a plastic tube. When did *that* happen?

Finally, a doctor who looks like she's still in medical school shows up. She asks you a bunch of questions and then tells you they're sending you for a CAT scan. When it's done, you find yourself once again abandoned in the corner of the ER.

After what seems like hours, a group of physicians arrives, and the one in charge—who looks only slightly older than the first one—starts peppering you with questions. Any history of cancer in your family? Are you a smoker? Are your arms or legs weak? Have you ever had any trouble with your speech? Finally, you build up the courage to ask, "What did the CAT scan show?" You see the look of concern on their faces. Then you hear the words: "Well, we don't have all the information yet, but it looks like you may have a brain tumor."

The words sink in.

Time stops. In fact, there is no time. There used to be time. But from this moment on, there is no longer time in the way you once knew it. There is no longer you. Everything has changed. You are now a diagnosis, and your single focus is your new persona. Your illness is your identity. The once clear road ahead dissolves into a fragmented blur. Certainty, you realize, was an illusion. It's all chaos now, punctuated by questions and fear— a deep fear that lingers in your gut.

I specialize in the surgical treatment of brain tumors. I see patients like this almost every day. I am, sadly, only too familiar with this story.

Brain tumors are rare, with a lifetime risk of about six-tenths of one percent. Still, this means that one out of every 161 people will develop a brain tumor at some point in their lives. If you believe evolutionary anthropologist Robin Dunbar, who claims—based on the size of our brains and the average population of inhabitants in ancient villages—that any one person can maintain meaningful relationships with roughly 150 different people, then one person you know well will develop a brain tumor at some point in your lifetime.

My first encounter with brain tumor patients generally occurs a few days after they've received the news, so it's still raw and not yet processed. Sometimes they've seen another neurosurgeon before me. Sometimes I'm the first. Either way, we always have a lot of ground to cover.

Most people think a brain tumor is a death sentence. I'm glad to report that most of the time this is not the case. The 2016 WHO guidelines identify 145 different varieties of brain tumor, and at least 70 percent of them are benign. Benign. This means that the tumor remains in one location, grows slowly, and is often curable with surgery. Over 90 percent of people with a benign brain tumor will still be alive five years later; and that even includes elderly patients with huge tumors, who may die of some other disease along the way or who are too frail to undergo surgery. Some may even refuse treatment altogether. So the actual survival statistics for most people with a benign tumor is even better.

In contrast, the average five-year survival period with a *malignant* brain tumor is around 36 percent. Not so good. But depending on the exact type of tumor, some malignant brain tumors can be cured. Brain metastases, for example, are the most common malignant brain tumor, and since they don't infiltrate deep into the brain, they are also eminently treatable.

THE CASE OF
LANCE ARMSTRONG

After winning the 1996 cycling world championship, Lance Armstrong was diagnosed with advanced testicular cancer. He was twenty-five. The tumor had already spread to his abdomen, lungs, lymph nodes, and brain. Although his type of cancer, embryonal carcinoma, is potentially curable, his prognosis was not hopeful, given the tumor's extensive spread. Armstrong was treated first with chemotherapy: toxic chemicals injected into the bloodstream through a vein. A few weeks after his diagnosis, Indiana

University neurosurgeon Scott Shapiro removed two metastatic brain tumors through two separate openings in Armstrong's skull.

Given his unusual level of fitness and determination, Armstrong began competing again two years after surgery and went on to win seven Tour de France titles as well as a bronze medal in the 2000 Summer Olympics. Unfortunately, Armstrong's return to success, which first depended on lifesaving drugs that fight cancer, eventually ended with a reliance on prohibited ones that enhance performance—a revelation that marred his otherwise remarkable athletic career.

Armstrong founded the Livestrong Foundation, whose mission is to raise awareness, support patients, lobby government agencies, and raise money for research to fight cancer. With its signature yellow bracelets, Livestrong, at the time of this writing, has raised over $500 million, 81 percent of which has gone directly to funding cancer research. Although Armstrong's career was derailed by his illicit strategy to outrace his opponents, his ability to outrace his cancer diagnosis remains an inspiration to countless patients facing a similar challenge.

Metastases form when cancer cells located somewhere else in the body spread to the brain, usually through the bloodstream. For a tumor to grow, it requires a constant blood supply to bring oxygen into each new cell as it replicates. This ever-increasing mass of oxygen-hungry cells must create new blood vessels to keep itself alive, which it does quickly and somewhat haphazardly, like a foreman on a job site given an unrealistic deadline. These hastily constructed channels provide a conduit for the tumor cells, which detach from the primary tumor and enter the bloodstream, spreading to other locations in the body. Once in the bloodstream, cancer cells can, in principle, go anywhere, but the brain is a preferred location. Arriving en masse, these crab-grassy cells lay down roots, sometimes in more than one location.

Cancer that has spread beyond its site of origin is called stage 4, meaning that it's advanced to its most deadly level. Depending on the type of cancer—whether it originated in the breast, lung, testicles, or elsewhere—the prognosis will be determined by its growth rate and its sensitivity to treatment. Not all cancers, I should note, are equally likely to spread to the brain. Lung, kidney, breast, melanoma, and colon cancer make up almost 80 percent of brain metastases. In other words, not only was Armstrong's testicular tumor uncommon in someone his age, but it was also extremely unusual for such a cancer to spread to the brain.

Most cancers in the body are treated with either chemotherapy or targeted immune therapies, but when tumors enter the nervous system, they become difficult to manage because the brain is screened off from the bloodstream by a protective barricade called the blood-brain barrier.

A fine filter, developed over eons of human evolution, the blood-brain barrier is like a moat around the brain, a way of defending itself from the onslaught of toxic chemicals our ancestors might have ingested. This barrier is not impenetrable and allows certain essential elements, like oxygen or glucose, to pass through its filtration system. Metastases have figured out ways to bypass the blood-brain barrier and sneak into the brain to take root, which is what makes them so difficult to treat, since they remain hidden behind the very same fence the brain has erected to protect itself.

As such, chemotherapies that might be effective against cancer cells in other parts of the body are often unable to pass through. In this situation, there are two options. The first is to have a neurosurgeon operate and physically remove the tumors. The second is to treat them with radiation, since X-rays can pass through skin and bone to reach virtually any location in the body.

Surgery to remove a brain metastasis, such as Lance Armstrong's, is almost always successful. Armstrong had not one but two tumors, which were removed through separate craniotomies. But if a patient has dozens of small tumors, surgical removal of all of them becomes impossible, since the risks multiply with each intervention. Moreover, surgeons can remove only the ones they know about. Sometimes, when there are several visible tumors, it means the brain has been showered with cancer cells, so there are probably more microscopic ones concealed below the radar. A surgery that removes only the visible ones won't be effective. Eventually these scattered tiny tumors will grow full-sized. Some brain metastases can also take root in difficult-to-reach places, rendering surgery too risky. On top of all that, patients with cancer are often frail and may not tolerate multiple brain surgeries. This is where alternative number two—radiation—comes in.

A few decades ago, brain metastases were mostly treated by giving ten doses of radiation to the entire brain. Bathing the whole brain with radiation guaranteed that even the small unseen tumors were treated. Not surprisingly, so much radiation was not great for the healthy brain cells, the innocent bystanders that also got bombarded. Patients' cognitive abilities suffered. Their memory failed and their concentration dimmed. Moreover, presumed invisible micro-metastases were not as common as previously imagined. Dousing the entire brain in toxic radiation for the sake of treating a few small tumors was the equivalent of burning your whole house down to treat a termite infestation. It might be effective, but it was overkill—a Pyrrhic medical victory.

Today, very few patients receive whole-brain radiation because of a new device invented in the 1950s by a brilliant Swedish neurosurgeon named Lars Leksell. Leksell created an elegant method for delivering high doses of radiation to a small area in the brain to minimize any collateral damage. His invention, the Gamma Knife, led to the formation of an entirely new field of neurosurgery.

Like Cushing before him, Leksell began his medical career administering anesthesia—which at the time consisted of dripping chloroform on a cloth—for the great Swedish neurosurgeon Herbert Olivecrona (who, to no one's surprise at this point, trained under Harvey Cushing). As Olivecrona's apprentice, Leksell was also responsible for ensuring that enough blood was available for transfusion during his mentor's more complex operations. This process generally consisted of accessing the veins of family members lined up outside the operating room while the operation was underway. According to one of his students, Leksell fell behind on more than one occasion with disastrous consequences. It was this experience that motivated him to conceive of a less invasive way to perform brain surgery. Leksell also had extensive battlefield experience, and his desire to remove buried bullet fragments from the brain inspired him to imagine a device that could attach itself to the head and reach in and grab embedded shards of shrapnel.

For such a concept to work, Leksell devised a method to calculate the entry site and trajectory required to reach any target anywhere in the brain. He figured out that if he could take an X-ray of the head with the frame in place, he could make the necessary calculations. The methodology, called stereotaxis, was already being developed in the United States at the time, albeit using a slightly different concept. Nowadays, stereotaxis relies on CAT scans and MRIs to achieve much greater precision. But it was the marriage of the stereotaxis concept with radioactive sources that ushered in one of the first great revolutions in minimally invasive neurosurgery—the invention of stereotactic radiosurgery.

STEREOTAXIS

The word "stereotaxis" derives from Greek, combining *stereo*—dealing with three dimensions of space—and *táttein*—to place or to position: basically, the ability to accurately place something anywhere in three-dimensional space. Say you were a neurosurgeon living in the 1950s and you had a patient with a tumor deep in the brain. You might want to do a biopsy of the tumor to see if you could treat it with chemotherapy or radiation. To perform this biopsy, you would need to know three coordinates: where to stick the needle through the skull, the angle of entry, and the depth to get there. Unfortunately, none of this information was obvious, and if you tried to just guess, you were likely to be off by quite a bit, resulting not only in harm to the patient but also an unsuccessful biopsy. The ability to deliver treatment to a precise location in the brain is critical not only for tumor biopsies but for many other fields of neurosurgery, including the treatment of Parkinson's disease and epilepsy, which rely on the precise insertion of electrodes into the brain.

Stereotaxy was first devised by British neurosurgeon Victor Horsley and his engineer partner Robert Henry Clarke. Horsley, considered the father of British neurosurgery, predated even Cushing. Clarke was more the mathematician in the partnership. As legend has it, Clarke was gazing

up at the stars while convalescing after a bout of pneumonia he'd contracted during a trip to Egypt, sometime in the 1890s. Something he saw on
that starry night allowed him to conceive of an apparatus that could be
attached to the skull and used to define a three-dimensional space around the
head using the trio of X, Y, and Z coordinates to define any point in space.
For those of you who remember Cartesian space from tenth-grade geometry,
the idea was to leverage that concept, described by the French philosopher
René Descartes back in the seventeenth century, to locate a single point in
the brain. (Coincidentally, Descartes himself had come up with the idea of
Cartesian space while lying in bed, watching a fly zip around his room.)

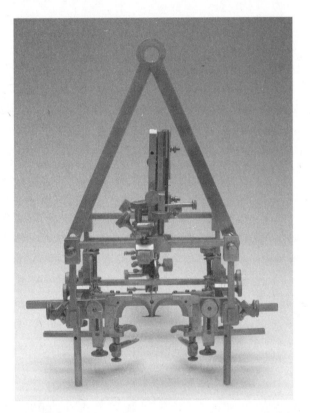

The Horsley-Clarke stereotactic boxlike frame attached to
the head and localized a point in space using X, Y, and Z
coordinates.

Science Museum Group

In 1905, Clarke approached Horsley with his idea, and together they built the first stereotactic device, designed for experimental use in monkeys. Alas, the Horsley-Clarke apparatus, which relied on external skull landmarks, was never quite ready for prime time, and so they never had a chance to try it on patients. In fact, it wasn't until 1947 that neurologist Ernst A. Spiegel and neurosurgeon Henry T. Wycis, working at Temple University in Philadelphia, figured out how to modify the Horsley-Clarke idea to assemble a practical device that could be brought into the operating room to treat brain diseases in real human patients.

Spiegel, a Jew from Vienna, saw his scientific funding dry up as Austrian sympathy for the Nazi movement swelled during the buildup to World War II. To his good fortune, he and his wife were allowed to emigrate, and they landed in Philadelphia. Wycis, a New Jersey native and semiprofessional baseball player, began working in Spiegel's laboratory on his way to becoming a neurosurgeon. Together they modified the Horsley-Clarke apparatus to rely on internal rather than external landmarks and created a working prototype, which they began using in living patients.

Spiegel and Wycis could not have appreciated the far-reaching benefits of their invention. Their motivation was simple: to find a better way to perform frontal lobotomies, considered at the time the most effective treatment for mental illness. The lobotomy was an inelegant operation, involving the blind insertion of a butter knife–like instrument into the frontal lobe, where it was swept back and forth to disconnect it from the rest of the brain. Stereotaxis, simply put, was devised to be a lobotomy upgrade.

Once they'd developed the stereotactic tool, however, Spiegel and Wycis quickly realized its potential and rapidly changed course, using their system to target the problematic neurons that caused the tremors in Parkinson's disease. The history of science has repeatedly shown that innovations that are developed for one application are frequently adapted into other areas where they prove more effective. Viagra, for example, was created to treat high blood pressure and chest pain . . . that is, until its other use was discovered. And it is in this tradition that stereotaxis was soon repurposed to treat other diseases for which it was better suited. For now, we will focus on its application in the treatment of brain tumors and leave lobotomies and Parkinson's disease for later.

Although Leksell was aware of Spiegel and Wycis's invention, his insight was to add a unique twist to the concept that made it even more powerful. Rather than think of the space around the head as a box—with X, Y, and Z coordinates—he thought of it as a sphere.

Why a sphere? Because if you can define a sphere around a target in space, then a line drawn perpendicular to the surface of that sphere will always hit the geometrical center—namely, the target. And since the radius of a sphere is fixed, the depth to the target will always be the same.

Imagine a knitting needle that measures exactly half the diameter of a basketball. If you place the needle through the wall of the basketball perpendicular to its surface, it will hit the geometric center of the basketball every time, no matter where you insert the needle. Leksell took this concept and ran with it, shaping it into a new stereotactic device. But instead of knitting needles, Leksell used beams of radiation—several hundred of them, in fact—to create a tool we now call the Gamma Knife. In the Gamma

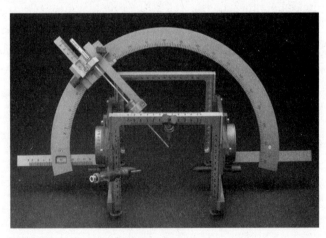

The Leksell arc- or sphere-based system, conceived of the space around the head as a sphere, rather than as a cube.

Science Museum Group

Knife, Leksell not only built a better mousetrap but also pioneered a brand-new field of neurosurgery.

FANTASTIC VOYAGE

Stereotactic radiosurgery comes close to achieving the neurosurgical holy grail: to deliver energy deep into the brain without opening up the skull. That energy can take one of several forms, either mechanical (delivered via a surgeon's hands), electromagnetic (delivered via radiation), optical (delivered via laser beam), or acoustic (delivered via ultrasound).

The concept is captured vividly in the classic 1966 movie *Fantastic Voyage*, in which a team of scientists shrink a group of doctors and their submarine ship, then inject them, ship and all, into the arm of a patient with a life-threatening blood clot. The doctors travel through the body, using the bloodstream as a conduit to reach the clot, which they obliterate with a laser gun. The treatment is minimally invasive, and the destructive energy is delivered directly to the problem. Normal blood flow is restored. Collateral damage is minimized. Stroke averted.

Stereotactic radiosurgery, like the nano-sized doctors from the movie, aims to deliver energy to a target inside the skull without harming anything else in its the path. The science behind it can be understood through this thought experiment: Imagine you are in the wilderness trying to cook dinner, and all you have is a magnifying glass. So you find a dry leaf in the hope of shining the sun's rays onto it through the magnifying glass to start a fire. But what if it's overcast? The heat provided by the magnifying glass would probably not be sufficient. However, imagine that you were not alone in the wilderness but you happened to have brought along twenty of your closest friends, and each of them had their own magnifying glass. If everyone was to stand in a circle around that same dry leaf, each holding a magnifying glass that could focus its rays on the same spot at the same time, the combined energy would have a better chance of igniting your fire. Although one beam might not be enough to kindle a flame, twenty beams would probably do the job. The accumulation of power would occur instantly since the energy converges not only in space but in time.

Now imagine that, instead of light, these magnifying glasses could focus individual beams of radiation, and nearly two *hundred* magnifiers were lined up inside a metal helmet that encircled a patient's head. If a brain metastasis were placed in the geometric center of the helmet, all the radiation rays would focus onto the tumor and obliterate it. That's precisely how the Gamma Knife and most other forms of stereotactic radiosurgery work. The tumor at the focal point is destroyed, and the rest of the brain remains unscathed.

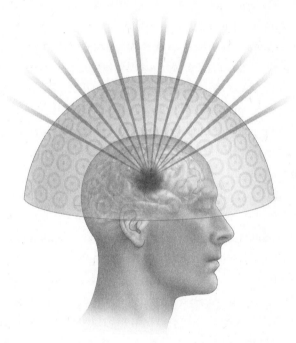

The Gamma Knife delivers 192 separate pencil-thin beams of radiation through a spherical helmet to a focal point within the brain.

Although stereotactic radiosurgery is effective, it's also imperfect. No matter how precise the delivery, some normal structures—either brain tissue or another nearby structure—will receive a bit of unwanted radiation.

Worst-case scenario, this can lead to a dramatic form of brain swelling called radiation necrosis. Sometimes the radiation doesn't work at all, and the tumor continues to grow. Nevertheless, for a brief time, stereotactic radiosurgery was the closest neurosurgery came to reproducing Hollywood's *Fantastic Voyage*.

Once radiosurgery was married to advanced imaging techniques like CAT scans and MRIs, neurosurgeons began to use focal radiation to treat a variety of brain diseases, including benign and malignant tumors, Parkinson's disease, epilepsy, arteriovenous malformations, and mental illness.

While stereotactic radiosurgery seems an ideal, elegant, noninvasive tool, many brain tumors still require surgery, since they are often too large or too close to important structures to be safely treated with radiosurgery. The good news is that traditional neurosurgery, the kind where the skull is cracked open, is also changing and becoming less and less invasive. The idea is to be like a cat burglar: Get in and get out. Try not to disturb anything. Leave no clues that you were there. Since many brain metastases are now treated with stereotactic radiosurgery, the jewel that we neurosurgeon-safecrackers are most commonly trying to nip from the skull's vault is a different tumor, a benign one called the meningioma.

SOMETIMES A HEADACHE IS JUST A HEADACHE

THE CASE OF
KATE WALSH

Kate Walsh is an American actress best known for playing Dr. Addison Montgomery, Derek Shepherd's ex-wife on *Grey's Anatomy*. In 2015, when she was forty-seven, Walsh began feeling tired and having trouble concentrating. She was also experiencing headaches, trouble with her balance, and a feeling that she would "dip" when she put weight on her right side. Her language became clumsy. "I would reach for words or thoughts, and I just couldn't finish them," Walsh said in a 2017 interview with *Cosmopolitan*.

She was referred for an MRI. It showed a 5-centimeter meningioma pushing on her left frontal lobe as well as edema (swelling) in her brain. She was placed on an anti-seizure medication and within three days underwent surgery to have the tumor removed. After her surgery, she took some time off to recover but quickly resumed her intense pace. Walsh is now considered cured, although she has periodic scans to monitor her brain in the unlikely chance of recurrence. After her experience, she and Patrick Dempsey, who played her on-air ex-husband, neurosurgeon Dr. McDreamy, spoke out publicly about her ordeal to raise awareness about the importance of annual checkups and medical self-advocacy.

Meningiomas are the most common benign brain tumors. Unlike metastatic tumors, they don't arrive in the brain from anywhere else in the body, nor do they spread. They pop up like tulip bulbs along the inner surface of the brain's thick membranous covering. Their name, "meningioma," was conferred by Harvey Cushing based on where they blossom: from the meninges, the outer lining of the brain and the thickest part of the dura.

One of the first successful removals of a meningioma was done by Cushing in 1910. The patient was General Leonard Wood. Wood, a Harvard-trained physician, was the personal doctor to presidents Cleveland and McKinley. Equally renowned for his ferocious skills in battle as for his healing abilities, Wood earned a medal of honor for his bravery in the campaign against Geronimo's Apaches and commanded the Rough Riders alongside Teddy Roosevelt. He went on to serve as the governor of both Cuba and the Philippines. At one point he was only a few votes shy of clinching the presidency of the United States.

A controversial figure on account of his fierce, merciless fighting spirit, Wood noticed his left arm and leg weakening while slaughtering a tribe of Filipino Muslims in the name of American expansionism. He sought treatment and, given his connections, ended up in Cushing's clinic. Suspecting a malignant tumor, Cushing brought Wood to the operating room. What he encountered, upon opening the general's skull, was massive bleeding— sufficiently profuse that he was forced to abort the operation, fearing for Wood's life. Five days later, Cushing gathered his courage and tried again.

This time he removed the cauliflower-shaped mass, which to his surprise was a benign tumor that he later christened the meningioma.

While Cushing's surgery was trumpeted a success and greatly contributed to his reputation as America's foremost brain tumor surgeon, he made a fateful error, one for which he cannot be blamed, since little was understood back then about meningiomas. Cushing failed to remove the tumor's roots within the dura, as well as the invaded adjacent skull. Although Wood survived the surgery, so, too, did a snippet of his tumor. Seventeen years later, Wood, along with the recrudescing lump in his brain, both found themselves back in Cushing's office. This time the general could barely walk. Cushing, now at the height of his abilities, made a less forgivable error, one common among surgeons when caring for acquaintances. He allowed his patient, who had become a friend, to orchestrate the operation's execution. Cushing agreed to perform this second surgery in one long session rather than in two, as he often did for his most difficult cases. Although he capably removed General Wood's tumor, the blood loss was catastrophic. Wood died the very next day. It is said that Cushing was so distraught, both at the loss of his friend, a man so highly regarded, and at his poor judgment in not following his surgical instincts, that he fell into a deep melancholy and refused to operate for weeks.

––––––

When I see a patient in my office with a meningioma, I immediately try to convey a few key messages. The first and most important? This is *not* cancer. Meningiomas, I tell them, are benign tumors. Not only will they not spread to any other location in the body, but in most circumstances meningiomas can easily be treated and often cured. Moreover, they generally grow slowly. While there are some exceptions to this rule, and some meningiomas can be considered *atypical* or *anaplastic* and grow more rapidly, the majority are benign. Had Cushing done a more aggressive surgery the first time, when Wood's tumor was small and less invasive, he would not have struggled against the more formidable recurrence. Wood's tumor was indeed curable.

The symptoms of any brain tumor are related to its location and to the function of the part of the brain being compressed. Kate Walsh complained of weakness on the right side of her body and trouble with her speech, so her tumor must have been pressing on the left frontal lobe. Leonard Wood, on the other hand, was weak on the left; thus, his tumor was on the right. Depending on their location, meningiomas can cause double vision, blurry vision, tingling, numbness, or seizures.

A seizure occurs when the surface of the brain is irritated by anything that shouldn't be there. As a result, the aggravated neurons respond with a burst of activity that spreads across the brain like a tsunami, leading to several minutes of uncontrolled limb flailing. For this reason, Walsh, like most patients with brain tumors, was given anti-seizure medication to keep her from seizing.

Walsh also complained of sharp, stabbing headaches. People with headaches often worry that their pain might be the harbinger of an undiscovered brain tumor. Such fear motivates a lot of unnecessary brain scans. Most headaches are *not* caused by brain tumors, so the odds were in Arnold Schwarzenegger's favor in *Kindergarten Cop* when he told those kids, "It's not a tumor!" But sometimes brain tumors do indeed cause headaches. So how can we know when a headache is—or, more important, *isn't*—just a headache?

Headaches are so common that almost everyone will have had a headache at some point in their lives. On the other hand, brain tumors are rare. Most doctors don't order an MRI when you complain of a headache. Yet, 50 percent of people with a brain tumor will complain of a headache as one of their symptoms. Meanwhile, only 10 percent of people with brain tumors will have *only* a headache and no other symptoms. That's why if a new or worsening headache is accompanied by nausea, vomiting, weakness, personality change, memory loss, difficulty with speech, or a seizure, an MRI scan is absolutely warranted.

Some headaches are particularly worrisome. A headache that wakes you up in the middle of the night, for example, may be more indicative of a tumor. Also, headaches that are worse in the morning but then get better as the day wears on are also potentially worrying, as are headaches that get worse with straining, coughing, sneezing, or going to the bathroom.

Why do these early morning and activity-related headaches raise a neurosurgeon's eyebrows? Because they indicate that pressure within the head may be increasing. When we stand or sit, the head is above the heart, so blood flows against gravity. During sleep, when we are lying flat, intracranial pressure goes up, since the heart's pumping force is less diminished by the pull of the earth. We also breathe differently when we sleep, and the amount of carbon dioxide in the blood rises ever so slightly. This causes blood vessels to dilate, which, in turn, delivers more blood to the brain, so pressure in the head rises. Similarly, coughing, sneezing, or straining of any sort leads to an increase in pressure in the abdomen and the chest, and this can also raise the pressure in the head.

If a brain tumor is taking up space and crowding the head, then there is, plain and simple, less room to spare. Anything that might further raise the pressure—lying flat, slowed breathing, coughing—tips the balance, resulting in headaches. One easy test that a neurosurgeon or an ophthalmologist can perform—to identify the kind of increases in pressure caused by a brain tumor—is to look through a patient's pupils to the backs of their eyes. Dilating the pupil with drops makes this easier and allows us to see the optic nerve, which carries vision from the retina to the brain. Swelling in the optic nerve, called papilledema, is a clear sign of long-standing increased pressure and warns of a problem.

The second key piece of information I try to impress upon my patients during our first discussion about meningiomas, to simplify our joint decision-making, is that there are only three treatment options: surgery, radiation, and the least invasive, observation. Observation is one of the most common ways we treat meningiomas, particularly those discovered by accident. Since MRI scans are now doled out like Botox at a Beverly Hills dermatologist's office, doctors frequently find meningiomas that are small and not causing any symptoms. In these situations, the best management strategy is observation, which usually involves checking an MRI once a year or so for a few years to see if the tumor grows.

When Sheryl Crow, the singer who also happened to have dated Lance Armstrong, was diagnosed with a meningioma, she was *not* offered surgery, since the tumor was so small. Crow had been complaining of memory loss, which is why she got the MRI in the first place. The scan uncovered a small meningioma, which was not responsible for her memory problems given the location and size of the tumor. How do I know? Because it wasn't located in the temporal lobes, the part of the brain that stores memories, and the tumor was too small to cause a problem.

Once a meningioma becomes big enough, however, observation is no longer prudent. Stereotactic radiosurgery provides one option for treatment—and an appealing one at that, since the alternative, surgery, requires a craniotomy. But radiation works well only for small meningiomas and is only an advantage if the tumor is difficult to reach. If the tumor is big or sitting near the surface of the brain, surgery is usually a better choice.

In some circumstances it's clear which of the two options, surgery or radiation, will be best for a particular patient. Larger tumors that can be easily removed in young patients are often treated with surgery. Smaller tumors deep in the brains of older patients receive radiation. Unfortunately, at least a third of the meningiomas I see in my office fall into that hazy middle ground. Each treatment option has its pluses and minuses, and there are no clear-cut guidelines that indicate which will be more effective.

Every neurosurgeon has their own individual algorithm regarding cases that they prefer to treat with surgery versus cases they treat with radiation. A patient can visit ten different neurosurgeons and find five who suggest radiation and five who favor surgery. Why so much ambivalence? Let's try to unpack the inherent ambiguities of the situation and hopefully understand a bit more about how neurosurgeons grapple with potentially life-altering decisions in the face of imperfect information. Without a crystal ball, neurosurgeons, like most doctors, must settle on a plan of action based on the best available evidence, which is often incomplete.

DECIDING WHEN TO OPERATE

Whether to choose radiation or surgery to treat a meningioma depends on a few quantifiable factors, such as the age of the patient, the size of the tumor, and its location in the brain. The age of the patient is important because, to state the obvious, we humans have limited time here on earth and an average life expectancy (in the United States in 2023) of 77.5 years.

So, for example, if an older patient comes in with a tumor that won't grow large enough during their remaining years to cause symptoms, surgery makes no sense. The risks of surgery also increase with age. After eighty, a patient's risk goes up fourfold compared with those under sixty. The surgeon's threshold for removing a meningioma in the elderly must therefore be higher than for a younger person, in whom a tumor will have more time to grow.

I often tell my young patients with meningiomas requiring surgery that the tumor is never going to be smaller, and they are never going to be younger, so my advice is to take it out now. Why? Because if the patient is going to need surgery at some point, it makes little sense to wait any longer than necessary. The larger the tumor grows, the more difficult it will be to remove later, and the risks of surgery will only increase with each passing month.

One might argue: Why risk hurting the patient now with surgery if they have so few symptoms? Why not wait until they're symptomatic and then remove the tumor in a few years?

The error of this logic has to do with the growth pattern of meningiomas. Over time, meningiomas not only invade into the brain, absorbing its blood supply, but also engulf nearby arteries, veins, and nerves. Picture the foam insulation injected into the walls of your house that surrounds the wires and pipes. Meningiomas envelop everything in their path like sap running down the trunk of a tree.

Unless you have sat for hours, peering through a microscope, painstakingly dissecting a meningioma away from a nerve or artery, and then found after the operation that your patient can no longer see, move a limb, or smile because of a decision you made, it's hard to fully understand the impact and ramifications of delaying surgery. When a neurosurgeon tries to remove a large, invasive tumor, the risk of a complication is higher than if that same tumor had been removed a few years earlier, when it was smaller.

Postponing surgery on an asymptomatic patient may make you *feel* that you are protecting a patient from potential injury; this type of reasoning can become a self-fulfilling prophecy. The delay, by giving the tumor time to grow, becomes the proximate cause of the very complication you are trying to avoid.

The best-case scenario for any brain tumor, whether a meningioma or another kind, involves a close collaboration between all the specialists involved—both surgeons and non-surgeons—at every stage, from diagnosis to each scan thereafter. Everyone should be in conversation regarding when it's time to intervene. For this reason, many hospitals have weekly tumor board meetings, during which cases are presented to a roomful of specialists: in neurosurgery, neurology, radiation oncology, and medical oncology. Each specialist weighs in on the case, providing their opinion and input until the group reaches a consensus.

Another critical factor to weigh when deciding how and when to treat a meningioma is the size of the tumor. Stereotactic radiosurgery works best for small tumors, generally less than 2.5 centimeters in diameter. Tumors larger than that will put pressure on the brain, which can be alleviated only with surgery. Radiation may halt or slow growth but rarely shrinks a tumor. Moreover, the efficacy of radiation is directly proportional to the tumor's size, since the dose must be distributed over a greater volume. Location also matters because some parts of the brain, like the optic nerves, are very sensitive to radiation. Tumors near these delicate regions are often referred to surgery rather than radiation because the latter may damage the nerves, causing further visual deterioration.

Based on these three criteria—age of the patient, tumor location, and size of the tumor—most neurosurgeons would probably agree on the best way to treat around 70 percent of meningiomas. However, the other 30 percent fall into a gray zone. When faced with shades of gray, how do surgeons settle on black-and-white decisions?

Let's use baseball as an analogy. If you were a runner on first base, how would you decide whether to try to steal second base? Part of the decision rests on how close you can get to second base before the pitch is thrown. The farther you can go, the less distance you need to cover. What about the conditions of the field? If it's raining, you won't be able to run as fast. How is the catcher's throwing arm? Strong? Weak? All these variables are both quantifiable and not debatable, just like the age of the patient, the size of the tumor, and its location.

But the runner also ponders factors that aren't necessarily measurable: *How good am I at stealing bases at this point in my career?* This is *somewhat* quantifiable but also open to interpretation. Let's say it's the pre-Moneyball era and no one has recorded your past performance statistics. Maybe you are also getting faster and better at stealing bases, so you imagine you'll do a slightly better job this time than you did last time, based on your increasing experience and optimism. You may also be inclined to steal more bases, since the coach has been grumbling that you don't steal enough. You may also be thinking about what happened the last time you tried to steal a base. Did you succeed or were you called out? How did your decision affect the outcome of the game?

Similar variables run through the head of a neurosurgeon when deciding whether to operate on certain meningiomas—or any tumor, for that matter. Just like the runner, who might go for second in one game and sit tight in the next, neurosurgeons are swayed by situationally dependent variables that are not quantifiable. Basically, we try to get a feel for our chances of success and then go with our gut.

When a difficult case presents itself, a neurosurgeon will run through a certain thought process. We begin with an "objective" assessment based on our training and our understanding of conventional neurosurgical wisdom developed by experts in the field. We like to think that we decide on *the right thing to do,* on what's in the patient's best interest. More often than we like to admit, however, our decisions are equally influenced by subjective, intangible factors—like the runner deciding whether to go for the steal.

This is probably the more impactful part of surgical decision-making. Here we remember other times we've attempted a similar case and remind ourselves of the outcome; with more recent cases, for better or worse, foremost in our memories. If a recent surgery went well, we might be more likely to recommend surgery. If it went poorly, we might want to choose a different approach or endorse radiation. But this pivotal set of circumstances is unique to that one surgeon and to that one surgeon alone.

If we are considering surgery, we then begin a process of visualizing how the operation will play out, picturing both the anatomy we will encounter as well as the potential obstacles we will face. We then ask ourselves: What is the level of difficulty of this surgery? What is our probability for success or failure? These hypotheticals help us recommend a course of action. If we are experienced, this process occurs rapidly, if not instantaneously. If it's early in our career, we might second-guess our judgment and run the case by a more senior surgeon for another opinion.

When it comes to the most difficult cases, the gulf between neurosurgeons widens. Some are particularly talented at removing the most challenging tumors. Others are not. What might be considered a dangerous surgery in one surgeon's hands might be regarded as safe in another's more experienced hands. The first surgeon might recommend radiation, while the second might recommend surgery. Both may be making the right decision for them and for their patients—because, depending upon whose hands are rooting around in your skull, you might be better off with one treatment than the other.

SEVEN

WHERE TO BEGIN?

He glided into my office in patent leather shoes—shiny, brown, and freshly polished. His socks, a bright mustard, perfectly matched his tie as well as his handkerchief, neatly folded in his left breast pocket. Light blue pinstripes ran vertically up his gray blazer, drawing my gaze upward toward his healthy, tanned face. No surprise, his teeth were ivory and straight, almost as white as his pants. Not a hair was out of place. He was charming. He was Italian. He lived a part of the year in New York but most of the time in Florence. His heavily accented baritone was rich and smooth but also cheerful and full of life. He sat down across from me, his wife by his side. They did not look their age—early seventies, if I had to guess. But I didn't have to, since his chart was open on the screen in front of me. As I sat there typing notes, my head bobbed up and down, alternating between making eye contact and doing my best to avoid hitting the wrong keys.

I tried to gently nudge the flow of the conversation toward the reason he was there: his symptoms. "When did the weakness start? Is it only in the foot or also the leg?"

The man had other plans in mind. He didn't have time for illness. He first needed to let me know that he had come from nothing. His success had been earned through hard work. His wardrobe was emblematic of that.

The beautiful fit and fabric of his shirt hugged his chest like Olympic gold medals, arranged for all to see. He boasted. He wanted me to know that he was not just any patient.

I wanted to know if he was right- or left-handed.

He told me what motivated him, what made him rise early every morning and kept him moving forward.

I asked him if he'd ever had a seizure.

He vividly described a memory from his childhood—why this memory at that moment, I could not fathom—in which he had walked past an old man sitting in the subway who was wearing worn, tattered clothes. In his outstretched hand the man held a tin cup full of pencils that he was selling. Pencils! Can you believe it? My patient swept his outstretched fist in a circle mimicking the beggar. He didn't want to end up like that, alone in the subway, selling pencils, he said. His eyebrows danced as he spoke. Then he smiled and paused, as if waiting for me to respond.

I politely excused myself to look at his MRI scan, which I was loading from a CD onto the computer down the hall. As I scrolled through the images, I knew right away what I was looking at. When you've seen as many malignant brain tumors as I have, you just know: the sharp contrast between the white outer border—the periphery of the tumor, highlighted by the contrast agent—against the dark inner core, devoid of anything except dead, necrotic cells. These tumors tear through the brain like a swarm of locusts devouring everything in their path, moving so quickly they outrun their blood supply, as if growth were more important than life itself. They say that sharks die if they don't keep moving. Malignant brain tumors are worse. They keep moving until *you* die.

I went back into the room and sat down. He was still smiling at me.

I thought: Where do I begin?

Glioblastoma multiforme might be the most terrifying diagnosis in all of medicine. GBM, as it's more commonly known, is one of the deadliest forms of cancer. Without treatment, the average life expectancy is around four months. This evil villain's superpower is its shape-shifting ability, which in biological terms means a rapid mutation rate that allows it to evade the entire arsenal of sophisticated weaponry at modern medicine's disposal, including surgery, chemotherapy, radiation, immunotherapy, and anti-tumor vaccines. GBM is the fourth and most nefarious stage of a tumor called a glioma, since it arises from the glial cells that normally surround, protect, and sustain the neurons, the cells that perform the computational work of the brain. Glial cells, when functioning normally, are nurturing caregivers to the neurons, attending to their every need like dutiful servants. But when they are angry and transformed into tumors, they spread through the brain like lava rolling down the lush green slope of a volcano, incinerating everything in its path.

Another name for certain glial cells is astrocytes, which provides these tumors with their other name: astrocytomas. The four stages of glioma each have their own name. Grade 1 is also called a juvenile pilocytic astrocytoma, a benign tumor more common in children. Grade 2 is called either a glioma or an astrocytoma. Grade 3 is an anaplastic astrocytoma—the word "anaplasia" roughly translates to a cell that has lost its way—and grade 4 is a GBM. The distinction between these four types of tumors was traditionally made by pathologists who examined the cells under a microscope and described what they saw.

Today, tumors are differentiated based on the specific genetic mutations found within their DNA. While Grade 1 tumors tend to remain grade 1, grade 2 tumors often progress to grade 3 and then grade 4 over a period of several years. Moreover, because of our ability to characterize the genetic code of these tumors, we can predict with better clarity which tumors will progress and how they will respond to treatment.

A few minutes into my morning rounds, I stopped by to see my Mediterranean patient. It was the second day after the operation, "post-op day two," as we call it. The operation had been "successful" insofar as such an operation could be. What I could remove of the tumor was out. The MRI scan appeared to indicate that it was all gone, but I knew very well that the tissue around the crater that I had excavated in his brain had been infiltrated with microscopic cancer cells invisible to an MRI—cells that were already beginning the inexorable death march that no surgery could arrest. Although the tumor was nudged up against the part of the brain that moved his arm and leg, luckily it was nowhere near the language-processing part of his brain, so at this point his mind and his ability to speak were intact.

He was lying in bed, his pale, frail body covered by rumpled sheets. His hospital gown, open in back, was a far cry from his usual snappy attire. I surged into his room, upbeat and smiling, trying to lighten the moment while also conveying a slight sense of urgency. I was hoping he might pick up on the fact that there were three other places I needed to be at that moment and forgive my haste. But as our eyes met, I saw that he was crying. No, more like bawling. I asked him what was wrong. He could hardly get the words out.

In a halting whisper he said, "I . . . don't want . . . to end up on the street, selling pencils." At that moment I suddenly saw him as he probably saw himself. He was facing his worst fears—the nightmares that woke him up in the middle of the night in a cold sweat and pushed him out of bed every morning with entrepreneurial urgency had become all too real. Was this where it all ended? The rest of my patients could wait. My paperwork could wait. I sat down at the foot of his bed, a consoling hand resting gently on his leg and just listened, joining his chorus of tears with my own.

FOUR POLITICIANS, ONE TUMOR

THE CASE OF
TEDDY KENNEDY

On May 17, 2008, Edward Moore Kennedy, the youngest of the nine Kennedy children and the Democratic senator from Massachusetts, had a seizure. He was rushed to Massachusetts General Hospital, where an MRI revealed a tumor in his left parietal lobe. The surgeons at MGH felt the tumor was inoperable: his biopsy revealed a glioblastoma multiforme (GBM). Two weeks later he went for a second opinion at Duke University Medical Center, where neurosurgeon Allan H. Friedman, chief of the division of neurosurgery, removed as much of the tumor as he could.

Kennedy was awake for part of the surgery so Dr. Friedman could map his patient's brain. Why? Because the left parietal lobe is high-priced cerebral real estate, critical for reading, calculation, spatial orientation, and higher-order thinking. Dr. Friedman had to be careful not to alter any of Kennedy's cognitive skills.

Following his surgery, Kennedy also received radiation and chemotherapy.

Later that summer, while he was still recovering, Kennedy paid a surprise visit to the Senate to cast a critical vote preventing cuts in Medicare fees to physicians. He then appeared once more at the August 25 Democratic National Convention, where he spoke out in support of Barack Obama. After Obama's victory, with Democratic majorities in the Congress, Kennedy devoted the rest of his years to shepherding the Affordable Care Act through Washington's convoluted system. He finally succumbed to his disease at age seventy-seven, fifteen months after his diagnosis. When Obama signed the Affordable Care Act into law seven months later, he wore a blue "Tedstrong" bracelet in Kennedy's honor.

THE CASE OF
JOHN MCCAIN

John Sidney McCain III, born into a military family, served as a pilot during the Vietnam War. In October 1967, his plane was shot down over Hanoi, where he was captured, held as a prisoner of war, and tortured for five years. Because of his family's connections, McCain was given the option for early release. He refused unless his fellow prisoners were also set free.

In 1981, he retired as a highly decorated war hero. He served two terms in Congress and then, in 1987, was elected a Republican senator from Arizona, a position he held over the course of six terms. McCain ran for president in 2008, famously—or perhaps infamously—choosing an inexperienced Sarah Palin as his vice presidential nominee. He was soundly defeated by President Obama.

While still serving in the Senate, McCain, unlike his good friend Ted Kennedy, voted along party lines and opposed the Affordable Care Act.

On July 14, 2017, eight years after delivering a eulogy for Kennedy, McCain began experiencing severe fatigue and blurry vision. Scans revealed some blood in his left frontal lobe. A few days later, surgeons at the Mayo Clinic in Arizona made a small incision in his left eyebrow to remove the clot. Careful examination of the evacuated specimen revealed an underlying tumor: a GBM, just like Kennedy's.

McCain was treated with radiation and chemotherapy and returned to work on July 25, to cast the vote that allowed the Senate to consider repealing Obama's Affordable Care Act, a bill the Republicans labeled "Obamacare." Then, two days later, in an unexpected turn of events—and a startling rebuke to his colleagues—McCain reappeared in the Senate chamber and brashly gave a thumbs-down, casting the deciding vote *against* the Republican effort to repeal Obamacare. Why? Was it his own dealings with doctors, his own brush with death? Not really. McCain said he wanted the law repealed, but he didn't feel that the partisan method was the best way to go about it. He preferred that the decision be debated with the hope of reaching bipartisan support for an affordable healthcare option.

McCain passed away on August 25, 2018, at the age of eighty-one, approximately thirteen months after his diagnosis.

THE CASE OF
BEAU BIDEN

Joseph Robinette "Beau" Biden III was the eldest son of President Joe Biden and his first wife, Neilia Hunter Biden. At the age of three, Beau and his brother Hunter were in a car accident that killed both their mother and infant sister, Naomi. Beau served in Iraq as part of the Delaware National Guard, for which he was awarded the Bronze Star. He was then elected Delaware's attorney general before serving as governor of Delaware beginning in 2016.

In May 2010, while still attorney general, Biden experienced sudden paralysis on the right side of his body and had trouble speaking. As quickly as these mysterious symptoms emerged, they soon resolved. The cause was never identified. The press reported that he had had a stroke, but in his father's book, *Promise Me, Dad*, the elder Biden clearly remembers that White House physician Kevin O'Connor thought Beau had what's called a Todd's paralysis, a temporary form of weakness precipitated by a seizure.

A few years later, Beau began experiencing both auditory hallucinations and panic attacks. The right-sided weakness and speech difficulty returned. These symptoms were, again, typical of seizures. It wasn't until August 2013 that the cause was finally recognized. He was diagnosed with a tumor in his left temporal lobe, yet another GBM.

Neurosurgeon Raymond Sawaya operated on Beau's tumor at the University of Texas MD Anderson Cancer Center. Dr. Sawaya, born in Syria and educated in Beirut before coming to America, eventually completed his neurosurgery training at Johns Hopkins on his way to becoming the chair of the department of neurosurgery at MD Anderson in 1990. Dr. Sawaya kept Beau awake for his operation so he, like Ted Kennedy's surgeon, could perform intraoperative brain mapping. Beau's tumor was close to the part of the brain that's critical for speech, in the left temporal lobe. Dr. Sawaya removed as much of the tumor as he could, trying to avoid harming Beau's ability to speak.

Following surgery, radiation, and chemotherapy, Beau received several investigational treatments, including immunotherapy and an anti-tumor vaccine meant to ramp up his immune system. These two treatments were designed to create potent antibodies to destroy the tumor. Unfortunately, these efforts failed. Beau died on May 30, 2015, at age forty-six, five years after his earliest symptoms and twenty-one months after his first operation.

Some seven months later, President Obama, along with Vice President Biden, announced a new Cancer Moonshot program, allocating a billion dollars over seven years to the National Institutes of Health to find a cure for cancer.

Back on July 9, 2008, when Ted Kennedy walked into the Senate to cast his vote, having just recovered from his own brain tumor surgery, one of the senators who rose to give him a standing ovation was then senator Joe Biden, at the time completely unaware of the events that were about to befall his eldest son. McCain, pre-diagnosis, might also have been present but was in fact absent, having spent the day campaigning in Pennsylvania and Ohio. The coincidence and overlapping circumstances of these men's disparate stories highlight the indiscriminate devastation wrought by this unforgiving tumor.

Malignant tumors don't care about your politics. They don't care if you're wealthy, famous, or powerful. They will grow and likely kill you all the same. I'd like to think that McCain, post-diagnosis, chose to stand with his opponents on the other side of the aisle at that moment because he, in the face of his own impending doom, realized how united we are in frailty and susceptibility to the ravaging effects of a grave disease.

In an even more bizarre case of tumor-in-the-Senate-chamber coincidence, when Ted Kennedy was in his first term, he bore witness to the passage of the Civil Rights Act of 1964. The bill, conceived by his brother John F. Kennedy just prior to his assassination, marked the culmination of the civil rights movement. The deciding vote was cast by Senator Clair Engle, who had to be wheeled into the Senate chamber that day, a victim of a GBM in his left frontal lobe that had been removed for the second time six weeks prior. Though he was paralyzed on his right side and unable to speak, he cast his "aye" vote by pointing to his right eye, making his voice heard both that day and then again one last time, when, a month shy of his death, he nudged the Civil Rights Act over the finish line.

Four politicians, four GBMs, all connected in an eerie timeline of tragedy, and all with tumors on the left side. Is there any sense to this coincidence? Probably not. Tumors don't strike politicians more commonly than members of any other profession, and they do not appear any more frequently on one side of the brain than the other.

———————

In 2017, the *New York Times* ran an article by Jeré Longman entitled "The Brain Cancer That Keeps Killing Baseball Players," which raised the question whether there was link between the artificial turf in Veterans Stadium and GBMs. What motivated that investigation? After the death of former catcher Darren Daulton of a GBM at age fifty-five, his team, the Philadelphia Phillies, realized that he was one of a series of four players with the same diagnosis, all of whom played on that turf between 1971 and 2003. A cluster of brain tumors also felled several members of the Kansas City Royals when they, too, played on a similar artificial turf.

No link was ever found.

In 2022, a husband, his wife, and one of their siblings living in New Jersey were all diagnosed with brain tumors. They began investigating a possible environmental link. They turned up over one hundred cases, all from students and staff who had worked at or graduated from Colonia High School. Environmental experts were brought in to search for a cause. These cases occurred over a forty-year period. In 2021, Colonia High School contained 1,335 students, or 333 students per class. Over forty years, we'd expect 13,350 graduates. If 1 in every 161 students develops a brain tumor—the known incidence in the general population—then we would expect 83 brain tumors coming out of Colonia High School, which is not very far off from what was observed. If you include the administration, teachers, and maintenance workers over that same period, it more than makes up the gap.

It's human nature to look for causality when it comes to illness. Finding a cause for meaningless tragedies makes us think we can stay safe from them, or so we tell ourselves. We don't want to accept the unsettling fact that disaster lurks around every corner—for all of us—no matter how carefully we try and avoid it. There is often no rhyme to our body's treason. It's neither punishment for bad behavior nor retribution for unpopular opinions. Sometimes it's just bad luck.

Another important takeaway from these cases is that the single best predictor of life expectancy is the age at which you are diagnosed. Beau Biden's initial symptoms were unquestionably the first manifestations of his brain tumor. Since grade 4 tumors can progress from lower grade ones, he might have been harboring a small tumor for several years before it was found. The fact that his seizures caused the same symptoms that would eventually be caused by his GBM cannot be a coincidence. Had the tumor been discovered earlier, prompt surgery might have delayed the progression of his tumor, but it's unlikely he could have been cured. Even the low-grade versions of gliomas can disseminate microscopic tumor cells to distant locations, where they can progress years later and explode into more malignant tumors. Because Beau was forty-six, he lived five years after his symptoms first appeared, but still only twenty-one months following his GBM diagnosis. Meanwhile, Kennedy, diagnosed at seventy-seven, lived fifteen months. McCain, at eighty-one, got only thirteen.

Although surgery cannot cure GBMs, neurosurgery plays a critical role in mitigating the swiftness of the disease's progression. The goal of surgery is to remove as much of the tumor as possible without causing harm. GBMs, unlike benign meningiomas, are not encapsulated. They infiltrate the surrounding brain much like the scattered shards from a broken crystal vase consume a floor.

In 1923, neurosurgeon Walter Dandy, Cushing's most famous pupil and the inventor of the batter's helmet, tried to cure a GBM by removing not only the tumor itself but also the entire half of the brain where the tumor originated. This Hail Mary desperation surgery, called a hemispherectomy, was the most neurosurgery had to offer—one last-ditch effort to halt the disease. It proved ineffective. The tumor simply recurred on the other side of the brain.

Since surgery cannot cure a GBM, and long-term survivors of GBM are rare, the primary goal of surgery is to preserve the patient's quality of life for as long as possible. Meanwhile, life expectancy is also directly related to the surgeon's ability to remove as much of the tumor as safely possible. In each case, the neurosurgeon faces a dilemma: whether to remove too little, which may limit longevity, or to remove too much, which may cause paralysis or speech difficulties that will impair the patient's remaining time. This Sophie's Choice calculation is weighed constantly throughout the operation, not only for malignant tumors but also for the benign ones.

But before we get caught up in a more philosophical discussion of intra-operative judgment, let's examine how neurosurgeons map the brain during surgery to better understand why Kennedy and Biden were kept awake under local anesthesia for their operations while McCain was asleep under general anesthesia for his.

NEVER SAY "OOPS!"

The areas of the brain dedicated to language processing are different in every individual. Unfortunately, we haven't yet developed a noninvasive test that can reliably map language zones with enough certainty that a neurosurgeon can fully depend on it when planning an operation. Functional MRI scans, which show blood flow changes in the brain associated with language, do provide some data, but the mapping is indirect and not always accurate, since blood flow doesn't always correspond with neuronal processing.

If I'm removing a tumor that I suspect may sit next to a part of the brain that controls speech, I need to be able to precisely define the outlines of that speech area. If I accidentally damage a module of the brain critical for language, the patient will wake up either completely mute, unable to understand what others are saying to them, or capable only of producing a string of unrelated nonsensical words. Such an outcome is devastating for everyone involved—mostly for the patient and their family, of course, but also for the surgeon, who must live with the knowledge that their error in judgment or technique led to grave harm. Such a catastrophic event must be avoided at all costs. For this reason, we neurosurgeons sometimes require that our patients be awake in the operating room so we can map out the parts of the brain dedicated to creating and deciphering language.

Most patients are terrified at the prospect of being awake during brain surgery. The images and sounds that come to mind—blood spurting, saws whirring, and victims screaming—are straight out of a horror movie. So even though we need our patients to be alert for the mapping, we keep them asleep and comfortable for other parts of the operation. The goal is for them to be alert for as short a time as possible. Generous quantities of local anesthesia along with rapidly reversible intravenous sedation help make the whole experience quite tolerable.

The brain itself has no pain receptors, so surgery on the brain is not felt. The brain is completely unaware of itself as a physical organ in space. We are as oblivious to what's happening inside our skulls as we are to what's going on in our spleens or in our livers.

If you could reach into your skull and touch your brain, it would just feel like touching a sponge. But there would be no sensation inside your head to alert you that your brain was being touched. Headaches arise from irritation to the membranes *around* the brain, such as the dura, the blood vessels, or the periosteum, the thin layer of tissue that covers the skull. Brain tissue itself cannot be a source of pain. It simply lacks pain or pressure receptors.

Neurosurgical brain mapping is based on the principle that when you stimulate the brain—or any nerve—with an electrical current, you can either activate or deactivate it depending upon how and where the stimulation is performed. For example, if you stimulate the part of the brain that moves the hand, the hand will move. If you stimulate the part of the brain that processes vision, the patient will see flashing lights. However, when you stimulate the part of the brain that's critical for language function, the patient does not blurt out sentences. Rather, they will suddenly be unable to speak.

The difference between *triggering* a brain function—like hand movement—or *blocking* a function—like speech—depends on complexity. Movement, for example, is a binary on/off phenomenon, meaning that either you can move your limb or you can't, so stimulation is sufficient to activate those circuits. Language, on the other hand, requires the sequential activation and deactivation of a complex pattern of neurons within a complicated network. These neurons must fire in a precise sequence, which cannot be easily recapitulated with a single electrical pulse applied to the surface of the brain. The bottom line: when a neurosurgeon touches an electrode to the brain in an awake patient, depending on the location of the stimulation, we have the capacity to instantaneously alter another person's ability to move, feel, speak, and understand language.

If I activate the part of the brain that moves your hand, your hand will move *every single time*, regardless of whether you want it to. If I trigger the part of your brain that processes sensation on your leg, you will feel as if something were touching your leg, even when you know the source is coming from within your brain. Why? Because sensations *always* come from inside your brain, even if a feather is tickling your leg. You don't really feel the feather or its tickle; you experience the neurons in your sensory cortex firing, which subsequently tricks you into thinking the sensation is happening in your leg.

Now, if you're speaking to me—maybe telling me a story about where you went for dinner last night—and I touch an electrode to the region of your brain that processes language, although you will no longer be able to speak, you'll still be able to think, and you'll have the sensation of knowing exactly what you want to say, but the words won't form in your mouth. This same stimulation in a different part of the language processing system can have a completely different effect. It might, for example, prevent you from understanding what I'm saying to you, as if you were suddenly a foreigner who's just arrived in a new country where the words sound like gibberish.

It's hard to imagine that such a drastic and sudden change can occur in our perception of reality and what it might be like to experience this unnerving event, but the patient undergoing brain mapping is not as much afraid as surprised. They'll say things like "That's so odd: for a moment I couldn't quite get the words out" or "Can you repeat that, Doctor? I couldn't quite hear what you said." There is a casualness to the experience, as if this has happened to them before under different circumstances. The truth is, it *has* happened before. We've all had the experience of having trouble finding the right words or understanding someone else's meaning.

Our brains are the substance of who we are and how we interact with the outside world. Yet they are also biological organs that don't always function at 100 percent efficiency. We are accustomed to brief glitches. Nevertheless, this familiarity doesn't undermine the basic fact that a neurosurgeon's ability to interact with the brain during surgery, and thereby alter another person's reality, has profound philosophical implications regarding the nature of free will, a subject we will explore in detail in later chapters.

When patients are anesthetized—the usual condition in a neurosurgical operating room—the environment is surprisingly casual and relaxed. When the patient is awake, however, the tenor of the OR transforms. Think of the difference between a cocktail party and a sacred gathering: flippant comments, frivolous conversation, or displays of anger are not just strictly forbidden, at least in my operating theater; they can interfere with the patient's well-being and therefore the outcome. I happen to specialize in awake brain mapping and perform this procedure a few times a month. My goal is to make my patients as comfortable as possible during this strange but necessary experience. They should feel not only that everyone in the room is focused on them and their surgery but also that technical or procedural issues are of no concern.

If equipment is missing, we ask politely and wait until it arrives. If the patient's brain looks swollen or bleeding and requires immediate attention, we work to fix the problem in silence, without any expression of alarm or concern. I advise my residents, only half-jokingly, that when they are operating on an awake patient, they should never say "Oops" lest the patient think there is a problem.

Each case begins with the anesthesiologist giving an IV cocktail of sedating medications. In other words, the patient is not totally out of it, but they won't remember what is about to occur. If you have ever had a colonoscopy, it's the same idea. Then I perform a scalp block, which means I inject a band of lidocaine around the head. This numbs the crown. I then open the scalp and skull in the same way I would if the patient were asleep because, for all intents and purposes, they are. Not only are they heavily sedated but the local anesthesia has kicked in as well.

The dura is very sensitive to pain, so before opening it I directly numb this as well. Once the brain is exposed, I must immediately rouse the patient, which can take up to twenty minutes. The key is to start waking them up well before you need them fully awake, to avoid waiting for them to come to. It's a careful dance: if you wake them too early, they may feel the painful slicing of the dura, which will require more sedation and a longer wait until it kicks in. It's critical for the patient to be comfortable if the mapping process is to be successful.

At this point the patient is lying on their back but with their head turned, facing the anesthesiologist, while I'm standing at the head of the bed, looking down at the brain. The surgical drapes must be placed properly, likes a nun's habit, so the patient can see the anesthesiologist but not the surgeon. With their head clamped into position and straps holding them in place on the operating table, the patient cannot move, even if they panic. I always tighten the head screws with extra force in these awake cases. Why? Just imagine the horrible prospect of a patient jumping out of bed in a panic and running down the hall with their brains hanging out. Yikes!

Such a scenario has, thankfully, never arisen, and I don't think it ever will. But my dread of even the *idea* of it forces me to apply extra caution and focus, in the same way I make sure my alarm is set multiple times before going to bed when I need to catch an early flight.

When waking up a patient whose brain is exposed, the first order of business is to remind them where they are. Sedating drugs wear off slowly, and patients are often confused as they come to. They may not recall, for example, that they fell asleep in an operating room, about to undergo brain surgery.

The neuropsychologist, who sits face-to-face with the patient, will start to speak in a loud voice at first, to penetrate the pharmacological fog. "You're in the operating room. Please don't move. Your head is fixed in place. That is why you can't move it." The patient's whole body begins to rustle upon hearing this, but they are immediately met with the restraints with which we have bound them to the operating table.

Eventually, they will recall where they are, having been prepared by us beforehand for this moment, and then they can relax, ready to proceed. I'm always amazed at how calm they are, as if having one's brain exposed to the air is not new to them. It's probably another example of the bravery that we all possess, rarely accessed when facing more trivial daily stressors. I've seen people become more anxious because they thought their waiter gave them caffeinated coffee and not decaf.

After my patient awakens, I try to keep the conversation as natural as possible. I ask them about their life, the ages of their children, what they did over their last vacation, and their favorite movies—anything to take their mind off their unnatural and uncanny predicament. I also talk a bit about myself, as if we were meeting for lunch, to help them understand that the current situation, as unusual as it may be for them, is just another workday for me.

WILDER PENFIELD

The history of brain stimulation began in 1786 when Italian physiologist Luigi Galvani showed that an electric current applied to a nerve running down the leg of a frog could make it twitch. Galvani's nephew, Giovanni Aldini, performed more gruesome experiments a few years later by stimulating the brains of recently decapitated criminals to reanimate their facial movements. Not only were such macabre demonstrations, held in town squares throughout Europe, crowd pleasers, but they also inspired Mary Shelley to write her famous novel *Frankenstein*.

The first neurosurgeon to stimulate the living human brain was the American doctor Roberts Bartholow. In 1874 he was called in to consult on Mary Rafferty, a woman at death's door. Her heartbreaking medical history was typical of healthcare at that time. As a child, Rafferty had a small patch of hair burned off that never grew back. The wig she wore to cover this defect was attached to her head with a rounded piece of whalebone. The constant pressure from the bone on her scalp slowly ate away the skin, exposing her skull, which became infected. Without antibiotics, she was doomed. The infection progressed to the point where it eroded through her skull, leaving a gaping hole. Her brain was now unprotected and exposed to the outside world. Bartholow saw, in Rafferty's dire circumstances, an opportunity to investigate the prevailing theories of brain organization. He proceeded to use her as a test subject for his experiments, stimulating her brain with a needle electrode to see what would happen. By delivering a shock directly to her cortex, he was able to elicit involuntary movements on the opposite side of her body, thus confirming the brain's role in causing the limbs to move. More disturbingly, he also triggered several long seizures, which ultimately precipitated her death.

When Bartholow formally presented his results to his colleagues, which he imagined would earn him their respect and admiration, he was instead sharply criticized and his ethics questioned. Instead of advancing the practice of brain stimulation, this event led to the immediate passage of a resolution by the American Medical Association mandating that all human experimentation be restricted to lifesaving procedures.

Bartholow claimed that he had obtained Rafferty's permission, but the details of the consent process and her ability to comprehend and willingly agree to his brain probing were challenged. Nevertheless, while Bartholow's accomplishment was not a high point in the history of neurosurgery, his work was a precursor to more thoughtful and ethical investigations performed during lifesaving operations by the greatest pioneer of awake brain mapping: the neurosurgeon Wilder Penfield.

Penfield was born in 1891 in Spokane, Washington. He studied at Princeton University, where he played football and even coached the team for a year after graduation. He received a Rhodes scholarship to study medicine at Oxford, devoting two years working under Sir Charles Sherrington, the same British neurophysiologist whom Cushing had visited several years earlier.

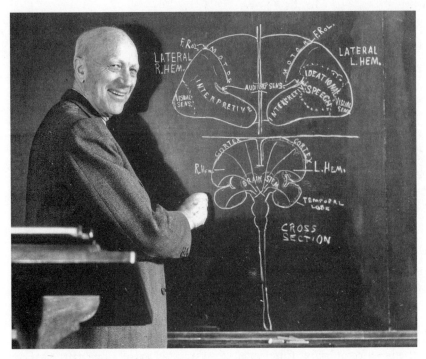

Wilder Penfield in 1963, sketching a cross section of the human brain.
Photo by Charles Hodge from the Osler Library, McGill University Library and Archives.
© Montreal Neurological Institute 2023

Penfield completed his medical training at Johns Hopkins and then spent a year as a surgical intern at the Peter Bent Brigham Hospital, where he met Harvey Cushing. Following this experience, Penfield once again found himself abroad, learning from the Europeans, just as so many other budding American neurosurgeons had done before him. In Spain he learned how to stain neurons and identify glial scars under the microscope in the laboratory of the renowned neuropathologist Santiago Ramón y Cajal. But it was in Germany that he was first exposed to the technique of safely stimulating the brains of awake patients during surgery, by watching the German neurosurgeons Fedor Krause and Otfrid Foerster.

In 1921, now back in the United States, Penfield was hired by Presbyterian Hospital in New York City, which had just combined with Columbia's

College of Physicians and Surgeons, the medical school of Columbia University. At that time, Presbyterian Hospital and Columbia University were not yet affiliated with the Neurological Institute of New York. Penfield was given privileges at both institutions and found himself caught in the middle of the contentious relationship between the neurologists and the neurosurgeons, who were vying for patients and power at the two centers.

In his autobiography *No Man Alone: A Neurosurgeon's Life*, Penfield tells the story of one of his first patients, a young child who was going blind from a brain tumor. Having realized that, without surgery, the boy would die, Penfield requested a consultation from the department of neurology, as he was unsure of the exact location of the tumor. Frederick Tilney, the head of neurology at the time, saw the boy late in the evening and left a brief note in the chart stating that the surgery should not be performed, period. Penfield, frustrated by this unilateral decision, called Tilney to discuss the matter. Tilney responded but was rude, curt, and dismissive.

Rather than relying only on Tilney's dictum, Penfield traveled to Johns Hopkins to learn how to perform a new test—the ventriculogram—recently invented by neurosurgeon Walter Dandy, the same man who went on to invent the batter's helmet and who tried to cure GBMs by removing half the brain.

Penfield, following Dandy's instructions, injected air into the child's brain and took an X-ray, which revealed the outline of the tumor deep within the third ventricle—an area that at the time was considered too risky to approach safely. Thus, Penfield confirmed that, yes, surgery would be too dangerous, but he made the decision on his own terms and with data to back it up, rather than simply following the mandate set forth by Tilney.

Penfield resented the fact that neurology and neurosurgery should be at odds with one another. Neurosurgeons were treated as technicians back then, their role diminished by what Penfield considered the arrogance of neurologists, who believed themselves to be more adept at making complex decisions about brain diseases than the surgeons, whom they viewed as mere "cutters." Penfield dreamed of uniting neurology and neurosurgery, alongside neurophysiology and neuropathology, under one harmonious roof. Realizing that his ambitious plan was unlikely to be realized in New York, he moved to Montreal.

Through the force of his dedication and charisma, Penfield was able to convince the Rockefeller Institute to support his vision. With their financial assistance, he founded the Montreal Neurological Institute, or the MNI, as it was later known. As mentioned earlier, the MNI was where the first Black American neurosurgeons learned their craft, since they weren't able to find a welcome home in any American programs.

Penfield is best known for developing a neurosurgical treatment of epilepsy, which became known as the Montreal procedure. He would anesthetize his patients with local anesthesia, keep them awake, and stimulate their brains with an electrode to map not only their normal brain functions but also the source of their epilepsy, which he would then try to remove.

Penfield eventually became somewhat of a celebrity in Canada. At one point he was dubbed "the greatest living Canadian," despite his U.S. origins. Penfield's first major contributions to the field of neuroscience were his detailed maps of the human brain, specifically which brain areas moved which parts of the body. When Penfield began his career, his German mentors, Krause and Foerster, had already established that small groups of neurons in specific parts of the brain separately controlled different parts of the body. One area was dedicated to moving the arm, another would move the leg, and so on. Less clear, however, was *how* these islands of neurons were organized. Did they look exactly like the human body, with the foot area below the knee area below the hip, etc.? Were the parts of the brain devoted to each body part the same size, or did larger parts of the body take up more space in the brain?

Penfield answered these questions by stimulating the brains of hundreds of his patients during surgery, creating a map of the organization of the neurons that control movement, which he called the "homunculus," meaning "little man." But the homunculus is simply a blueprint of the *layout* of these neurons. There is no Lilliputian gnome sitting inside our skulls, pulling the strings and controlling our movements like a miniature puppet master. Nor is there another, smaller homunculus within the brain of that homunculus, controlling its movements like a Russian Matryoshka doll.

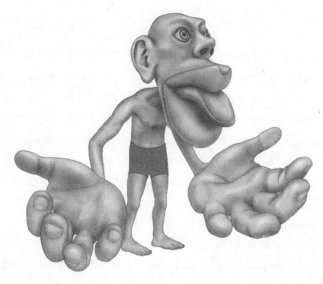

The homunculus is a figurative representation of how the brain maps the body from "real" space into "brain" space. The hands, fingers, lips, and tongue appear larger, since they are controlled by the greatest number of neurons.

The homunculus, then, is a schematic for the arrangement of the neurons that control movement, and, based on the relative size of each island of neurons devoted to each body part, we can learn a few important points about the brain's priorities. As is evident, the parts of the brain devoted to moving the hands, fingers, lips, and tongue are the largest. The parts moving the legs, feet, torso, and forehead are much smaller. What explains this distorted representation of the body? The larger the area of brain devoted to each body part, the more neurons are dedicated to that ability. Our distinctly human capacities to manipulate tools and produce speech, for example, depend upon the ability to perform intricate movements with our hands, fingers, lips, and tongue, so the brain devotes more neurons to those faculties. Wiggling our toes just doesn't give us much of an evolutionary advantage. In the monkey brain, on the other hand, the area devoted to the feet and toes as well as the tail are, in a relative sense, much larger. This expanded cortical real estate gives them greater control over their feet and tails, which they need to climb trees.

The brain also has another homunculus for sensory functions. In fact, there are multiple sensory homunculi. In the sensory homunculus, the index finger takes up the most space. Compare this with the motor homunculus, where the thumb is the largest. If you think about it, it makes sense, since the index finger is critical for touching objects, while the thumb is important for holding them. The mouth is also strongly represented in both the motor and the sensory homunculi, but for different reasons. In the motor homunculus, the tongue and lips are large, since they're both critical for language production. In the sensory homunculus, they are again both important, but here for touch and for taste, not movement. In one sense, the homunculus recapitulates human evolution. But in another, more accurate sense, the homunculus reflects the brain's attempt to impose its will on the existing body parts bestowed on us by evolution.

While the morphology of our bodies is mostly fixed by our DNA, our homunculi are not. Plasticity plays a role. For example, studies have shown that musicians may have larger areas of their brains devoted to finger movement. Thus, the left hand of a cello player—the hand whose fingers rapidly dance along the neck—takes up a larger area of brain than the right hand, the one that merely holds the bow. When we diligently repeat the same movements, as a musician who spends hours a day practicing does, we literally change the wiring of our brains. When we stop, these recently constructed pathways dissolve.

Clearly, the homunculus looks nothing like our actual bodies. But, depending upon your perspective, you might view the brain's dysmorphic representation of the human body not as a distortion of our physical bodies but rather as a truer depiction of *who we really are*. In other words, our physical body's configuration is not an accurate representation of the self.

The homunculus of a cellist will have a huge left hand and a shrunken right one, but their physical limbs will be the same size. If their musicality and cello-playing abilities are core aspects of their being, as they surely are for professional musicians, then their homunculi reveal something about them that is not otherwise evident.

What is common to all human homunculi, and perhaps most epitomizes humanity, is the overrepresentation of the mouth and the hands. Our civilization is a product of our ability to communicate and to build. At our most basic level, we tell stories, and we make things.

It is the brain, not the body, that is the priority. The body, after all, is nothing more than an elaborate scaffolding for the brain. Why are our legs so long and why do we stand upright rather than crouch down on all fours? Long legs don't help us run faster. The fastest animals run on four legs, not two. So what's the explanation? Standing upright gives our eyes a higher vantage point, allowing us to see farther. As far as brain real estate is concerned, we are mostly eyes.

Of all the five senses, the most dominant sense in the human brain by far is vision. How dominant is vision? Nearly one-third of the brain is devoted to processing it. This explains why the human brain wants us to stand upright—to see farther rather than run fast. Dogs, on the other hand, have a proportionally larger portion of their brain devoted to smell, which is why they keep low down and probe the world—and each other—with their noses.

Human vision, however, is not organized like a homunculus; hearing and smell are not, either. Each has its own structure, with neurons specifically tuned to process features that make up the building blocks of each of those sensory experiences. The smallest computational modules in the visual cortex process lines oriented in different directions. Think of the spokes on a wheel. If you want to drive your visual cortex crazy, try this: Without moving your head, look out a moving car window at a series of vertical lines passing by, such as tree trunks or telephone poles. In the auditory cortex, the units of measure are tones, with adjacent groups of neurons responding only to certain pitches and not to others.

———

P enfield, in addition to contributing to our understanding of motor and sensory function, also performed detailed mapping of human language and memory. In his groundbreaking 1959 work, *Speech and Brain-Mechanisms*, he established himself as the leading cartographer of the brain's language faculties. At the time, the brain was understood to have two important regions devoted to language. The first, sitting just in front of the motor portion of the brain, in the lower frontal lobe, was called Broca's area, named after French neurologist Paul Broca. We will take a deeper dive into Broca's contributions, but for now we need to know only that the area of the brain named after him is important for the production of speech. In the back of the temporal lobe a second area was identified, named after the German neurologist Carl Wernicke. Wernicke's area is

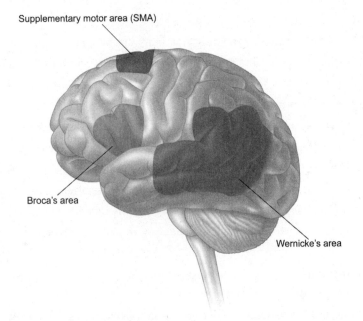

Penfield confirmed the location of an anterior language area named after Paul Broca, a posterior language area named after Carl Wernicke, and a third area devoted to the planning and initiation of verbal and motor output, which he termed the supplementary motor area.

important for speech comprehension. These two areas are intricately connected though the deep white-matter tracts of the brain.

Penfield not only identified a new area important for speech, called the supplementary motor area, but also showed that only a small portion of Broca's and Wernicke's areas are critical for speech. In other words, Broca and Wernicke grossly overestimated the sizes of the regions of brain that process language. Penfield found that language areas were small, each one about the size of a dime, and they reside within the larger regions defined by Broca and Wernicke.

Soon after moving to Canada, Penfield operated on a patient with a large tumor in her right frontal lobe. This tumor, called an oligodendroglioma, arises from a different type of glial cell—an oligodendrocyte—instead of the GBM's astrocyte. Tumors of this type have a better prognosis. Although they can also transform into malignant tumors, the transition generally occurs more slowly, over several years.

Penfield performed the surgery with the patient awake. He removed her entire right frontal lobe, not only to treat the tumor but also to control her seizures, which were triggered by the tumor irritating the adjacent brain. As he worked, he stimulated her brain and identified the parts dedicated to movement because removal of too much of the frontal lobe would have paralyzed her. In effect, he used mapping to determine a safe margin for his surgery. At the time, removal of so much of the frontal lobe to treat a tumor was considered somewhat heretical, since the impact on the patient's cognitive abilities was not well understood.

The patient recovered quickly, with no discernible alterations in personality. She lived disease-free for several years until her tumor recurred and was later operated on again, this time by Harvey Cushing. Penfield later published his technique for performing a complete right frontal lobectomy to treat brain tumors, a strategy still used today when operating in this location.

Penfield showed his bravery by pushing the boundaries of brain surgery with this operation, but what made it the more extraordinary was the patient's identity. She was his older sister, Ruth. Imagine it: not only operating on one's sibling, who lay awake throughout the entire operation, but also planning and executing such a risky and largely experimental surgery on a close family member. Lucky for those of us who have followed in Penfield's footsteps, his sister's surgery was so successful that it didn't just buy her more time but has also helped countless other patients with tumors of the right frontal lobe.

NEXT SLIDE . . . NEXT SLIDE . . .

After Penfield, the language-mapping baton was handed over to another neurosurgeon, Dr. George Ojemann, who worked in Seattle only a few hundred miles from Penfield's birthplace. Ojemann adopted and then extended Penfield's mapping techniques to explore with greater precision how language was organized in the brain. He discovered that the language modules first described by Penfield are almost never located in the same place in any two brains. Unlike movement, sensation, and vision, which are reliably found in roughly the same spot, language's home in the brain's architecture is unpredictable. In other words, just as no two people have the same speech mannerisms, word selections, phrasing, or tone, the locations of these speech-controlling and speech-absorbing areas of the brain are equally inconsistent and unpredictable. Think of it this way: the location of language in the brain differs the same way height, hair color, shoe size, and facial features differ. A range exists within which most people fall, but each brain is unique.

Ojemann's discovery is what makes brain mapping so critical when removing tumors. In fact, the only surefire way to unambiguously identify where each brain's language modules are located is to map them during brain surgery. And it's because of this variability that Ted Kennedy and Beau Biden had to be awake for their surgeries. McCain's tumor, on the other hand, wasn't near any language areas, so his surgery could be performed while he was asleep under general anesthesia.

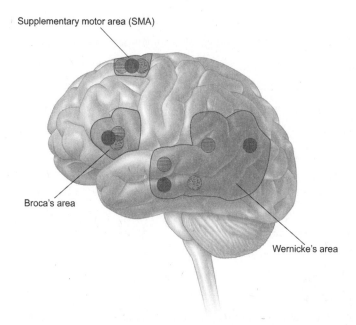

Supplementary motor area (SMA)

Broca's area

Wernicke's area

Penfield and Ojemann showed that the brain's modules most critical for language processing are small, roughly the size of a dime. While language modules are commonly found within the larger regions defined by Broca and Wernicke, they are distributed differently in every individual. This example shows the locations of the language modules in three different people, each shaded with a distinct pattern, superimposed on the same brain.

Between my third and fourth years of medical school, I elected to take a year off to work with Dr. Ojemann. Having graduated from college with a degree in philosophy and English, I was keen to learn more about how the brain's neurons code for language. Ojemann's research seemed like a perfect fit. I was able to secure some funding to pay my expenses and drove across the country in my parents' old Buick station wagon to spend a year in Seattle—a year that forever altered my life's trajectory.

Ojemann, a high school debate champion from Iowa, trained in Seattle with Arthur A. Ward, one of Penfield's residents. He was tall and wiry, with a slender frame dutifully maintained via early morning rowing excursions on Seattle's Puget Sound. He wore thick rectangular glasses to correct his myopia, likely exacerbated by reading the hundreds of scientific papers that lay stacked in towering piles on his desk, each one consumed but never discarded.

During my year with Ojemann, I spent many afternoons watching him in the operating room. He had retained his midwestern drawl and would speak to his patients in a calm pilot-addressing-the-passengers voice that never revealed the slightest hint of anxiety. When he mapped his patients' brains, he worked not with a neuropsychologist but rather with a warmhearted EEG technician and jack-of-all-trades from Egypt named Ettore "Hector" Lettich, who spoke several languages and had been assisting Ojemann with his research for over a decade by the time I arrived there in 1992.

Ojemann would methodically probe the brain with the bipolar stimulator that now bears his name—essentially a two-pronged electrode that passed a small current between its tips, just enough to interrupt the brain circuitry from working but not enough to trigger a seizure. As he carefully moved the electrode from one spot to another, Hector would prompt the patients from beneath the drapes, showing them pictures of objects to name or short phrases to read. This was before the days of computers, so the images and words were displayed using slides held in a carousel that would drop them one by one to be projected onto a screen at the same level as the patient's vision so they could be easily seen.

Awake in the operating room, their brains exposed, the patients would name each object: "This is a key. . . . This is a telephone. . . . This is a car. . . ." The moment Ojemann's electrode touched an important area, we could tell because the patient would suddenly hesitate: "This is a . . . it's a . . . ummm . . . ummm . . . ," at which point Ojemann would place a marker on the brain, usually a small cutout square of paper with a unique number or a letter on it to tag the location as an area critical for language. At the end of the mapping session, the brain would be covered with tiny labels, signposts warning of hazards up ahead. The whole process, start to finish, would take about half an hour.

One of Ojemann's most critical if disturbing discoveries—which I had read about as a medical student and which prompted me to fly across the country to work with him—was that it was possible, when mapping a bilingual patient, to knock out their ability to speak in one of their languages *without affecting their second language*. I was astonished that the brain would be organized in such a way, with separate languages finding their homes in different neighborhoods in the brain.

One day, Hector was out sick and Ojemann asked me to fill in. I was both nervous and excited. My job was to make sure that the slides were arranged in the carousel in the proper order, that the screen was visible to the patient, and that the slides would advance one at a time while Ojemann stimulated the brain. The first few slides slipped perfectly into place. Everything seemed to be running smoothly. Then the inevitable occurred, as it often did with slide carousels: one slide got stuck halfway down and refused to fall all the way into the projector's lightstream. Then the mechanism that pushes the slide back up into the carousel also jammed.

With the slide stuck halfway in the carousel and no way to advance, we, too, were stuck. I started to panic. If the mapping couldn't be done, the surgery would have to be aborted, and then the patient would have undergone a craniotomy for nothing.

I heard Dr. Ojemann asking in his even-tempered voice, ever so slightly escalating in impatience, "Next slide. . . . Next slide. . . . Next slide, . . ."

I tried to keep my cool as I told him what had happened, fully aware that the patient was also listening. Ojemann talked me through the corrective steps, as if dictating the landing procedures to a passenger who had just taken over the controls following the pilot's heart attack. "Twist the locking disc off the top of the carousel. Grab the slide. Remove it. Lift up the whole carousel. Put the slide back in place. Whatever you do, do *not* turn the carousel upside down, since without the locking disc—"

It was too late. The slides began cascading onto the floor of the operating room with the cacophony of a drum set falling down a flight of stairs. Slides were now scattered everywhere: under the drapes of the operating room table, beneath the feet of the scrub nurse . . . A few had even escaped out the door and into the hallway.

Ojemann never raised his voice. He never scolded me. He never let on to the patient that anything was amiss. He simply requested that I collect the slides and put them back into the carousel in the proper orientation so we could proceed. After this seemingly endless delay, we continued as if nothing out of the ordinary had occurred, and the patient's surgery unfolded without another hitch. I don't remember exactly how long it took, but I do remember that no matter how many times I've seen him since, he's never once mentioned this experience.

EIGHT

THE HARDEST PART IS
KNOWING WHEN TO STOP

A t some point in every brain tumor operation, I'm faced with the decision of how aggressive I should be. In an ideal world, I take out the entire tumor, leaving nothing behind. Unfortunately, many tumors sit extremely close to parts of the brain that are critical for abilities such as movement, navigation, and speech. Others are wrapped around small nerves and blood vessels that, if damaged, can cause double vision, blindness, deafness, or an inability to swallow.

Every case is different, and the scenario changes based on a few factors. How old is the patient? How malignant is the tumor? How devastated will they be if I make a mistake? What are the alternatives if I leave a piece behind? Most operations last several hours. Usually, somewhere between hours three and four, just as fatigue begins to set in, the moment of truth arrives when such lingering decisions demand attention. When faced with a fragment of tumor stuck to a nerve, or one resting dangerously near an area known to move some part of the body, I must decide, right then and there, how to proceed.

The patient, on the other hand, is unconscious, unable to affect the outcome of this momentous decision. Sure, if they were awake, we could discuss what they want me to do, but we often keep our patients asleep because it's generally safer. The brain is less tense, and if an awake patient has trouble breathing, the anesthesiologist will have a very hard time intubating them mid-surgery. In one version of their future, they are cured of their tumor, living as if nothing had happened, their operation but a distant memory. In another version, they are paralyzed or deaf or maybe blind, their normal lives now a distant memory, replaced with one beset by disabilities. Which future will unfold? It depends entirely on the experience, judgment, and technical abilities of their surgeon, which, if you are lying on my table, ends up being me. Because we brain surgeons must, at some point, balance quality of life with *amount* of life, sometimes the hardest part of our job is simply knowing when to stop.

THE CASE OF
EUGENE O'KELLY

Eugene Desmond O'Kelly was the CEO of KPMG, one of the largest accounting firms in the world. One morning only a few years into his tenure as CEO, O'Kelly's wife noticed a slight drooping in his right cheek. An MRI revealed a multifocal GBM on the left side of his brain, meaning it had already spread to several different locations and was just starting to impact his functions: speech, motor, and visual. While trying to decide how to proceed, O'Kelly sought the counsel of two neurosurgeons. The first, at Memorial Sloan Kettering, recommended a debulking surgery. He would perform a craniotomy but take out only a part of the tumor, since it had invaded O'Kelly's brain to such an extent that it could not be removed entirely without causing significant harm. Recovery after such a debulking would take at least six weeks.

A day later, O'Kelly showed up in my office. After listening closely to his story and unraveling his priorities, I recommended a biopsy, noting that the risk of removing it far outweighed any possible benefit, as it would not increase his life expectancy. Taking a tiny sample via a biopsy, on the other hand, would be safer and sufficient to make the diagnosis. Furthermore, the biopsy would not put any of his faculties in jeopardy and would allow him to begin radiation and chemotherapy sooner, which might extend and maximize the quality of his remaining life.

Given these two options, O'Kelly chose the biopsy. Then he made another choice that not many other patients make. He refused chemotherapy. He didn't want whatever time he had left to be consumed, either emotionally or physically, by the debilitating ravages of the treatment.

O'Kelly lived for one hundred more days, and during that time he wrote his *New York Times* bestselling book *Chasing Daylight: How My Forthcoming Death Transformed My Life*.

In this inspirational account of his final weeks, he described, with both clarity and sensitivity, how he translated the win-at-all-costs mentality of a CEO into the language of dying with dignity, optimism, love, and grace. He strove for presence. He found closure in each of his relationships and created perfect moments with his family and friends. This calculation—to forgo aggressive treatment—allowed him to take control of his disease and to die on his own terms.

Sometimes it's not the doctor but the patient who knows when to stop.

THE THING WITH FEATHERS

When a malignant brain tumor first sprouts in the brain, it arrives unexpectedly and makes its presence known indirectly. A subtle feeling of weakness might arise, a dimming of peripheral vision, or just a vague sense that something is not quite right. These symptoms are often ignored, attributed to lack of sleep, stress, or maybe age. As evidence mounts, acceptance does not always follow. Even the unambiguous image that appears on the MRI scan can be shrugged off as a possible misreading or a mistake: *"Couldn't it be something else? How do you know it's a tumor?"*

The morning before every brain tumor surgery, I get a new MRI scan, which I load onto a computer and use for intraoperative navigation. I cannot tell you how often I am asked by my patients whether the tumor is still there—as if somehow, it might have magically disappeared in the interval between diagnosis and surgery.

When I emerge from the operating room and talk to the family after the operation, any fantasy of disappearing tumors also disappears. After my close encounter with the alien invader, the family's first question is usually "What did the biopsy show?" During an operation, we always send at least two pieces of the tumor to the pathologist. The first, called the frozen section, or just "the frozen" for short, is evaluated immediately and provides rapid information that we use to determine how to proceed with the rest of the surgery. Occasionally our intuition about what we are seeing with our own eyes is wrong. Sometimes a seemingly benign tumor reveals malignant features. Occasionally a feared cancer appears more indolent. While we always hope that what looks like a GBM on the MRI scan is really an infection or perhaps some oddball benign tumor that merely mimics the appearance of a GBM, after years of operating on brains, I'm sorry to say that looks are usually *not* deceiving. The frozen usually confirms what we already knew.

The second specimen, called the "permanent," is the larger of the two, and it gets stained, scrutinized, and submitted for comprehensive molecular and genetic testing. This more rigorously examined piece gives the surgeon and oncologist the final diagnosis—the one that will determine not only the patient's prognosis but also what additional therapy might be needed, either chemotherapy, radiation therapy, or (more often) both together.

The permanent may take up to a week to come back, so at the end of the operation the surgeon still can't be completely sure of the identity of the tumor. All you can go on is your firsthand experience of what you saw in the operating room and the frozen, which is correct about 95 percent of the time. So the dilemma faced by the surgeon upon encountering the family in the waiting room after the operation is whether to reveal the results of the frozen right away or hold back. Why on earth, you ask, would this information ever be withheld? Two reasons. First, can you imagine telling the family, and then the patient, that they have a fatal disease with a year-and-a-half life expectancy and then finding out a week later that you were wrong? Not the best way to strengthen the doctor-patient relationship, to say the least.

The second reason not to discuss the frozen is that having this conversation *is really hard.* No one likes to give bad news. We surgeons want to come out of the operating room and tell our patients that the surgery was a success and that the tumor was completely removed—or at least that as much as could *safely* be removed is now gone. We want that hug of appreciation for all the hard work we just put in. To dodge what will inevitably be a challenging and emotionally wrenching conversation, some surgeons will evade the issue and tell a family that the frozen can't always be trusted—that it's better to wait for the permanent to come back. Some will entirely defer the conversation, leaving it to the neuro-oncologist, who won't sit down with the patient for another week or two, after the pathology report has been finalized.

Frankly, I can't imagine withholding this information, *particularly* if the tumor is malignant. This is where trust is built, and I view it as my responsibility to reveal as much as I know, when I know it, and not to hide facts or hard truths. If the frozen is consistent with my interpretation of the MRI scan combined with what I encountered during surgery, it's time to let the family know that, despite their inability to see the asteroid in the sky heading toward earth, this cataclysmic planet-destroyer is not just a blip on someone else's radar. It has arrived. It will hit, and the effects will be devastating.

This is when the tone of the conversation shifts from the breezy "The surgery went well!" to the more sobering "But here's what we're dealing with in the days and weeks ahead." And so begins the next stage of the process. The people in the waiting room are often the patient's closest relatives and friends, their support group. The sooner they can be involved in their loved one's care, the better. If the tumor is malignant, I let them know that the sum of the evidence is now leaning in that direction. That said, I am also always careful to add that we cannot be 100 percent sure until the final report comes back.

I try to gauge by their expressions their level of understanding of the difficult news I've just imparted. Those who have faced a GBM in the past know exactly what I've just told them: their loved one has limited time left to live. Most people sitting in that waiting room, however, do not. Whatever it is, they think, they will fight it. They've read about the miracles of modern medicine. They've seen the movies, read the stories about terminal patients who prevail. "What about Lance Armstrong?" they say. "He had a brain tumor, right? He went on to win the Tour de France, didn't he?"

In these moments the subtleties between a brain metastasis and a GBM are usually lost on my patient's family. My job is to hold their hands, both literally and figuratively; to answer their questions; and to let them know that we are in this together: I will not be leaving their side. Although the family might ask my advice about how to break the sad news to the patient, since the family will see them in the recovery room before I do, they almost never take on that burden. Instead, I'm the one tasked with having the frank conversation with my patient the next day, after the anesthesia has worn off, and they have rested and are ready to listen and absorb the information.

The truth is I've already started preparing the patient for this moment from their first visit to my office. I've removed almost 10,000 brain tumors and reviewed at least twice as many scans. The diagnosis is almost never a surprise: the MRI tells the story, like a crystal ball that shows the future with crisp, brutal clarity. I know a GBM when I see one.

The initial office visit, in fact, can be surreal. At this early stage, the patient is often minimally symptomatic. They are obviously aware that something is growing in their brain—they've sought out medical care, after all—and they know that it needs to be removed. Maybe they've done a little research or they've had a family member with a brain tumor, which may or may not have been similar. They are also often scared and unsure of what lies ahead or what it all means.

Commonly, they are frequently somewhat oblivious to the gravity of the situation. This is all new to them. But as I listen to their questions, I see things they are not yet capable of seeing, let alone processing. I see the mother of three young children who will not make it to their high school graduation. I see the father and sole provider for a family of teenagers with college payments looming who will not be walking his daughter down the aisle. I see the hedge fund manager who is sitting on top of the world, planning his retirement and next lavish vacation, who will soon be closing his fund. He's about to lose not only his long-anticipated opportunity to spend his money but his ability to bathe and feed himself.

And yes, thinking of others' deaths can be debilitating to even the most hardened of us surgeons: giving bad news, seeing families crumple from the oncoming train bearing down on them. As I stare into the void, imagining their future, I want to stand up and scream at the top of my lungs or collapse on the ground in a flood of tears. I do none of this, of course. My job at this moment is to fight this battle with every fiber in my body and shepherd these victims of nature's callous and indifferent design.

I believe in revealing the truth of my patients' prognoses at a slow and deliberate pace. But I also never, ever take away their most powerful weapon: hope. We're not talking about false hope, as in "We're going to beat this thing," but rather, *true* hope, a concept introduced by Jerome Groopman in his book *The Anatomy of Hope: How People Prevail in the Face of Illness*. True hope sounds more like "There are a small group of long-term survivors and I'm going to do everything in my power to give you the best chance of being one of them." Or even "Your remaining days with your family can be beautiful. Maybe even more beautiful than all the days that have come before."

So, how does a doctor walk this tightrope between truth and hope?

At the first office visit, I begin by focusing on the upcoming surgery, which is the initial psychological hurdle. Most people fear the unknown, so I take them through each step of the procedure. I describe what will be done to them like a tour guide: "The anesthesiologist will put a mask over your face, and you will go to sleep. You won't feel anything after that. Then I'll make an incision behind your hairline, which you won't see once the little bit of hair I have to shave grows back. Once the skin is opened, we will re-move a piece of the skull . . ." and so on. The vague and terrifying becomes concrete and simple when presented step by step.

We then discuss the possible complications of the surgery. I generally stick to things that could reasonably (if infrequently) happen, like an infec-tion or a bleed, rather than one-in-a-million calamities like the ventilator breaking or the anesthesiologist having a heart attack.

If we are operating near the optic nerves, for example, then I must pre-pare them for a possible loss of vision. If we are encroaching on the lan-guage areas, they may wake up with speech difficulties. Basically, any faculty in the vicinity of the surgical corridor is at risk of being impaired. This is the essence of neurosurgery: navigating the narrow boundary be-tween causing harm and doing good.

In my experience, emphasizing the remote possibility of disaster is not helpful. Think of a pilot explaining the odds of the plane crashing as the wheels leave the tarmac: most of us would rather *not* know this statistic at that particular moment. It just creates unneeded anxiety. As Groopman wrote, "Don't let fear overwhelm hope." At the same time, I will not lie or deliberately hide things from my patients. If the patient wants to know ev-ery possible wrong turn their surgery can take, I'll go there with them.

At this point, my job is more psychoanalytic than surgical. I read their faces, try to figure out how much they really want to know. If the tumor I'm expecting is a GBM, the brain surgery itself should be the least of their worries. What's more important right now is processing the news of the tumor's existence and preparing them for the rapid and relentless progres-sion of the disease.

Which is why, at this very first visit, I always introduce the *possibility* that the tumor could be malignant. Even if I'm often confident it's a GBM, sometimes—rarely—scans can be misleading, and my initial suspicions can be mistaken. Hitting a patient over the head this early by telling them that there is a high likelihood that they have a malignant tumor is, in my opin-ion, insensitive to them and to their family, and it does not promote a proper mindset going into surgery.

It's critical for the patient to show up on the day of surgery with both hope and optimism that things will go well. I also tell them that I'll do everything I can to ensure that the procedure unfolds as seamlessly as possible and that I'll be there for them every step of the way, no matter the ultimate diagnosis. I want them to know they have a seasoned veteran as their ally.

How do I break bad news to the patient after the surgery? I take my cues from them. I usually start the conversation with a clear presentation of the facts. I may say that the preliminary diagnosis showed what we feared: that the tumor is malignant. I prefer to use the words "we" and "us." I also emphasize whatever positives I can. The good news is that the surgery went extremely well and we got out as much tumor as could safely be removed: "Although it's a tough tumor to beat, the surgery puts us in the best place going forward to attack the microscopic disease invariably left behind."

I then tell them they will likely need radiation and chemotherapy—the standard of care in treating GBMs—and that we will find them the most experienced neuro-oncologist to help coordinate the next stage of this process. While our neuro-oncologists at Cornell are some of the best in the world, patients often want second opinions, so I let them know we will help them get their records together to send them wherever they like. Patients often express a fear of telling you they want a second opinion, as if they're cheating on their spouse or insulting a relative. You never want anyone looking back as the end approaches and feeling that they didn't do everything in their power to find the right treatment, didn't explore all the options, or left a stone unturned.

I have witnessed only a handful of medical miracles in my career: tumors that miraculously shrank without any treatment, long-term survivors of fatal diseases. What's the explanation? We don't know. But these cases do provide some room for hope. The patients I have treated who are still alive five, ten, or even fifteen years after a GBM diagnosis are a rare reminder that my degree and years of experience go only so far. What makes these long-term survivors so special? What did they do to beat the odds? Were they in some incredible new trial of a groundbreaking drug, or did they eat nothing but kale and quinoa and exercise every day? Nope. They were each treated the same way we treat everyone, and they ate whatever they wanted.

Which brings us to the last part of the conversation: clinical trials. With easy access to the internet, patients often hear about new treatments and trials for GBM, but the quantity of material out there can be overwhelming. It's nearly impossible for the layperson to sift through the dozens of ongoing and future trials and know which, if any, are appropriate; which are somewhat reasonable, perhaps; or which are too dangerous, with little likelihood of success. My general advice to my patients is that they get no more than three opinions and then go with their gut. Find a trustworthy neuro-oncologist and follow their advice. I also remind them that, were there a magic bullet to cure GBMs, we'd all know about it and already be prescribing it.

The odds of success for any new trial therapy, given the track record of clinical trials for GBM, are disappointingly low. All too often I hear from patients who wish they'd spent less time pursuing ineffective treatments and more time enjoying their remaining days with loved ones. That said, I do encourage my patients to enroll in clinical trials if they sound reasonable, don't require too much travel, don't drain too many resources, and don't take away too much time from family and friends. Clinical trials are the only way medicine advances, the only way we will eventually defeat this disease.

RADIATION, RINGWORM, AND CELL PHONES

Another frequent question my malignant tumor patients ask is "Why me? Was it anything I did?" It's human nature to attempt to find cause for suffering, to create order out of chaos, to shake their fist at the randomness of fate. Often my patients will place blame on environmental exposures such as smoking, power lines, or toxic chemicals released by a local factory. They also worry that their brain tumor might have been inherited or will be passed on to future generations. Both fears are somewhat legitimate, since most cancers arise from a combination of a genetic predisposition and an environmental trigger. But unfortunately the root cause of most brain tumors remains frustratingly unknown.

The National Institute for Occupational Safety and Health lists over 130 substances as potential carcinogens. Yet the brain has evolved to protect itself from most known toxins via the blood-brain barrier, which filters out those that might cause harm. And the few genetic diseases shown to increase the risk of acquiring a brain tumor, such as neurofibromatosis or Li-Fraumeni syndrome, are very rare.

Most brain cancers are triggered by some random and little-understood series of events that either alters the DNA within the nucleus of brain cells or misaligns the careful balance of proteins that promote and suppress cell growth. I therefore try to emphasize to my patients that they did nothing to bring this upon themselves. There is no one to blame or resent, and there's no reason to feel guilty that their children might be at higher risk of the same fate. As scientifically unsatisfying as the answer may be, the cause for most brain tumors is just plain old bad luck.

The only environmental exposure known to cause brain tumors is radiation. X-rays were discovered in 1895 by German scientist Wilhelm Conrad Röntgen and hailed as a powerful tool for gazing inside the body. It wasn't until the late 1920s, however, when their harmful effects became clear. Marie Curie—the only woman to be awarded two Nobel Prizes for her research on radiation—was unaware of radiation's risks until it was too late. She ultimately succumbed, dying of aplastic anemia.

It took years for the dangers of radiation to be appreciated. Radium, a naturally occurring source of radiation, was initially thought to be therapeutic, a panacea prescribed to treat, for example, pelvic pain in pregnant women. Before 1960, irradiating the scalp with X-rays was also the treatment of choice for ringworm, a type of scalp fungus. And while this treatment was at one time offered worldwide, the practice was most common in the newly established State of Israel.

Approximately 20,000 Israeli immigrants—particularly children—had their scalps irradiated for ringworm, with devastating if now predictable results: between 1948 and 1960, the years in question, brain tumors began popping up with alarming frequency in people who had been irradiated. It wasn't until 1974 that an Israeli study conclusively demonstrated that there were 10 times as many meningiomas and 2.5 times as many gliomas in those who had been irradiated as in those who hadn't been. The practice was eventually abandoned once an effective antifungal medication was discovered. As if the persecution of the Jewish people at the hands of their enemies weren't bad enough, imagine the anguish of the doctors who prescribed the treatment when they realized that they'd been welcoming refugees who had narrowly escaped the gas chambers and then bathing them with a harmful dose of radiation.

The link between radiation and carcinogenesis was further bolstered by the fallout—both literally and figuratively—from another man-made calamity: the nuclear bombs dropped on Hiroshima and Nagasaki at the end of World War II. Survivors living within a 1.5-mile radius of the blast had an increased risk of brain tumors (among their other chronic ailments), the most common being meningiomas and acoustic neuromas—the latter a benign mass that grows from the nerve in the inner ear that mediates hearing.

Radiation is now one of the few accepted environmental carcinogens unequivocally linked with an increased risk of developing a brain tumor. Benign tumors seem to be the more common sequelae, but a link also exists between radiation and malignant tumors. Though rare, what these radiation-induced tumors tell us is that sometimes the most effective treatments for one cancer can, in a cruel twist of fate, seed an even deadlier one years later.

THE CASE OF
JOHNNIE COCHRAN

Johnnie Lee Cochran Jr., an American lawyer born and raised in Louisiana, was inspired by his hero, Thurgood Marshall, to pursue a career as a civil rights attorney. Cochran later made his name and reputation in Los Angeles in several high-profile cases defending wealthy clients, including O. J. Simpson. "If it doesn't fit, you must acquit," he repeated during his closing argument, a phrase about O.J.'s gloves that would enter the legal lexicon of infamy.

According to Cochran's wife, her late husband's first symptoms were memory loss and speech difficulties. He was eventually diagnosed with a tumor on the left side of his brain, near the parts important for language and memory processing. His neurosurgeon, Dr. Keith Black, fearing imminent damage to his patient's famed debating skills, elected to do a biopsy and diagnosed Cochran with a GBM. That was in December of 2003. Four months later, Dr. Black performed another surgery to stave off further disease progression. Despite these heroic measures, Cochran passed away after another eleven months. He was sixty-seven years old. To honor his memory, the family established a brain tumor center in his name at Cedars-Sinai Medical Center in Los Angeles.

During his illness, Cochran claimed that cell phone use caused his tumor, as he always held it tightly against the left side of his head. His family took the same stance. In 2006, Dr. Black appeared on *Larry King Live* and reiterated this claim: "My own belief," he said, "is that there probably is a correlation between the use of cell phones and brain cancer, even though there's no scientific proof."

On May 27, 2008, after Teddy Kennedy was diagnosed, King once again asked Dr. Black to appear on CNN to discuss the possible link between brain tumors and cell phones, but this time he was joined by a few other guests, including Sanjay Gupta. Black restated his opinion that, in the absence of proof, the safest thing was to wear an earpiece. Gupta posited that, though current studies did not show a definitive link, long-term studies, particularly in children, were lacking, and therefore the cumulative effects of cell phone use over many years were simply unknown. I also got the call to appear. To prepare, I voraciously read all the studies I could find on the subject. When I added them together, the sum did not support a link between cell phone use and brain tumors. The data, I cautioned on the show, was inconclusive. Lack of proof that there is *not* a link is not proof of anything.

The uncertainty about the safety of cell phone radiation bred fear in an America still emotionally scarred by the lies of omission from cigarette manufacturers, who promoted their product as safe even as study after study—some of which they deliberately hid from consumers—proved otherwise. The cell phone industry, like the tobacco industry, is a large and powerful business with a mandate for profitability. No one would be surprised to learn that damaging data had been suppressed for the sake of the bottom line. But such was not the case with cell phones, perhaps only because duplicity wasn't needed.

The parallel between cigarettes and cell phones is weak at best. Almost every epidemiological study, from the 1950s onward, showed a link between smoking and lung cancer, while studies that try to link cell phone use with brain tumors have always been indeterminate. The number of articles showing that cell phones have no impact on or even *reduce* the risk of brain tumors is equivalent to the number revealing an increased risk. But we don't hear about these cell-phones-might-be-good-for-you studies, since they don't make for anxiety-provoking, attention-grabbing headlines.

Today, more than twenty years after Cochran's death, longer follow-up studies are finally available, including research specifically on children. No evidence as yet has been found to link cell phone use with the development of brain tumors.

The other big difference between cigarettes and cell phones is that the former are packed with literally dozens of proven carcinogens. But you might ask: Don't cell phones emit radiation? If radiation can cause brain tumors, like the X-rays given to treat ringworm, why can't cell phone radiation also lead to cancer? To understand the difference between these two forms of radiation, let's take a quick trip back to high school physics. (And relax: there won't be a test.)

NOT ALL RADIATION IS THE SAME

When we think of radiation, we generally think of what scientists call ionizing radiation or, more precisely, X-rays and gamma rays. The word "ionizing" refers to the ability of high-energy radiation to dislodge electrons as it passes through matter. A molecule that loses an electron also gains a positive charge and is called an ion, which we know can damage DNA. This explains why Marie Curie developed a deadly blood disease after her exposure to X-rays and why Bruce Banner, for all my fellow Marvel fans, turned into the Hulk after he was flooded with gamma rays.

Radiation comes in different forms that can be measured along a scale called the electromagnetic spectrum, since both electricity and magnetism are created by the movement of electrons. The electromagnetic spectrum extends from dangerous ionizing gamma rays and X-rays on the one end to non-ionizing and innocuous cell phones and power lines on the other. In the middle of the electromagnetic spectrum is visible light.

Exposure to what the human eye sees—visible light—doesn't cause cancer. Ultraviolet radiation, which lies between the harmless rays of visible light and the damaging energy produced by ionizing radiation, is, however, potentially carcinogenic. This is the component of sunlight that not only makes us tan but also increases our risk of skin cancer. As we move to the opposite end of the electromagnetic spectrum, the safer side, we pass through infrared radiation, a form of non-ionizing radiation that can be used to heat things up, like the red lights used to keep your food warm in a restaurant. If we keep going further in that direction, away from ionizing radiation, we get to microwaves, which can also be used to heat food, and then cell phones, televisions, and finally power lines. These forms of non-ionizing radiation, below the infrared spectrum, are *not capable of breaking DNA bonds* and thus are not capable of causing cancer. For this reason, I use my cell phone without a headset. So, too, do my children.

Despite the rapidly increasing use of cell phones in this country, the incidence of malignant brain tumors, according to the Central Brain Tumor Registry of the United States, has not increased over the last twenty years. You would expect that, if cell phones were causing brain tumors, we'd be undergoing a full-on epidemic at this point.

We're not.

Meanwhile, 60 percent of Americans admit to using a cell phone while driving, and the incidence of distracted driver fatalities since the advent of cell phones has increased by 30 percent, which precisely mirrors the increase in cell phone subscriptions. While cell phones are clearly a public health issue, they're not a brain tumor issue. Our money and scientific attention would be better spent preventing the thousands of deaths occurring every year because of distracted drivers rather than wasting our time worrying about what, at best, might amount to a trivial role in the generation of brain tumors.

A HOPE IN THE UNSEEN

Neurosurgery training is like the marshmallow test,* but instead of waiting fifteen minutes to eat the marshmallow, you wait eleven years to finish your training. You'd think that after four years of medical school and seven years of residency, I'd be eager to begin my career. Not me. Rather than jump right into clinical practice, I decided to put off real life a bit longer and sink another year into my education, the first six months of which I decided to spend in a scientific laboratory doing research in Munich, Germany. Had it been given to me as a child, I would undoubtedly have crushed the marshmallow test.

One day in the lab, someone mentioned in passing that, with my interest in brain imaging, I might want to visit Walter Stummer, a neurosurgeon working at a nearby hospital. Stummer had developed a new technique, I was told, that makes malignant brain tumor cells fluoresce, meaning they would light up in the operating room to help surgeons find and remove them.

Cancer cells and normal brain cells appear almost identical to the naked eye. This often leaves the surgeon in the uncomfortable position of not being sure where the diseased brain ends and the healthy brain begins.

---

*While many variations exist, the popular conception of the 1972 Stanford marshmallow test involved giving a child a choice between eating a marshmallow immediately or waiting fifteen minutes, in which case they were rewarded with an additional marshmallow. Supposedly, the child's ability to delay gratification predicted success later in life.

Stummer's solution, which seems obvious in retrospect, was to find a dye that could identify which cells were tumor cells and which were not. Enter 5-aminolevulinic acid, or 5-ALA for short, a potion the patient swigs just before the operation like a shot of whiskey to settle their nerves. After getting absorbed by the gut, 5-ALA travels through the bloodstream, sneaks through the blood-brain barrier, and parks itself inside the glioblastoma cells. A few hours later, these cells fluoresce bright pink when illuminated with a blue light. This allows the neurosurgeon to differentiate the GBM cells from the surrounding normal brain.

At that stage in my career, I'd never even heard of 5-ALA. In retrospect, this was not so surprising, since the drug was still experimental and no one in the world was using it outside of this one operating room in Munich. I'd randomly stumbled into Stummer's OR only a few months after his first patient received the drug.

Peering over Stummer's shoulder that day, I watched the cocktail work its magic. All the lights in the operating room were extinguished, leaving the surgeons, nurses, and me in complete darkness. Stummer pushed a button on his custom-made microscope, which bathed the surgical field in a deep blue light. Suddenly, out of the darkness, a light pink island of tumor cells, as if flying over the lost city of Atlantis on a cloudy day, slowly came into view. At first, the color was vague. But once my pupils dilated, the faint salmon glow brightened into a brilliant red, vividly highlighting the tumors cells against a sea of deep cobalt. I was astonished, both at this apparent feat of magic and at the clarity of the image. I knew, even then, that I was witnessing something special, a sneak peek at the future of brain tumor surgery.

The drug 5-ALA was approved for use in Europe in 2007, but only after a randomized controlled study showed that it was not only safe but increased the amount of tumor that surgeons could remove by a whopping 30 percent. However, it was not until 2017—eighteen years after I first watched Stummer apply 5-ALA in Germany—that the drug was approved in United States.

So, what took so long?

The FDA walks a fine line between the too-rapid approval of a potentially harmful drug and a too-long delay of the release of a potentially beneficial one. As an organization, they generally err on the side of caution, due in no small part to the hasty release in Europe of the drug thalidomide, which caused severe birth defects in tens of thousands of babies—a biomedical disaster that was mostly averted in the United States because the drug was never approved here. The FDA's Dr. Frances Kelsey stood firm against mounting pressure from the pharmaceutical companies, who wanted to bring the drug to market as quickly as possible. In 1962, John F. Kennedy awarded her the President's Award for Distinguished Federal Civilian Service as a token of his appreciation for the lives she saved.

While stringent criteria are obviously important to prevent harm, the protracted process of drug approval has been described as an invisible graveyard slowly filling with the bodies of those deprived of potentially lifesaving treatments.

The issue for 5-ALA was not safety. Stummer's trial had already addressed that concern. The issue for the FDA was efficacy. Did it work? The FDA was considering 5-ALA as if it were a therapy for cancer, like chemotherapy. Before approving it, they requested another large multicenter trial be undertaken here in the United States to prove that patients whose surgeons used 5-ALA lived longer than those whose surgeons didn't. Such a trial would have been both incredibly expensive and difficult to perform, never mind the absurdity of even attempting to make it a double-blind study. The surgeons could never be blinded as to whether the drug was being used, since they were looking right at it!

In the end, researchers had to convince the FDA that 5-ALA was an intraoperative diagnostic aid, not a therapy. Its value, the FDA was told, would be to help surgeons *visualize* the tumor during surgery, like the contrast given before a CAT scan. It took only seventeen years, but this new strategy proved successful.

In 2021, I had the opportunity to become the first neurosurgeon in the United States to use a newly modified headlight that makes the 5-ALA fluoresce almost ten times brighter than what I had witnessed back in Germany all those years before. Rather than filter the light through the microscope, which was the norm at the time, this new device gets strapped onto the forehead like a spelunker's headlight so that everywhere the surgeon looks, the fluorescent light follows. This makes surgery much easier to perform, and the increased brightness makes the dye easier to see.

I now use 5-ALA in all my GBM surgeries and, as a result, am a better surgeon for it—able to remove more malignant cells. Unfortunately, surgery alone will never cure GBM. Malignant cells invade deep, well beyond the limits of what can safely be removed. Despite our best efforts with chemotherapy, radiation, immunotherapy, and cancer vaccines, the cure for GBM remains elusive. The good news is that hundreds of scientists are working to develop new therapies.

One possibility would be to create a dye that, like 5-ALA, selectively enters tumor cells. When light hits them, instead of producing fluorescence, it would trigger a chemical reaction that simply kills the cells. This so-called photodynamic therapy would need to depend on deeply penetrating infra-red light to be effective at addressing the rogue cells that migrate deep into the brain beyond surgery's reach. A similar chemical sensitive to high-frequency sound waves would be even more effective, since ultrasound can penetrate brain tissue even deeper than infra-red light.

Our understanding of the basic biology of glioblastoma is expanding rapidly. I truly believe that it is only a matter of time before science triumphs over this scourge once and for all.

NINE

JOURNEY TO THE CENTER OF THE BRAIN

L ike the peak of Mount Everest or the Mariana Trench, there are places on this planet so inhospitable and unwelcoming that it can seem humankind was never meant to explore them. Similarly, there are locations in the brain where tumors can lurk, deep in its innermost chambers, hidden from all but the most intrepid of adventurers. Neurosurgeons who specialize in operating in these buried compartments—of whom I am one—are called skull base surgeons, since the bottom of the skull sits beneath the brain, protecting it, like Smaug the dragon perched atop his mountain of gold.

Few neurosurgeons choose to specialize in skull base surgery. It requires a certain personality. Like rock climbers or cave divers, we embrace the challenge of long and tedious operations fraught with danger that require careful planning and meticulous execution to avoid failure. The hidden territories into which we enter are named accordingly: Meckel's cave, Dorello's canal, the cavernous sinus, and—the sanctum sanctorum—the third ventricle. This latter place, which sits at the center of the brain, is a chamber roughly the size of a quarter that is so difficult to reach, an entire textbook with over 1,000 pages, published in 1987, was required to help surgeons tunnel there safely.

If there is a geometric center of the brain, it's undoubtedly the third ventricle. More a cavity than an object, the third ventricle is part of the ventricular system through which cerebrospinal fluid (CSF) flows. The ancient Roman physician Galen posited that CSF housed our vital spirit, like the liquid computer in the movie *Rollerball*: an erroneous idea that endured well into the seventeenth century. The third ventricle is located so deep in the middle of the brain, in fact, that no single best way to reach it exists since all paths must traverse an equally long distance through a field of land mines. As a result, neurosurgeons have devised literally dozens of different ways to get there, each with its own inherent advantages and disadvantages.

From the earliest days of neurosurgery, attempts at reaching the third ventricle—and the tumors contained within it—almost always ended in failure. Of Cushing's famous series of two thousand brain tumor operations, roughly twenty were directed toward the third ventricle. He never made mention of their outcomes. Those results were recently unearthed, exposing a shocking mortality rate of 27 percent! Compare this with the 8 percent he achieved with his other cases or with the modern rate, which is far less than 1 percent.

Several early neurosurgical pioneers attempted third ventricular surgery, but the first to firmly plant his flag there was Walter Dandy. Dandy, who we've come across already through his invention of the batter's helmet and his attempt to cure GBM by removing half the brain, was one of Cushing's residents at Johns Hopkins, and their relationship was considered one of the most contentious rivalries in modern surgery. Dandy was Cushing's Oedipus, who sought affection through figurative patricide. He was irreverent and challenged Cushing at every turn. Cushing was abusive and dismissive of his young apprentice. While Cushing came from a long line of blue-blooded, wealthy physicians, Dandy was raised in the small mining town of Sedalia, Missouri, the son of working-class English immigrants. He was their hope, and he was hungry to break into American society. Rumor has it that Cushing once scolded Dandy when he tried to use his left hand while assisting Cushing: "Use your right hand, Dandy, you're clumsy enough with that!"

The more Cushing abused and ignored Dandy, the more the younger surgeon's zeal grew to show up his master. When Cushing left Hopkins to start his neurosurgical department at Harvard, he didn't take Dandy along, abandoning his young protégé. Dandy not only rose to the occasion but elevated neurosurgery to new heights with his talent and dexterity. While Cushing would perform one surgery a day, plodding along at a meticulous pace, Dandy was known to complete five or six operations in the same period of time with astonishing agility.

While Cushing's goal was safety, Dandy strove for efficiency. Cushing made neurosurgery dependable; Dandy made it more effective. Cushing wanted to ensure the patient survived the operation. Dandy strove for a cure. In response to Dandy's brash demeanor, Cushing wrote to one colleague: "Dandy is young and somewhat radical, and time has a way of curing both of these things—youth and radicalism."

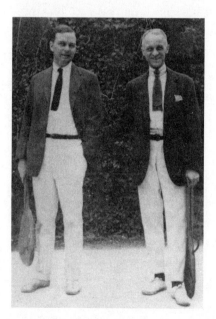

Dandy (left) and Cushing after one of their tennis matches. Supposedly, Dandy won this one.

The Chesney Archives of Johns Hopkins Medicine, Nursing, and Public Health

One of Dandy's many contributions was that he figured out the pathway by which CSF flows through the brain. At the time, the circulation of blood was well-understood. Powered by the heart's rhythmic pumping, blood was known to flow out by way of arteries and back toward the heart via veins. In contrast, no one quite understood where CSF was made or by what route it traveled through the brain before being reabsorbed. By obstructing the outflow of CSF from the bottom of the third ventricle, Dandy demonstrated that the CSF would back up, causing a ballooning of the ventricles, which in turn raised the pressure in the head, a condition called hydrocephalus, Greek for "water on the brain."

Dandy then took his discovery and applied it to create a new way to see inside the brain. Since air is less dense than both brain tissue and CSF, he realized that if he could inject air into the ventricles to replace the CSF, an X-ray of the skull would reveal the contours of the ventricles as air-filled silhouettes. If a tumor was distorting them, the air cast would reveal it. He called this technique "ventriculography" and it provided neurosurgeons with the ability to localize tumors prior to surgery, freeing them from their dependence on neurologists, whose detailed physical examinations had previously been the only way to predict a tumor's location. Like throwing paint on the invisible man, the outline of the trespasser could be rendered visible, and what had been a blind search-and-destroy mission became more of a fair fight. Wilder Penfield, as you recall, traveled down to Johns Hopkins from New York to learn how to perform ventriculography from Dandy to find the tumor that was growing deep in that little boy's head.

Before the ventriculogram, surgeons often performed entire operations only to discover that they'd missed the tumor completely and had to back out empty-handed. (Cushing, ever prideful, was dismissively slow to appreciate Dandy's contribution and refused to adopt ventriculography until late in his career.) The MRI scan, which arrived on the medical scene in the mid-1980s, had a similar impact on the field. So transformative was the MRI that one of my neurosurgery professors used to say half-jokingly that he would trade a stadium full of neurologists for one MRI scanner. Dandy's ventriculogram, the MRI of his era, allowed him to become one of the first surgeons to safely remove tumors of the third ventricle, which he detailed in his book on the subject, *Benign Tumors in the Third Ventricle of the Brain: Diagnosis and Treatment.* Published in 1933, his book appeared a full fifty years before the modern 1,000-page tome mentioned above.

Dandy was also one of the first pioneers of a concept that is, some hundred years later, only now being fully realized—that of minimally invasive brain surgery. As early as 1920, he attempted to access the brain's ventricles through a small corridor using a speculum and a headlight, which he ultimately abandoned since the technology of his day was not sufficiently advanced and the visibility was poor. In modern neurosurgical operations, the third ventricle can now be approached using any one of several minimally invasive approaches: one through the nostrils, which requires no incisions whatsoever, and another through a small hole the size of a dime, drilled at the top of the head. The key piece of equipment that makes these surgeries possible is the endoscope, a modern version of Dandy's speculum and headlight, essentially the same idea now enhanced with sophisticated optics: high-resolution digital cameras and flat-screen monitors. An endoscope is a pencil-thin rod that houses a light and lens on its tip, like the fiber-optic devices FBI agents place under a door to look around a room before a raid. With an endoscope, a surgeon can work through tiny holes in the skull, or even through the nose, to perform delicate operations that reduce our surgical footprint.

A MOST FORBIDDING TUMOR

THE CASE OF
MRS. X

Mrs. X had worked assiduously over the course of her career, rising to become one of the top designers in the world. By her early fifties, she was almost a household name and frequently appeared on TV. Accordingly, her image was critical to her marketing. But something unseemly was happening. Her weight had ballooned at an alarming rate despite valiant attempts to control it. She was also waking up in the middle of the night to go to the bathroom and becoming increasingly irritable and moody with her colleagues and family. She attributed this to her sleep deprivation and her frustration at losing the battle with her scale.

But it wasn't until Mrs. X began noticing that her vision was starting to blur, making it harder for her to do her design work, that she finally sought medical care. She booked an appointment with an ophthalmologist. At their initial visit, the doctor was concerned enough to order an MRI, which revealed a brain tumor growing in the middle of Mrs. X's third ventricle. The tumor was pushing on her optic nerves as well as her hypothalamus, the part of the brain that regulates how much food we eat before we are satisfied. So that explained her symptoms. But what to do about it?

When the MRI report came back, the diagnosis at the top of the list was one the doctor had encountered only once or twice before in her career: a craniopharyngioma.

Mrs. X had both the wealth and connections to consult with a few top neurosurgeons not just in New York City but around the country. The first one told her that she needed a craniotomy, which would have involved making a long incision behind her hairline, then completely dismantling the bone of the forehead and the side of her face, and finally dissecting around her brain to reach the tumor. He told her that he might be able to get it all, but he wasn't sure; if any were left behind, she would need radiation to prevent regrowth. The reconstruction of her skull would make the surgery hardly noticeable once everything healed, but it was possible that her forehead might look a bit asymmetrical.

The second surgeon told her that there was no way this tumor could be completely removed safely because of the large cysts that were also stuck to her hypothalamus. Removing them, he said, would cause irreversible brain damage. This surgeon recommended a stereotactic biopsy—basically, a computer-guided procedure—followed by injection of a radioactive liquid into the center of the cyst to control its growth. If this failed, she could try stereotactic radiosurgery, or focused radiation, which was also somewhat effective at stopping a tumor from growing. Cosmetically, she would have no noticeable scar, but the radiation could possibly damage the adjacent brain, causing further weight gain and possibly long-term memory loss.

Reeling from this second opinion, Mrs. X showed up in my office. She'd heard that I'd developed a new, minimally invasive technique, using endoscopes, that offered some promise for removing this type of tumor. At the time, I was two decades younger than the other surgeons she'd visited. They were both the chairs of their respective departments. I was still an assistant professor, just five years from finishing my fellowship. However, I had one advantage: my youth and open-mindedness had pushed me to become an early adopter of a new paradigm for performing minimally invasive skull base surgery.

And did I mention that craniopharyngiomas of the third ventricle were the ideal candidate for this new technique?

———

When I began practicing at Cornell, I was tasked with building a brain tumor program in arguably the most competitive medical environment on earth. In fact, Manhattan has the highest density of hospitals per square mile of any major city. Though we are approximately one-thirtieth the size of London, we have only half as many hospitals. And each major hospital has one or more well-respected neurosurgeons treating brain tumors, many of whom had been in practice for decades.

In other words, the ease with which patients in New York can obtain second and third opinions made my ability to thrive as a young surgeon quite difficult. Why choose me when you could choose any one of several other neurosurgeons who were not only older and more experienced but also very good at their jobs? In the face of such fierce competition, I felt like an unknown pony at a racetrack, going up against Secretariat, Seabiscuit, and War Admiral. It was proving more difficult than I'd imagined convincing new patients, facing life-and-death decisions, to bet their futures on my as-yet-nonexistent track record. But necessity, as they say, is the mother of invention. If I wanted to build my reputation, I needed to offer a unique service, something that could differentiate me from the other excellent surgeons in New York.

Then I read an article by a neurosurgeon in Naples who had teamed up with an ear, nose, and throat specialist (better known as an ENT) at his hospital to adapt and repurpose the endoscopes, formerly used to treat nasal sinusitis, for the removal of pituitary tumors—benign tumors that sit at the base of the skull, which also happen to be at the back of the nasal cavity. I had originally been trained to do this type of surgery—called transsphenoidal surgery—using an older method, which involved making an incision under the upper lip and peeling the gums away from the teeth to create a cavity big enough to insert a large retractor like a speculum. Since this type of surgery was performed with a microscope, if you wanted to see anything, you had to crank open the speculum wide enough to let the light in, which would invariably fracture the nasal septum. It was an inelegant way to operate, and it was also easy to get lost, so we used X-rays to help us find our way, which, in turn, necessitated wearing lead vests and skirts throughout the procedure, making the whole endeavor both hot and uncomfortable.

Transsphenoidal surgery was developed by an Austrian surgeon named Hermann Schloffer. Slicing the face vertically just off midline, from brow to upper lip, Schloffer flapped the nose over like a page of a book and created a corridor into the nasal sinuses through which he could expose the tumor. First successfully employed in 1907, this disfiguring surgery was performed in three stages, each done—wait for it—*under local anesthesia!* Schloffer appropriated this idea of traversing the nose and the nasal sinuses to reach the pituitary gland from the Egyptians, who used long, hook-like instruments inserted into the nose to soften and remove the brain during the mummification process. The Egyptians deemed the brain unnecessary in the afterlife, believing that the seat of the soul was in the heart. The brain, they thought, was only the source of nasal secretions. (I guess spending an eternity in the afterlife without a runny nose seemed like a good idea to them!)

The endoscope changed the whole landscape. Transsphenoidal surgery could now be done through the patients' nostrils—no incisions, no fracturing of the septum, no getting lost. All this to say that, twenty years ago, few neurosurgeons were using endoscopes to remove pituitary tumors, let alone complex craniopharyngiomas, and the concept of minimally invasive neurosurgery was very new and not yet widely accepted. Essentially, all surgeons felt they were performing minimally invasive surgery because, in their minds, the holes they drilled into the skull were already as small as they could possibly be to get the job done.

Endoscopes back then were generally relegated to simpler surgeries on the knee, gallbladder, and prostate; they had never really found their way into neurosurgery, since our procedures were felt to be too technically challenging to perform through small holes without the binocular vision provided by a microscope.

Endoscopes project their images onto a two-dimensional monitor, like a TV screen. By contrast, the human eye and surgical microscope see the world in three dimensions, which provides a sense of depth considered critical for avoiding injury when dissecting around small blood vessels and nerves. Just two decades ago, it seemed impossible to imagine such fine and delicate work being done without binocular 3D vision. Moreover, the ENTs, who were already using endoscopes to treat sinus disease through the nose, were forced to operate with one hand, since they needed to use the other hand to hold the endoscope. But a neurosurgeon operating with one hand? No way. Impossible.

I dredged up all the articles I could find on surgical endoscopy, trying to find out more. I soon discovered that a few brave neurosurgeons had published a handful of cases in which they worked *alongside* an ENT to remove a pituitary tumor by threading an endoscope through the nostrils to reach the bottom of the patient's brain. The ENT would not only open the passageway to get the neurosurgeon to the pituitary gland but, once there, would hold the endoscope in place so the neurosurgeon could operate with both hands. Seeing what I thought was the future of pituitary and skull base surgery—and my opportunity to get there before most of my colleagues—I decided to become an early adopter of the endoscope in my practice. The pioneers of this type of surgery were in Italy, so in 2003, I flew to Bologna to learn the technique. The rebirth of endoscopy for operating on the skull base, like the Renaissance, took root in Italy, which proved yet again to be a fertile ground for creative thought.

The course took place in a small hospital called Bellaria. The schedule was typically Italian and, for this non-smoker, quite comical: a few lectures in the morning were followed by an espresso and a cigarette, then a few more lectures, with another break for lunch, then more espresso and more cigarettes, and then—finally—we headed into the operating room to watch the first surgery. Once completed—surprise, surprise—it was time for yet another espresso and a cigarette, then back to watch a second surgery, more espresso and cigarettes, and then back to the hotel to shower off, followed by an elegant dinner, and one last espresso and a cigarette. Despite an overdose of secondhand smoke and caffeine—or perhaps because of the latter—I learned quite a lot on that trip.

Back at Weill Cornell, I found a like-minded and talented ENT named Vijay Anand. Together we started a new program in endoscopic pituitary and skull base tumor surgery that quickly took off. As we started to get more comfortable operating together, like a Rodgers and Hammerstein song (but somewhat less catchy), the sum was greater than the parts. Soon after the start of our collaboration, we realized that by using the natural openings of the nostrils and the nasal sinuses as corridors, we could reach a variety of different locations at the base of the brain. And just like that, the stars aligned, and I found myself at the right place at the right time with the ideal partner at the launch a new neurosurgical subspecialty.

When Mrs. X walked into my office, I took note not only of her elegant dress and well-coiffed appearance but also—after inspecting her MRI scan—of the enormous tumor ensconced in the center of her brain. I had no doubt that this was a craniopharyngioma, a benign tumor consisting of cysts and calcified nodules with a tendency to stick to everything around it.

The term "craniopharyngioma" was first coined by neurosurgeon Charles Harrison Frazier, a contemporary of Harvey Cushing. Frazier had also spent time studying in Europe and honed his skills on the battlefield during World War I. He then rose to become the premier neurosurgeon at the University of Pennsylvania.

It was Cushing, however, who popularized the name and summarized his feelings on the challenge these tumors pose. To quote him: "These cases offer the most baffling problem which confronts the neurosurgeon; and the fact that the mortality which accompanies radical attempts to

JOURNEY TO THE CENTER OF THE BRAIN

extirpate a large-solidified tumor must approximate 100% probably accounts for the few reports of these lesions other than by pathologists." Elsewhere he described them simply as "the most forbidding of the intracranial tumors." Frazier came to a similar conclusion and recommended treating craniopharyngiomas with just a biopsy followed by radiation. In fact, it's highly likely that the little Italian boy whose surgery was deemed too risky by Penfield and Tilney harbored a craniopharyngioma in the center of his brain.

In Mrs. X's case, the at-risk structures surrounding her tumor included the nerves for vision, the pituitary gland, her hypothalamus, critical components of the circuitry that forms new memories, and, finally, several hair-thin arteries that shuttle blood to the parts of the brain that moved her arms and legs. Basically, just about everything that makes Mrs. X Mrs. X.

Instead of suggesting the craniotomy offered by the first doctor or the stereotactic instillation of radioactive liquid advised by the second, I told Mrs. X that I thought I could remove her tumor through her nostrils without making any incisions whatsoever. My hope was to eradicate the tumor entirely and cure her of it once and for all: no additional radiation would be necessary. Although I had performed this surgery a few times before, with excellent results, in Mrs. X's case I would be tackling by far the largest tumor to date.

Very few people in the world were doing this type of surgery at the time, and if anything went wrong, my choice of surgical approach would be harshly criticized by the more senior neurosurgeons in my department. My reputation and my confidence were at stake, not to mention my patient's life and her career.

A few days later I got a call from Mrs. X. She'd gone back to see one of the other neurosurgeons, just for a reality check. She was curious about why no one else had offered her the minimally invasive transnasal approach that I was offering. I still remember what he told her, word for word: "Whatever you do, do *not* let Dr. Schwartz take that tumor out through your nose." (Welcome to New York neurosurgery!)

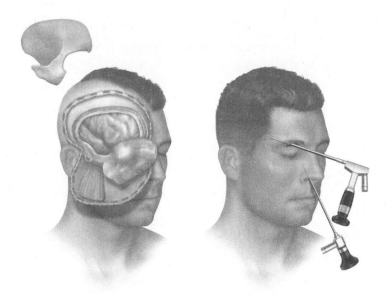

The more traditional method for exposing the anterior and middle skull base is through an approach called an orbitozygomatic craniotomy (left). Compare this with the less invasive endoscopic approaches through the nose or the eyelid (right).

Though shocked by this other surgeon's forthrightness, I also understood where he was coming from. I probably would have said the same thing a few years earlier. But times were changing—fast—and I had a front-row seat to the future of our specialty. I explained to Mrs. X the basis for our differing opinions and alleviated her fears. Then I called up my ENT partner and we set a date. The next thing I knew, Mrs. X was on the OR schedule for the following week.

GETTING IN THE ZONE

While some aspects of neurosurgery resemble other disciplines, such as playing music, sculpting, or competing in a sport, in many respects some of our long, complex, and dangerous operations have no parallel. If you mess up a note in a sonata or miss an extra point, no one dies. Not so for neurosurgery, a life-and-death technical exercise in which the surgeon must exert his or her will on the external world, working at the bottom of a deep, narrow corridor with a margin of error measured in millimeters.

Think of it this way: most of the ships in a bottle you see in souvenir shops are built first, before inserting them into the bottle. Imagine having to assemble the ship, piece by piece, by working through the neck of the bottle with the bottle intact.

The key to success relies not just upon a detailed understanding of the brain's anatomy but also on careful preparation, including the mental rehearsal of every step. The analogy to a mountaineer is apt. The equipment is laid out in advance. Every piece of gear is examined for weakness, and each step is rehearsed again and again until it becomes rote. The night before a complex operation, like Alex Honnold preparing to free solo El Capitan, I will often review a few textbook chapters, then revisit the anatomy to make sure I have a perfect mental vision of the upcoming assault on whatever summit I will be tackling the following day.

After a few hours of sleep, I often find myself staring up at the ceiling at 4:00 a.m. My internal alarm is unrelenting, telling my body to begin preparing for the day ahead. At this early hour I am usually not thinking so much about the *who* of the operation. I focus more on the *what* and the *how*. While it may sound callous, I don't want to be distracted by any emotional attachment that might cloud my judgment. I knew one neurosurgeon, in fact, who refused to even look at his patients in the twenty-four hours leading up to their operations. At the end of the day, while the doctor in me requires deep wells of empathy and heart, the surgeon in me must be able to turn *off* the heart and focus solely on one thing: flawless execution.

Operating deep in the brain, whether through a microscope or an endoscope, requires intense, sustained focus in which the eyes and hands must work together seamlessly. No matter how much preparation you've done, until you are there, seeing the relationship between the tumor and the distorted anatomy, all bets are off. For this reason, the first move is always just to look around. You try to compare what you *thought* you were going to see with what you *are* seeing. Then you come up with a game plan—a blueprint for altering the anatomy to accomplish your goal. Even at this early stage, what you imagined you would do and what you now realize you need to do might be completely different.

You begin by making a series of minute finger movements to manipulate long, thin instruments whose sharp tips gently begin to dislodge the spaghetti-like nerves and hair-thin arteries from the tumor's surface. Some of these blood vessels are so threadlike, it would seem the red cells must pass through single file. As the tips of your instruments first brush up against the capsule of the mass, you give the beast its first poke and watch it rise from its slumber. Its bloodshot eyes slowly open as it prepares for the battle ahead. You pause for a moment to see how it will react. Sometimes it starts as a slow ooze; sometimes it's an eruption, as if you've angered the gods with your hubris. *Just what do you think you are doing?* Either way, your focus shifts to controlling the bleeding, which you do by rolling your thumb over the teardrop-shaped opening in the suction to increase the aspiration. Too much force and those angel hair strands carrying the fuel of life will be damaged. Too little and the rising crimson tide will become overwhelming.

At this stage in my career, I've seen pretty much everything—and multiple times at that—but experience has taught me never to become complacent. Each case is different. Not only is the normal anatomy of every human variable and unique, but every tumor has its own configuration that distorts the terrain into which it has dug itself in a slightly different way. Inevitably, the reality we encounter differs from our expectations of what we thought we would find. So the game plan subtly shifts, requiring a new set of movements, a reappraisal of the anatomy, and ultimately the formulation of a new plan of attack. All with the clock ticking.

Anatomy textbooks depict an idealized version of reality, like the map that appears on your navigation screen before you leave the driveway. Neurosurgical operations are more like driving with the Waze app. You might set out thinking you are going to take the Bronx River Parkway, but if the traffic gets heavy—or, heaven forbid, there is an accident or a flood—you may need to take the next exit ramp and get on the Major Deegan. And, yes, accidents and floods happen in neurosurgery, too.

During critical movements, when the tips of the microscissors are cutting adhesions that attach small but crucial vessels to the walls of a tumor, I'll take in a deep breath and hold it until the maneuver is accomplished. This control of my breathing allows me to minimize any tremor in my hands, as does bracing my wrists or my pinky or some part of the instrument I'm holding against a rigid structure, like the edge of the skull.

Operations unfold like a three-act play or a performance. The opening of the skull and the approach to the tumor are the setup. The exposure of the pathology raises the stakes as the tension builds. Inevitably the complexity of the situation increases. It seems that the villain is gaining the upper hand. The tumor may be firmer than anticipated, the anatomy more complex, the normal structures just too stuck to allow safe removal. You may start to wonder whether the surgery is even feasible. Self-doubt may set in: Wait, maybe I chose the wrong approach?

Over time, an obstacle that appeared insurmountable is overcome, a corner is turned, and we reach the climax of the operation. As the stakes finally abate, it's time to exhale. The last move is to cauterize any small capillaries that may still be oozing and evacuate any blood that may have pooled in secluded locations. At this point it's time to close everything up and exit stage left. Sometimes I even take a bow.

A few of the most terrifying moments in brain surgery occur when we need to remove the bone overlying certain critical structures such as the carotid artery, which carries most of the blood supply to the brain, or the optic nerves, which transmit visual information from the eyes to the visual cortex. Each of these structures passes through a small canal encased in bone, which must be shaved away to expose the relevant anatomy. The best way to remove this bone is with a power drill. Shaving the eggshell-thick encasing away from a gossamer nerve or tenuous blood vessel with a 2-millimeter ball-shaped diamond drill bit, rotating at 10,000 rpm, requires a combination of practiced skill, confidence, and delicacy—not to mention constant irrigation with cold saline to minimize the heat created by the friction, which would otherwise cause thermal damage, even if the task were performed flawlessly.

Ideally, we execute every move as we visualized it earlier. But what about when you're working down a deep, narrow hole and you can see only partially that last tiny bit of tumor because it's obscured by a small piece of bone, or by an unexpected artery that was too small to have been visible on the MRI? Is it worth the risk to pull that last bit out blindly, or do you leave it behind, knowing that it will only grow back and require yet another risky surgery in the future? What if that last bit of tumor is stuck to another artery or a hidden nerve? Is it worth the risk of damaging those structures to get that last remaining piece? How much manipulation can the nerve tolerate before it loses its ability to transmit information? Decision after decision after decision, with so much on the line . . .

We try to make each determination objectively, but should these choices be the surgeon's sole responsibility? Well, yes and no. No, because it's not my body, and if I make an error, I don't suffer the consequences. In some sense, I have no right to make these kinds of decisions for someone else. And yet who else can or will? Ultimately, it comes down not to a simple yes or a no but to the plain fact that the decision is going to be made either by the tumor or by me. So better it be me.

In these moments, the fact is that no one in that operating room, aside from me, can make those decisions at that very moment about that particular artery, adhesion, or tumor fragment. Moreover, the patient has temporarily relinquished their rights over their body for the duration of the procedure. And since I've done this surgery thousands of times before and seen the ramifications of each choice I've previously made, I am, at that moment, by default, the most qualified person in the room to make those decisions. This aspect of neurosurgery, at first the most intimidating, quickly becomes, admittedly, the most intoxicating.

Most patients, I've learned, will never acquire enough information or experience to make a truly informed judgment when faced with a complex neurosurgical predicament like a brain tumor. Although we try our best to educate and obtain informed consent, studies have shown that patients retain no more than *one-fifth* of the information presented in a doctor's office. Sometimes, frankly, their choices are almost nonsensical, as in "I don't care if that little tumor is not causing my problems; I just want it out of my head," or "I know I need surgery, but unless you can guarantee me that there are no risks, I'm not interested," or even "I don't care if I end up paralyzed: just take it all out." Although we serve our patients, we also need to be able to make some executive decisions based on our experience, training, and perspective.

We generally decide together that if I think I can get it all out, and I judge that the risk is not too great, I should go for it. If I think the risk of collateral damage is high, however, it's usually better to be conservative. As much as this *sounds* like I am empowering the patient to get involved in the decision-making, in the end it leaves me right back where I started. Ultimately, I must weigh the potential risks and benefits of each move and make the decision I would want made for myself if I were lying on that table.

M rs. X's surgery went flawlessly. Now, twenty years later, she remains cured. She has since sold her business and retired to Florida. Meanwhile, I've done thousands of similar operations, sometimes tackling tumors even larger and more complex.

Once I realized that some skull base tumors could be removed through such small openings, I began looking for new ways to access other difficult-to-reach places. I now use small incisions in the eyebrow and even the eyelid, as I described in the opening pages of this book. The removal of skull base tumors through the nose, eyebrow, or eyelid is no longer considered reckless but rather routine. The endoscope has become an essential piece of neurosurgical equipment, both as critical and as unremarkable as a spelunker's headlight, illuminating our perilous expeditions into the dark, inner chambers of the brain.

Yet, I also must say, with appreciation for Mrs. X's bravery and the trust she gave me, that her surgery was a pivotal moment in my career, a moment

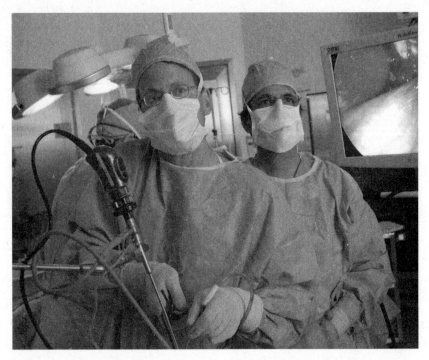

That's me, on the left, performing an endoscopic skull base operation. The endoscope can be seen in the foreground, held by a metal bar. Dr. Vijay Anand, the ENT with whom I work, is on the right.

when I decided to push forward and risk confronting a difficult tumor with a new approach, hoping that my instincts would prove correct. If the surgery had gone poorly, well, such a failure so early in my career would most likely have delayed or even prevented me from adopting the minimally invasive endoscopic brain tumor surgeries that now make up a substantial part of my practice.

CUSHING'S GLAND

The area of neurosurgery where the endoscope has had the biggest impact is unquestionably in the removal of tumors of the pituitary gland. The pituitary hangs down from the brain into the back of the nasal sinuses. If you were to lift the brain out of the skull and gaze up at it from below, the gland would look something like a tiny punching bag the size of a pea, hanging by a thin pedicle, called the stalk, through which it communicates with the brain. Weighing in at just 0.5 grams—the weight of a raisin or a paper clip—this gland secretes *ten different hormones*, making it, pound for pound, arguably the most powerful organ in the body.

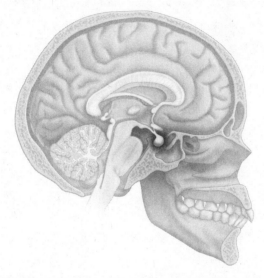

The little pituitary gland, highlighted in black, sits underneath the brain at the back of the nasal sinuses.

The so-called master gland of the endocrine system, the pituitary not only orchestrates human growth, development, and reproduction, but also regulates body temperature, maintains blood pressure, coordinates the immune system, equalizes fluid balance, governs hunger, regulates stress, and influences our moods.

The brain controls the body on a millisecond-by-millisecond timescale through the firing of neurons. If you want to get up and take a walk, you're quickly on your way. If you want to pour yourself a cup of coffee, you make it happen. However, when the brain needs to exert its influence more gradually, over hours, days or weeks, it resorts to hormones.

Hormones are chemicals released into the bloodstream like slow-release capsules. The pituitary gland can thus be seen as our body's internal apothecary. But while the pituitary gland is your friendly corner pharmacist, carefully doling out the medicines you need to get better or stay well, a pituitary tumor is the drugstore cowboy, pointing a gun at the pharmacist's head and demanding they give you, an innocent bystander, massive doses of the wrong medications.

Tumors arising from the pituitary gland are remarkably common. Some studies have estimated that as many as 10 percent of the population will develop a pituitary tumor at some point in their lives, although only a small number of those will ever need treatment.

Two types of tumors affect the pituitary gland: those that make hormones and those that don't. The so-called non-hormone-producing ones can grow quite large and, as they expand, they push on the optic nerves, causing a slow loss of peripheral vision called tunnel vision. Visual decline can be so gradual, in fact, that most patients barely notice. By the time they arrive in my office, many have already been in a few car accidents, undergone unnecessary cataract surgery, and purchased at least three progressively larger TV sets before an astute ophthalmologist picks up the problem and orders an MRI scan.

The other half of patients with pituitary tumors—those with tumors that *do* produce hormones—have profound problems with their endocrine systems. Their tumors pump out massive amounts of hormones, which throws the body's physiology out of whack. Of the ten hormones secreted by the pituitary gland, only four are made in excess by certain pituitary tumors. One of these tumors, which overproduces thyroid-stimulating hormone, is extremely rare. The other three types, which secrete either cortisol, growth hormone, or prolactin, are more common.

Tumors that make prolactin are often treated with medications, not surgery. Therefore, I will set those aside and focus on the tumors that need surgery: namely, those that make cortisol, which causes Cushing's disease (since it was discovered by Harvey Cushing), and those that make growth hormone, which causes a disease called acromegaly.

Let's begin with Cushing's disease.

In the history of world, only a handful of people have gained notoriety merely for being ill. Despite their untimely deaths, they live on both in medical textbooks and in our collective psyche. Take Typhoid Mary, whose given name was Mary Mallon. An immigrant from Ireland, Mary served as a cook in the homes of several wealthy families, where she infected not only her employers but also their families with typhoid fever. Moving from house to house, staying one step ahead of the health authorities, Mary was responsible for infecting no fewer than fifty people. When she was finally caught by medical detective George Soper, Mary was forced into quarantine for the last half of her life, where she remained isolated from friends, family, and any future victims.

Gaëtan Dugas gained notoriety as the alleged patient zero of the AIDS epidemic. Dugas, a Canadian flight attendant, was suspected of having acquired the HIV virus in Africa, then spreading it to several of the earliest victims in North America. He was consequently vilified by Randy Shilts in his book *And the Band Played On: Politics, People, and the AIDS Epidemic*.

Despite their demonization in the press, Mary Mallon's and Gaëtan Dugas's stories contain more nuance than is widely known. Dugas, for starters, was recently absolved of his inaccurate moniker after retroactive genetic analyses of blood samples showed that he was much closer to patient several thousand than to patient zero. And Typhoid Mary was not actually the most egregious spreader of typhoid. That distinction goes to Tony Labella, who infected over twice as many people. Yet Mary was sentenced to spend her life in isolation, while Labella and other carriers roamed free.

Like Mary and Gaëtan before her, Minnie G has been enshrined in the annals of neurosurgery with a similarly canonized but oversimplified story. In 1910, Harvey Cushing described a twenty-three-year-old patient whom he called Minnie G but whose real name was Maita. A dressmaker from Brooklyn, of Russian Jewish descent, Maita was referred to Cushing for severe headaches and an ill-defined glandular problem. Standing only four feet nine inches, she weighed 140 pounds and her round face was covered in stubbly hair. She'd also stopped having periods in her late teens. According to the Johns Hopkins medical records, her body was deformed by two large mounds of fat growing above her clavicles, and her abdomen was crisscrossed with thick purple stretch marks. She complained of excessive fatigue and swollen ankles. She was admitted by Cushing to the hospital, where she stayed for thirty-three days, until she was finally discharged, receiving neither diagnosis nor treatment.

Upon leaving the hospital, Maita continued to write letters to Cushing describing her situation: persistent weight gain, worsening headaches, and constant exhaustion. Cushing saw her again two years later and admitted her for surgery to the Peter Bent Brigham Hospital, where he was now the chief of neurosurgery. In the operating room, he performed a surgical decompression by removing part of Maita's skull, believing that her symptoms were due to increased intracranial pressure. During the surgery, suspicious that the origin of her problems might lie in the pea-sized but potent pituitary gland, he attempted to expose it, to no avail. He just couldn't create enough room to shine light down into the undersurface of her brain to get a good glimpse.

Nevertheless, Cushing hypothesized that Minnie G had a problem with her pituitary gland, and he included her case, along with a few others, in a treatise on a new syndrome he believed he had discovered, one caused by an elevated level of cortisol in the blood. Cushing hypothesized that the source of the hypercortisolemia was the pituitary gland, and Minnie G was his exemplar. When his theory was eventually proven correct, the disease was anointed with his name, even though he was never able to uncover any definitive proof that Minnie G in fact harbored a pituitary tumor. Even more curious, Cushing later mentioned that Minnie G's symptoms mostly resolved on their own, which would be highly unusual if Minnie G truly had a pituitary tumor. Ironically, it's unlikely that Minnie G—whose case formed the basis for Cushing's greatest discovery and arguably his defining achievement—ever truly had the disease she has come to epitomize.

Modern medicine has proven Cushing correct with regard to the primary cause of hypercortisolemia, the medical term for increased blood levels of cortisol. Some 80 percent of such cases are caused by a tumor in the pituitary gland that secretes abnormally high levels of adrenocortico-tropic hormone, or ACTH. This ACTH is then absorbed by the adrenal glands, triggering them to pump out large quantities of the stress hormone cortisol.

Imagine having a ten-year anxiety attack but not being able to get up off your couch to do anything about it. The disease also transforms the body, leading to increased fat deposition, muscle atrophy, and stretch marks. The skin becomes paper-thin and fragile. Infections are common. In women, hair grows thick and covers large areas of their body. Men become impotent. Additional symptoms include fatigue, depression, anxiety, and irritability, not to mention high blood pressure and diabetes.

Another famous patient with Cushing's disease may have been King Henry VIII. The British historian Robert Hutchinson has proposed that undiagnosed Cushing's disease might explain Henry's massive weight gain later in life. Henry also displayed other symptoms of the disease, such as the so-called moon face and buffalo hump caused by inconveniently located fat deposits. He also had several jousting wounds that failed to heal, and his body was eventually covered in boils and pustules. He became impotent and increasingly irritable, bordering on paranoid and psychotic. Henry grew so massive that he required mechanical devices to help him get around. Still, there's no definitive proof that Henry VIII had a pituitary tumor, and it's unlikely his body will ever be exhumed from St. George's chapel in Windsor to ascertain the truth. Despite Henry's possible diagnosis, we cannot blame his predilection for wives and beheadings on a presumed pituitary tumor.

Another remarkable fact about Cushing's disease is that these insidious and devastating symptoms arise from a tumor so tiny that it's often invisible on an MRI scan. In fact, the biggest challenge when operating on a patient with Cushing's disease is simply finding the darned thing. We make the diagnosis from blood and saliva tests, since almost a third of the tumors are so small, it's impossible to see them. Those of us who operate on such tumors are faced with the daunting prospect of trying to locate something the size of a pinhead inside an organ the size of a raisin.

Nevertheless, we pituitary surgeons have developed a systematic method for exploring the gland. We make fine cuts in specific locations, at certain angles, that will hopefully not damage the gland's function but will expose the tiny culprit. It's kind of like a game of Battleship: we guess and explore until we get a hit. And, yes, as far as modern medicine has developed, we still have no better way to locate these needle-sized tumors hidden in the pituitary haystack.

The good news is that surgery for Cushing's disease is usually successful, and the life-transforming result is nothing less than miraculous. In the first few days after surgery, we check the patient's cortisol levels every six hours. I usually get updates on my phone, sent by the residents, as the cortisol levels start their dramatic downward trend.

Unless the number gets below 2, the patient is probably not cured, and the risk of recurrence is high. The first measurement is usually still elevated since the half-life of cortisol is several hours. The night after surgery, for example, if I get the first value, and it's 54, I am not concerned. The next morning I'll wake up and it'll be down to 21. Later that day it might be 14, then 6, then 4, then 4 again. This is when I start to question myself. Did I leave a little behind? Should I have removed that area off to the side that looked suspicious? Why wasn't I more aggressive?

I visit with the patients daily, sharing the lab values with them, sweating out the numbers like a stock trader who has just bet his client's life savings shorting the price of orange futures. The next morning, if the text from the resident tells me it's 1.9, I breathe a sigh of relief. At this point we must begin replacing the patient's cortisol, since they're no longer able to make the hormone on their own. Without adequate levels of cortisol, the body's vital functions will collapse.

A year later, when they return to my office, these patients are barely recognizable. Thin, happy, energetic, they've morphed into completely different, rejuvenated human beings. When I see this, I always marvel at how *who* we are and how we behave—the very nature of our selves—is not as immutable as we think, but rather the product of the chemicals coursing through our bodies at any given moment.

SHREK'S SYNDROME

Perhaps the most beloved character in the wildly popular movie *The Princess Bride* was Fezzik the Giant. Though he is known as a fearsome colossus, Fezzik is kind and fair. He prefers entertaining people with his rhymes rather than hurting them. (*Anybody want a peanut?*) He wants to be liked, not feared. Fezzik is reminiscent of another famous giant, the ogre Shrek, whose massive size and grotesque appearance engender fear in the pitchfork-carrying townsfolk, who don't know him like we do: as the irreverent, sarcastic, fun-loving dude who'd rather be hanging out with his buddies, eating waffles, than devouring innocent children and using their bones for toothpicks.

What few people know is that Fezzik and Shrek have much more in common than just being misunderstood, massive man-children.

THE CASE OF
ANDRÉ THE GIANT

André René Roussimoff, aka André the Giant, was a professional wrestler and actor of Bulgarian ancestry who was born in France in 1946. Labeled the "eighth wonder of the world," André started off enormous and then grew even more so. He weighed 13 pounds at birth. By age twelve, he was already six feet three inches. At his peak, he grew to seven feet four inches, weighed 520 pounds, and wore a size 22 shoe. His battles with Hulk Hogan in WrestleMania were legendary. In 1988 he won the World Wrestling Federation World Heavyweight Championship.

André's other claim to fame was playing Fezzik in *The Princess Bride*. His massive frame, like the character he portrayed, contained an inner tender core. Alas, André was not as indestructible as he appeared on-screen.

He was eventually forced to retire due to declining health. Plagued with arthritis and cardiovascular issues, he self-medicated to alleviate his pains by consuming legendary quantities of alcohol. In 1993, at the age of forty-six, he died in his sleep of congestive heart failure.

André had a tumor in his pituitary gland. He knew about his diagnosis. He knew that his life expectancy would be greatly reduced if his tumor, which produced an overabundance of growth hormone, was not treated. But his size was critical to his identity, income, and success, so he refused therapy.

Acromegaly, as André's disease is known, takes two different forms: it strikes either before or after puberty, which creates a critical distinction between its victims. If the growth hormone excess begins before puberty, the disease is called gigantism, since patients grow unnaturally tall. Excess growth hormone also impacts many of the other organ systems of the body and can wreak havoc on a patient's physical health, causing an enlarged heart, diabetes, colon cancer, carpal tunnel, sleep apnea, and problems with sexual function. Most people with untreated gigantism rarely see their thirties.

If it hits after puberty, the patient's growth plates in their bones are closed, so they can't grow any taller. However, the parts of the body that *can* still grow, like the brow, nose, chin, tongue, hands, and feet, continue to enlarge, giving them a distinct appearance. The alteration in facial features is so characteristic that an experienced neurosurgeon can often make the diagnosis the second a patient walks into the office just by looking at their face.

Occasionally I'll see the same distinct set of features while gazing upon the countenance of a stranger sitting across from me on the train or in a restaurant. It takes all my inner restraint, and sometimes a few stringent warnings from my family, to prevent me from catapulting myself into the seat next to them, Sherlock Holmes–style, to alert them of their yet-to-be-diagnosed predicament.

Besides André, several other well-known professional wrestlers and actors have also leveraged their disease into a career. The acromegalic face is perhaps most widely recognized in the Disney character Shrek, whose facial features were modeled after those of the French wrestler Maurice Tillet, another acromegalic. Richard Kiel, the actor who played Jaws in the James Bond movies; Ted Cassidy, the actor who played Lurch in the TV series *The Addams Family*; and Dalip Singh, the Indian professional wrestler known as the Great Khali, also suffered from acromegaly.

———

Charles Byrne, another victim of pre-pubertal gigantism, was better known by his stage name, the Irish Giant. Born in Northern Ireland in 1761, Byrne stood over eight feet tall, which made him one of the tallest men in the world. Like André, Byrne self-medicated with alcohol and died young, at age twenty-two. His skeleton was purchased, against his wishes, by John Hunter, a famous British surgeon, who apparently bribed the undertaker, after getting him drunk, for control of Byrne's body. The skeleton became the centerpiece of Hunter's anatomy museum, which was then donated to the Royal College of Surgeons, where it remained on display for over a hundred years until Harvey Cushing stumbled upon it.

In 1909, when Cushing was first developing his theories on pituitary tumors, he befriended the curator of the museum and obtained permission to open Byrne's skull. He wanted to examine the bony cavity containing the pituitary gland, which is housed in an area near the base of the skull called the sella turcica, named for its resemblance to a Turkish saddle. Sure enough, Cushing found that Byrne's sella turcica, or sella for short, was enlarged and misshapen, presumably from the presence of an enlarged pituitary tumor, another piece of evidence in support of his theory.

But just because Byrne had a large sella didn't necessarily mean that it harbored a tumor. Without an MRI, Cushing had only two ways of confirming his clinical suspicion. Either he could find another acromegalic patient, convince them that their unnatural size was caused by a pituitary tumor, and then persuade them to have surgery, or he could wait until they died and perform an autopsy. Given that the link between acromegaly and pituitary tumors wasn't yet fully established, combined with the high risks of brain surgery back then, he took the latter course.

Cushing's opportunity arose while he was still at Johns Hopkins, around the same time as his encounter with the Irish Giant. John Turner, another 275-pound titan of a man with obvious acromegalic features, was admitted to the hospital, quite ill with the various maladies associated with his condition. Cushing was called in to see him. Turner's condition was so advanced that Cushing didn't think surgery would be of any benefit. Expecting that Turner might not have long to live, Cushing tried to force him to remain in the hospital until his death so he could procure his precious autopsy. After the nurses complained, Cushing was obliged to let the poor man return to his home in Washington, DC, to live out his final days.

Cushing kept a vulture eye on Turner, and his patience was rewarded six months later. As soon as the funeral was announced in the local newspapers, Cushing called the undertaker and offered him $50 to allow him to perform an autopsy, only to learn that the family had already forbidden it. Undaunted, Cushing sent two of his students down to crack open Turner's skull and retrieve its osseous underside, including the sella and its contents, which they did just before the funeral began. Cushing's minions craftily lifted Turner's brain from his skull and then brought it back for their master to examine in his lab. Sure enough, housed inside the enlarged sella, Cushing found a pituitary tumor, the source of Turner's deadly disease. Here was indisputable proof. In retrospect, it's hard not to deem Cushing insensitive, but his tenacity must also be admired.

In his book *David and Goliath: Underdogs, Misfits, and the Art of Battling Giants,* Malcom Gladwell explains how acromegaly might have been the reason that Goliath, the colossal giant and warrior from the Bible, suffered an unexpected defeat at the hands of the smaller, slingshot-shooting David. The idea was first proposed by David and Pauline Rabin, physicians at

Vanderbilt University Hospital. By their account, published in *The New England Journal of Medicine*, Goliath's gigantism was caused by a large growth hormone–secreting pituitary tumor that, in addition to producing his massive size, must have also been distorting his vision by pushing on the nerves that transmit visual information from the eyes to the brain, as these tumors are known to do. Had Goliath seen the rock coming, he would have ducked. Moreover, Goliath's inability to fend off David's unexpected attack might have been due to clumsiness, since acromegaly also makes its victims slow and uncoordinated.

This clumsiness can also explain why more acromegalics don't find their way into the NBA. While those with gigantism might have the soaring height so prized by coaches, teams, and owners alike, they simply don't have the speed and skill to compete. Take Sun Mingming, who had the height but not the moves. At seven-nine and 370 pounds, the Chinese basketball player and acromegalic was one of the tallest men to ever play the sport. After achieving some success in a few low-tier U.S. basketball leagues, he was too slow to make it in the NBA. Moreover, Mingming was plagued with physical injuries: arthritis, stiff joints, mangled, misshapen toes—all unwanted gifts of his acromegaly. To put things in perspective, Kareem Abdul-Jabbar and Shaquille O'Neal, two of the most dominant big men in the game, were both under seven feet two inches. Their heads would have barely made it to Mingming's shoulders.

Given the slow timescale of hormonal changes in the body, Cushing's disease and acromegaly are not typically discovered until several years after the onset of symptoms. Unfortunately, most physicians lack familiarity with these afflictions, leading to delays in making the diagnoses. One promising new technology that might speed up our ability to identify these pituitary tumors is facial recognition software. Using 3D facial analysis, combined with artificial intelligence and machine learning, researchers can pick up the characteristic changes in a patient's appearance by comparing their facial features with a database of normal ones. The computer's memory contains an extensive record of the range of standard-sized chins, noses, eyes, and brows. Thousands of data points on any new face can be instantaneously juxtaposed against the averages to find statistical deviations.

Someday the same facial ID processes used to unlock your cell phone could also alert you to the possibility of an unrecognized brain tumor. It could, in theory, even make you an immediate appointment with the local endocrinologist for confirmatory blood tests. One morning you wake up, you look at your phone, and it tells you that it's your best friend's birthday or that a hurricane is brewing in the Gulf and that you have an appointment at 2:00 p.m. with Dr. So-and-So at Such-and-Such Hospital to discuss your newly diagnosed pituitary tumor. Sound like Big Brother invading your privacy? You bet, but it could also save your life.

TEN

A TIME BOMB IN THE BRAIN

very neurosurgery resident looks forward with both anticipation and dread to a unique rite of passage when they go from masquerading as a neurosurgeon to really *feeling* like one. That Rubicon moment—as completing hell week might be for a Navy SEAL—is the first time you clip an aneurysm.

An aneurysm is a ballooning of the wall of a blood vessel that can rupture at any given moment. When an aneurysm bursts, blood floods into the space around the brain, also called the subarachnoid space, causing a rapid rise in intracranial pressure. This four-alarm fire is a life-threatening emergency like few others in medicine. The risk of instant death is about 50 percent; 10 percent die instantly and another 40 percent will eventually die, even if rapidly and expertly treated.

Although genetics and other risk factors, such as smoking or high blood pressure, can predispose someone to develop an aneurysm, they also arise in healthy individuals for reasons we don't yet fully understand. What starts out as a small bubble—picture your tire after your car has hit the curb one too many times—gradually expands into a balloon, whose thinning walls can no longer handle the constant pounding from the blood pulsing through the brain's arteries. That's when, all at once, it gives out.

Whereas tying knots, drilling burr holes, opening the skull, and even removing small bits of a tumor are all tasks that any surgeon in any specialty could probably perform, the surgical treatment of aneurysms takes a level of skill, confidence, and levelheadedness that requires years of specialized training to master. In one sense, the surgery could not be more straightforward. The goal is to isolate the aneurysm from the bloodstream by placing a spring-loaded clip across its neck—the base of the aneurysm— so called because its rounded dome resembles a head perched atop a body. Aneurysms tend to arise at division points in the circulation, so the inflow and outflow segments appear like a torso with arms extended as if waiting for a hug. Or, more aptly, surrendering at gunpoint.

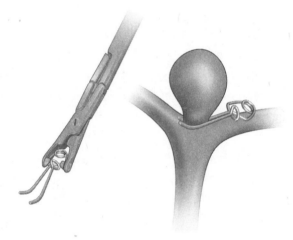

Aneurysm clips (left) come in different shapes and sizes and have a special clip applier. The goal is to place the clip along the neck of the aneurysm (right) to isolate the aneurysm from the circulatory system but keep the vessel open so blood can flow to the brain.

The opportunity to clip an aneurysm generally doesn't present itself to the neurosurgery resident until late in their training, around the sixth or seventh year. And the anticipation feels a bit like the night before a final exam, when fears of coming up short fill fitful sleep with dreams of failure.

That said, clipping an aneurysm as a trainee is not a free-solo endeavor.

The life-and-death stakes are too high. It's more like a driver's test, since there is always a more senior neurosurgeon standing by, taking them through the entire procedure, ready to intervene at a moment's notice. However, only one physician at a time can sit in the operating chair and gaze through the microscope, their elbows resting on the cushioned armrests to reduce tremor. There is only enough room for one physician to advance the clip toward the aneurysm neck, snuggle it down in just the right location, ensure that the nearby small blood vessels—called perforators—are not crimped, and then, ever so gently, release the clip into its final position.

Few neurosurgical procedures provide this kind of instant cure to an immediate problem. In fact, when a neurosurgeon releases an aneurysm clip into its final position, the relief in the OR is palpable, felt deep in the gut, as when the hero in an action film defuses a bomb and the audience finally exhales.

The trick is to place the clip just right so that neither the artery from which the aneurysm arises nor the dozens of small blood vessels—the perforators—that course around it become occluded. These tiny vessels can sometimes become quite stuck, not only to the neck of the aneurysm but also to the dome—the bulbous part on top—which often happens to be the precise region where a rupture is most likely to occur. If one of these minuscule vessels is accidently injured or caught in the jaws of the clip, this will deprive the brain region of the oxygen supplied by that vessel, causing it to die or leading to a stroke, which can, in turn, cause paralysis, loss of language, and/or blindness.

With enough grit, training, and practice, most neurosurgeons will attain a basic level of proficiency in aneurysm surgery. Mastery is another matter and requires an ability to both embrace risk and remain undaunted by the inevitable failures. And by "failures" I obviously mean deaths. Lots of them.

For early neurosurgeons like Horsley and Cushing, the only available treatment for aneurysms was to tie off the carotid artery, the primary conduit of blood and oxygen to the brain. While this strategy decreased blood flow into the aneurysm, it often led to a stroke. Without enough oxygen, the brain's neurons can't survive. Clearly a better solution was needed.

Aneurysms most commonly arise from a ring of blood vessels at the base of the brain called the circle of Willis, named after the British anatomist Thomas Willis, who described it in 1664. The circle of Willis creates a redundancy of flow: if one artery becomes occluded, the ring provides a backup source of oxygen. Nature, in its infinite wisdom, created a series of superfluous connections between several of the major blood vessels feeding the brain. Picture a traffic roundabout that moves cars through the heart of a city, only this roundabout shunts blood to where it's needed in order to prevent a catastrophic stroke.

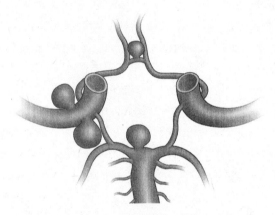

The circle of Willis provides redundant blood flow to the brain but also enables aneurysms (four of them shown here) to be perfused from several different sources.

Unfortunately, the same backup system that preserves flow to the brain also continues to shuttle blood into the aneurysm, even after the carotid artery is occluded. This is another reason why tying it off proved ineffective. Cushing alternatively tried to wrap aneurysms in muscle to fortify them against rupture, like stacking sandbags around a barricade, which also proved futile, as 50 percent of his patients still died. He did, however, develop the first clip made of silver that could be used to occlude the feeding artery, but he never had the opportunity to deploy it. That honor went to Cushing's acolyte and nemesis Walter Dandy. In fact, the clip used by Dandy was the very same clip designed by Cushing.

I am not currently a vascular neurosurgeon—the name given to aneurysm specialists—but I did train at Columbia-Presbyterian's Neurological Institute of New York, under the leadership of three renowned vascular neurosurgeons: Bennett M. Stein, Donald O. Quest, and Robert A. Solomon. We clipped roughly 150 aneurysms every year, and as chief resident, I made sure to scrub in to as many of those cases as possible.

By the time I started my first job at the University of Medicine and Dentistry of New Jersey, I had already decided to focus my career on brain tumors and epilepsy; however, like any young attending, I rotated through the on-call schedule. Gunshot wounds, subdural hematomas, and spinal cord injuries made up the bulk of our emergency surgeries, but every week or so, another ruptured aneurysm would roll into the emergency room, requiring treatment.

Studies show that 5 percent of the population harbors an undiagnosed brain aneurysm. That is a terrifyingly large number. Luckily, most of these aneurysms are quite small, with little risk of rupturing, at least not imminently. But even the thought of all those undiscovered aneurysms should give us pause. *Life is fragile!* aneurysms shout. More fragile than most of us are willing to admit.

Aneurysms are discovered in one of three ways. Sometimes they are picked up on a brain scan performed for an unrelated symptom, like dizziness or blurry vision. If these incidentally discovered aneurysms are large, they require treatment; if they are small, we just monitor them. What constitutes large and small in these cases is a matter of debate, but 4 millimeters is a reasonable cutoff above which rupture is more likely and thus treatment is recommended.

The second way an aneurysm is found is after a patient comes to us complaining of a thunderclap headache—often the worst of their lives. When we hear this, we always check for an aneurysm, because aneurysms occasionally will release a small quantity of blood into the brain without fully rupturing, hence the headache.

In the same way every first-year intern is taught to assume a heart attack whenever a patient says they feel like an elephant is sitting on their chest, first-year neurosurgery residents are told that if the patient describes the sudden onset of the worst headache of their lives, it's an aneurysm on the verge of rupture until proven otherwise. While most headaches are benign, if you are experiencing the worst headache you've ever felt and it came on all at once, get yourself to the nearest emergency room, pronto.

This event, the small leakage of blood from an aneurysm, is also called a sentinel bleed. It's akin to Paul Revere riding through the town square, shouting, "The hemorrhage is coming! The hemorrhage is coming!" When the aneurysm fully ruptures, which is the third way aneurysms declare themselves, the symptoms hit hard and all at once: the proverbial anvil dropped from on high. Intracranial pressure rapidly increases due to the torrent of blood escaping through the gaping hole in the aneurysm. This blood then envelops the brain like a fresh coat of paint applied with a power sprayer.

Clipping an aneurysm requires careful, meticulous dissection under a microscope. Aneurysms are buried deep in the brain, surrounded by other blood vessels that reside at the base of a narrow cleft nestled between the frontal and temporal lobes. This cleft is called the Sylvian fissure, named by a Dutch anatomist Franciscus Sylvius. Surgical exposure of most aneurysms can take twenty to thirty minutes of careful microdissection that requires prying apart the frontal and temporal lobes, a maneuver called splitting the fissure. This skill is one of the basic microsurgical moves learned during residency, part of the technical vocabulary of the discipline, like a double axel or a lutz might be to figure skating. By the time the aneurysm is encountered, the surgeon must manipulate their instruments at the bottom of a long, narrow corridor, visible only via a microscope—instruments, that is, that are six inches long and have tips the size of insect legs.

What makes aneurysm surgery so challenging is the sword of Damocles—rupture—that hangs in the air and provides an endless source of stress. The wall of an aneurysm at its weakest point is measured in microns, which is a unit three factors of ten smaller than a millimeter. One false move releases a fierce, continuous torrent of arterial blood that jets out under shockingly high pressure.

When an aneurysm ruptures, controlling the gush of blood is both crucial and seemingly impossible. In a normally functioning body, 20 percent of the heart's pumping force is dedicated to perfusing the brain. This prodigious force is now redirected along the path of least resistance: through the open wall of the aneurysm and directly into the surgeon's field of view, which is immediately obscured by a surging ruby wave that obliterates the anatomy you just spent the last half hour carefully exposing. The following three steps, done in rapid succession, are the only way to begin to deal with this situation with any hope of success:

1. Ask the scrub tech for the largest suction available and get it in there immediately to evacuate the blood so you can see what's going on.

2. Alert the anesthesiologist that a rupture has occurred so that the patient's blood pressure can be lowered quickly to slow down the bleeding.

3. Ensure that all intravenous lines are promptly opened to transfuse saline, blood, or any immediately available fluids to prevent imminent cardiovascular collapse from rapid blood loss.

If these three maneuvers are not successful, the situation becomes dire and the salvage strategies proportionately more extreme. Some surgeons will paint the patient's neck with Betadine and slice through it to get a clamp across the carotid artery. Another option is to administer a drug called adenosine, which will stop the heart for a few moments—just long enough to clear out the blood so the surgeon can see what's going on.

If any of these tricks work, the surgeon now has two options. The first is to place a clip across the neck of the aneurysm to stop the bleeding. However, the lack of visibility from the constant influx of fresh blood makes this nearly impossible, particularly if the surgeon has not yet adequately exposed the aneurysm, including its neck and all the small perforating vessels. The second option is to place a series of clips across all the arteries feeding the aneurysm. This latter procedure, called trapping, isolates the aneurysm from the rest of the circulatory system and prevents it from bleeding. Trapping, if done successfully, also allows the surgeon to clear the blood from the operative field so they can continue with the operation. This is usually the preferred tactic.

What does such an emergency feel like as it's happening? Imagine a bottomless pitcher of grape juice being poured continuously into a shot glass. At the bottom of the glass sits a BB held in place by a thread. With tweezers in one hand and a suction in the other, you must suck out the grape juice while simultaneously grabbing the BB. But wait! Your heart rate has also just shot up to 150 beats per minute, and your hands have begun to shake, because you are also acutely aware that if you can't tweeze that BB—which you can barely see—your patient will die.

If the surgeon is successful at trapping the aneurysm—by placing a series of lower-strength temporary clips on all the feeding vessels—then the bleeding will slow to a trickle. While this does provide a few stolen moments to gather your wits, the temporary clips shut off the blood supply not just to the aneurysm but also to the brain, and the brain can survive only a few minutes without oxygen. So once the bleeding is controlled, the surgeon's momentary relief is immediately replaced by the stress of having to clear out all the blood, expose the aneurysm neck, gently nudge aside all the surrounding critical tiny arteries that might inadvertently get pinched, place a perfectly oriented and well-secured clip on the neck, and then remove all of the temporary clips from the carotid to prevent a stroke—*all within minutes*. Tick, tick, tick, tick . . .

YOU'RE ON YOUR OWN!

About two months into my first job and about a year after the birth of our first child, I was sitting down for dinner alone with my wife—a rare

Saturday-night date night. Just as the appetizers appeared, my beeper went off. I rang the resident who was waiting for my call in the ER and listened to her bullet list description of the new case that just rolled in. *Fifty-two-year-old man. History of hypertension. Collapsed at home. Brought in by EMS. GCS 5T. Hunt-Hess 4. Fisher grade 3. CTA showed a 6-millimeter PCOM aneurysm.* This was neurosurgical jargon for a ruptured aneurysm with a description of the patient's neurological examination, the thickness of the subarachnoid blood, and the location and size of the aneurysm. Basically, this guy was in big trouble and had about a 50 percent chance of dying in the next twenty-four hours if not managed properly. This moment would be a test for me, as it would be the first aneurysm I had to face on my own.

If the aneurysm ruptured again, his chances of survival were almost zero. A few decades ago, neurosurgeons would wheel patients like this one into the operating room as soon as possible to clip the aneurysm as quickly as possible to prevent it from rupturing again. Since aneurysms don't always bleed during normal business hours, aneurysm surgeries were often performed in the middle of the night. In time, however, we learned that this was not the best approach. Using late-night operating room staff and relying on surgeons and anesthesiologists who'd been awakened from the depths of stage 4 sleep didn't always lead to the best outcomes. More critically, the risk of a re-bleed in the first few days turned out to be relatively low. These days, most aneurysm surgeries are performed the following day, and, as a result, the surgical outcomes are better.

At the hospital where I was working at the time, one of my partners, a more senior surgeon, had amassed decades of experience treating aneurysms. Out of respect for his expertise and in a gesture of collegiality, I gave him a call and told him I was taking this case to the OR the next day. Could I run it by him to get his advice? Or, if he was available to help, I would really appreciate it. Neurosurgeons tend to be territorial. As much as we have a reputation for self-confidence, this bravado masks a deep-seated fear of failure. Add to that the constant competitive pressure from our peers. Not to mention that every year, residency training programs churn out a stream of young, bright, talented new surgeons, one of whom might take our place. Or just take our patients.

No matter how skilled and successful the neurosurgeon, we sometimes face challenges that are so complex that failure, however infrequent, is inevitable. And failure breeds self-doubt. Could someone else have done a better job? We neurosurgeons measure our self-worth in several different ways. One is by the number of cases we've performed in the previous year; another is by our perceived expertise at doing certain cases better than the other neurosurgeons practicing in our zip code. So, when I heard my senior partner's response—"If you do this case, you are on your own," followed by the sound of a click and a dial tone—I was not that surprised.

Undaunted, I proceeded the next day. Luckily, the surgery went well— another small brick in the citadel of confidence I was slowly erecting.

The next five aneurysms I clipped flying solo went smoothly. The patients recovered and left the hospital quickly. I was feeling like Achilles before his little heel episode. My sixth aneurysm, however, ruptured during surgery, although calling it a rupture would be like calling Old Faithful a water fountain. It didn't simply rupture; the blood vessel from which the aneurysm arose seemed to disintegrate before my eyes just as I was trying to visualize the source of the bleeding and apply the clip. I was able to isolate the tear by placing temporary clips on either side, but I could neither safely secure the aneurysm nor reconstitute the fragile vessel. Although I had successfully stopped the bleeding, I had also permanently interrupted all the blood perfusing the poor patient's left hemisphere.

We managed to move her out of the operating room alive, but she died a few days later, as the damaged half of her brain swelled to unmanageable proportions. I was devastated and am still haunted by the memory. At the same time, a neurosurgeon on call does not have the luxury of grief. I was back in the operating room the next day, operating on another patient, who required all of my attention and focus. Naturally, I felt horrible for her and her family. Sadly, I had barely met her husband before I was forced to rush her into the operating room. I hadn't had the opportunity to speak with her at all when she came in, since she was unconscious at the time.

Emergency surgeries are very different from elective ones. In elective surgeries, the patient chooses you specifically to do their operation, and you develop a trusting relationship beforehand. For this woman's surgery, I was simply the surgeon on call the night she came in. It was my duty to take care of her and to let her family know the gravity of her situation. I told the husband that his wife would certainly die without surgery and that this operation, while extremely risky, was her only hope of survival. Afterward, when I told him what had transpired in the OR, he simply appreciated the fact that I had tried to save her life.

Neurosurgeons compartmentalize. We have to. It's a coping mechanism we develop that allows us to move from one tragic situation to the next without breaking down. But despite our heroic, steely faced efforts at repression, our complications continue to jolt us awake in the middle of the night with pangs of regret, no matter how many times we return to the scrub sink—with Lady Macbeth intensity—in a futile attempt to cleanse our hands of our, thankfully, uncommon errors in judgment. I know I did my best for her at the time. It's just that my best wasn't good enough. Could another, more experienced surgeon have done a better job? Possibly. But I was on call that night, and I was the doctor she got. Did she pick the short straw in the neurosurgeon's lottery? Although I was fresh out of training at the time, I was also better trained than most neurosurgeons, so maybe she picked the medium-sized straw? In any event, the urgency of the situation dictated my involvement.

This poor outcome, early in my career, was not the first nor the last time my fortress of confidence would be shaken. Sometimes brain surgery can seem like a Sisyphean game of Brick Breaker. Each time you fail, your only recourse is to go back a few levels and start all over again.

From that day on, I decided to leave the aneurysm clipping to the vascular neurosurgeons and focus all my energy instead on treating patients with brain tumors and epilepsy. While I might be able to get through an aneurysm surgery at this point in my career, a patient with an aneurysm would be better off in the hands of someone who has devoted their entire career to treating this one specific disease. Every aneurysm that is referred to me now gets promptly handed over to one of my vascular partners, and they, in turn, refer all their tumors to me. Unfortunately, it's impossible to be great at everything, and anything less than great, in my opinion, is just unacceptable when a patient's life is on the line.

THE ONE-EYED NEUROSURGEON

THE CASE OF
JOE BIDEN

In 1972, when he was only twenty-nine, President Joe Biden was elected the Democratic senator from the state of Delaware. That same year he suffered the unimaginable: he lost his wife, Neilia, and their one-year-old daughter, Naomi, in a tragic car accident, leaving him the sole guardian of his two sons, Hunter and Beau.

Sixteen years later, in February of 1988, Biden passed out in his hotel room. "Lightning flashing inside my head," he later wrote of this event, "a powerful electrical surge—and then a rip of pain like I'd never felt before." He flew back to Delaware and went straight to the hospital, where a lumbar puncture—also known as a spinal tap—revealed the presence of blood in his cerebrospinal fluid.

In this procedure, the physician advances a small needle into the lower back to access the fluid surrounding the spinal nerves. Because the CSF in the spine communicates with the CSF around the brain, you can sample the brain's CSF through the spine. The presence of blood in Biden's spinal tap indicated a temporary leak from a vessel, likely coming from his brain. The source of that leak became readily apparent after an angiogram showed that he had two separate brain aneurysms, one of which was large, irregularly shaped, and likely the cause of the hemorrhage.

As if one aneurysm were not bad enough, multiple aneurysms are quite common, found in almost 20 percent of all cases. The combination of elevated blood pressure and genetic factors that trigger the formation of one aneurysm also increases the risk that a second or third aneurysm will arise elsewhere.

Biden was rushed into surgery at Walter Reed Medical Center, where the first aneurysm was clipped by opening his skull via a craniotomy. "Doc, what are my chances?" Biden asked his neurosurgeon while he was being wheeled down the hallway to surgery, to which the doctor flatly replied, "Senator, for morbidity or mortality?"

Biden, none too pleased with that answer, thought about it and came back with "Let me put it this way. What are my chances of getting off this table and being completely normal?"

"Well," said his neurosurgeon, "your chances of surviving are much better."

So much for bedside manner.

Biden's operation was performed by Drs. Eugene George and Neal Kassell. Kassell was interviewed after the operation and explained that the aneurysm had ruptured during the surgery but that he and his partner were able to control the bleeding and successfully place the clip.

A few months later, Biden underwent a second surgery to secure the other aneurysm and prevent it from bursting. Prior to the operation, Biden looked up at Kassell and made a prescient joke: "Doc, do a good job, because someday I'm going to be president."

When asked what saving Biden's life meant to him, Kassell supposedly replied with a line from the Talmud: "Save one life, you save the world."

Much ado has been made about the possibility that Biden's cognitive abilities may be slipping, either from his age or his aneurysm surgeries thirty years ago. I have no opinion about the impact of age on Biden's ability to lead, other than to state—and broadly at that—that decision-making skills decline after a certain age in everyone, but the rate of decline is variable and unique to each individual, some becoming cognitively impaired earlier than others. Age alone cannot and should not be used as a metric of anyone's cognitive capacity. We also know that Biden has battled a stutter for most of his life and sometimes needs to talk around words that he has trouble pronouncing, which may give the illusion of impairment.

With respect to Biden's aneurysm, two potential aspects of this event might have affected his brain function. The first was the subarachnoid hemorrhage itself and the potentially harmful effects that such bleeding may cause. The second was the surgery to clip the aneurysm, along with the manipulation of the brain that inevitably occurs during such a procedure.

While a subarachnoid hemorrhage has the *potential* to inflict long-term difficulties with attention, memory, and decision-making, this is *not* a given. And even if the event causes some sort of decrease in mental abilities at the time of the rupture, dramatic improvements can occur over time.

The important but still unanswered question is whether any of Biden's abilities were permanently lost, but this is almost impossible to know. To answer with any degree of certainty, Biden would have had to undergo a detailed cognitive test *before* the hemorrhage as a baseline, and then he would have needed to be retested a few years later. Unfortunately, an aneurysm rupture is an emergency, so there's no time to obtain baseline testing before the event. All we can say is that Biden was probably not himself for the first few months after his subarachnoid hemorrhage, and that he was likely still improving for about a year. But again, these generalizations are made by averaging data from large groups and cannot be applied with any certainty to one individual.

We also know that brain surgery, in and of itself, when performed without complications, does not alter long-term cognitive abilities. And while the adage "You ain't never the same when the air hits your brain"—*When the Air Hits Your Brain* is also the title of an excellent book about neurosurgery by Pittsburgh-based neurosurgeon Frank Vertosick Jr.—has some truth to it, post-craniotomy personality changes have more to do with why the patient had the surgery in the first place—namely, the underlying disease itself. In other words, there is no evidence that routine, uncomplicated neurosurgery causes significant long-term changes in a patient's mental faculties.

In fact, if you take two groups of patients with ruptured aneurysms and treat half by opening their heads—that is, performing a craniotomy—and the other half by using a minimally invasive catheter-based technique in which the brain is not exposed to the air, the patient's long-term cognitive outcomes are roughly the same. If a craniotomy in and of itself caused harm, studies such as this would show it. Bottom line: while Biden's mental capacity might have been impacted by his aneurysm rupture and its treatment, it's also possible that these events had no long-term consequences. We just don't know.

Dr. Neal Kassell, Biden's neurosurgeon, has his own remarkable life story. He was born into limited means with a disability called microphthalmia in his left eye, a condition that left him with limited vision on one side. Because he grew up with only one working eye, his brain had plenty of time to adjust. He found other ways to create depth perception, so he never felt visually impaired. In fact, he told me that he plays squash and tennis, drives, and even skis without any problems.

Kassell also confirmed something that I found hard to believe until I heard it directly from him: he never graduated from college. So how is it possible that one of the nation's top aneurysm surgeons flunked out of college?

This is what he told me: For as long as he could remember, Kassell had always wanted to become a neurosurgeon. After he failed high school calculus, his parents decided that their boy needed some direction. They made a connection, through a family friend, with Dr. Thomas W. Langfitt, who would later go on to become the chair of neurosurgery at the University of Pennsylvania. Kassell began working in Langfitt's lab and would often assist him in the operating room. This was back when there were few neurosurgery residents training at Penn, so many of the operations had no assistant.

Kassell managed to right his ship and get accepted to the University of

Pennsylvania as an undergraduate, but he spent so much time working for Langfitt that he never fulfilled his graduation requirements. (He also failed a few classes along the way.) Nevertheless, he made such an impression at the hospital that he was basically guaranteed a training position. All he had to do was graduate from medical school. Having already secured a spot in the residency, and with more publications on his CV than most attendings, he was backdoored into Penn's medical school. Kassell went on to train with the great Canadian neurosurgeon Dr. Charles George Drake, one of the most renowned aneurysm surgeons of his era. Kassell then settled at the University of Virginia, where he had an illustrious career of his own. This highly unlikely path explains how a one-eyed neurosurgeon without a college diploma ended up saving the life of the future president of the United States.

Let's step back for a moment. How is it possible to operate with only one eye and see as well as someone who uses two? The brain relies on both eyes to perceive depth in the outside world. This is also called stereoscopic vision. With only one eye, depth perception is compromised, such as when we watch the 3D version of *Avatar* compared with the 2D version playing in the theater down the street. Endoscopes—the thin telescopes we use to operate through the nose or the eyelid—provide only a 2D representation of an operation, since they have only one lens, and then that image is projected onto a 2D monitor.

I can personally attest to the fact that operating this way, in only two dimensions, provides more-than-adequate information to perform delicate microsurgery deep in the brain despite the lack of stereoscopic vision. So Kassell's technical abilities are not that surprising. The brain uses other cues to create depth of field, such as the relative size of objects that lie closer to or farther from the eye, as well as the size of the tips of the instruments as they move in and out of the surgeon's field of view. Given the choice, most surgeons would rather operate in 3D than in 2D, but ultimately the most important factors are the combination of magnification, resolution, and illumination that allow surgeons to see what they're doing.

This conversation about seeing brings us to one of the greatest of all the twentieth-century revolutions in neurosurgery. As you may recall, Cushing operated in a room with large open windows that bathed the surgical field in natural light so he could see, back before operating rooms were fitted with ceiling-mounted lights. Walter Dandy, a few years later, devised a speculum with a light on its tip to see deep into the brain's ventricles. (This was before endoscopes were invented.) As the 1950s rolled around, another revolution was imminent. As with other, similar leaps forward, the technology for this one already existed. What was required was someone with the vision to see the future before anyone else could and to champion the cause with energy and aptitude. This someone, the neurosurgeon who introduced the microscope into neurosurgery, was credited with establishing the brave new world of microneurosurgery, which probably had as profound an impact on brain surgery as did Cushing himself.

SEEING IS BELIEVING

"When you change the way you look at things, the things you look at change," said Max Planck, the Nobel Prize–winning physicist who was the originator of quantum theory. Perception, in other words, results from an interaction between the information arriving through our senses and the brain's expectations about what it's going to see.

During my residency, one of my neurosurgery professors constantly reminded me, "You see what you look for, and you look for what you know." He was trying to help me see the anatomy and pathology as *he* saw it, so I could interact with the patient's problem in a more informed way. But before I could see what he was seeing, I first had to know what I was looking for. There is a chicken-and-egg situation when it comes to perception, where seeing and knowing are two sides of the same coin, with one constantly informing the other. But before you can see anything, let alone have a clue to what you're looking for, you need access to proper illumination and magnification. The tool that provides these critical abilities to the neurosurgeon is the surgical microscope.

Head-mounted lights and loupes, or magnifying lenses attached to glasses, were the first step forward, but such magnification was limited because even minimal head movements can cause rapid changes in the field of view, an effect that is extremely disorienting when the lenses become too strong. The obvious solution was to use a microscope, but no one thought to bring one into the operating room until well into the 1950s, and these early prototypes were relegated to surgery on the ears and eyes. Neurosurgery wasn't even a consideration.

Even after other specialties began using operating microscopes, neurosurgeons, accustomed to seeing the operative field with their bare eyes or with low-level magnifying lenses built into their glasses, had a difficult time making the transition. The early pioneers merely dabbled.

Then, in 1957, after practicing in a laboratory for an entire year, a USC neurosurgeon named Theodore Kurze became the first to use a microscope during a neurosurgical operation. One of Kurze's junior partners, Michael L. J. Apuzzo, told me that the credit really should have gone to Howard P. House, the famed otolaryngologist, who pushed Kurze to try the microscope.

The first brain surgeon to have the audacity to clip an aneurysm using a microscope was J. Lawrence Pool, the chief of neurosurgery at the Neurological Institute of New York. Pool, as you may recall, was one of the neurosurgeons consulted on RFK's case after his assassination. He was also a legendary Renaissance man in the tradition of Cushing—two-time U.S amateur squash champion, author of thirteen books on a variety of historical subjects, talented artist, and avid fly fisherman—who also, in his spare time, piloted his sailboat across the Atlantic.

But Pool's and Kurze's early test runs with microscopes were not enough to convince their colleagues that the instrument improved surgical outcomes. Microscopes back then were not really designed to be used in operating rooms. They were cumbersome and unwieldy. These were not the microscopes you remember from your high school biology class. Operating microscopes weighed over 500 pounds, sat on the floor on a five-foot-wide base, and required a complex system of counterbalances to suspend the eyepieces over the patient like a construction crane.

Kurze struggled with how to keep such a massive device sterile—a problem he attempted to solve by using plastic turkey bags and rubber bands, a less-than-ideal solution that nearly set his operating room on fire on more than one occasion when the hot lights melted the plastic.

As with the endoscope, the mere *idea* of the microscope was met with resistance among the older generation of neurosurgeons, who were conservative thinkers set in their ways. One neurosurgeon with whom I spoke remarked that he had heard his mentor make the myopic claim "Any vessel that you can't see with the naked eye is irrelevant." Back then, microscopes would be brought into the field and used for a short while, but when things got challenging and visualization became difficult, they were quickly abandoned so the surgeon could "see better."

For at least two decades, neurosurgeons resisted. Why? Partly because the microscopes of that age were poorly designed and partly because the instruments required for microsurgery had not yet been invented. But these were technical issues that would soon be solved. The real issue for neurosurgeons of that era was a basic lack of insight into a future they could not yet imagine. Unable to envision what they couldn't foresee, they didn't look for it.

Out of this miasma emerged a visionary who was not only able to make the necessary cognitive leap but also happened to possess remarkable operative skill. This neurosurgeon—who was credited with developing modern microneurosurgery and who was also named *the neurosurgeon of the century* by his colleagues—was named Mahmut Gazi Yaşargil.

Yaşargil was born in Turkey in 1925 but spent most of his career in Zurich, Switzerland. At the age of forty, after thirteen years in practice—during which he was relegated primarily to performing angiograms for his boss, the father of Swiss neurosurgery, Hugo Krayenbühl—he was sent to visit the only training center in the world dedicated to microsurgery, in bustling Burlington, Vermont. Established in 1958 by neurosurgeon Raymond Madiford Peardon Donaghy—or Pete, as he was better known—the world's first microsurgery research facility was dedicated to training aspiring surgeons in how to perform one basic skill: creating vascular anastomoses, which is the reattachment of small blood vessels using fine, threadlike sutures.

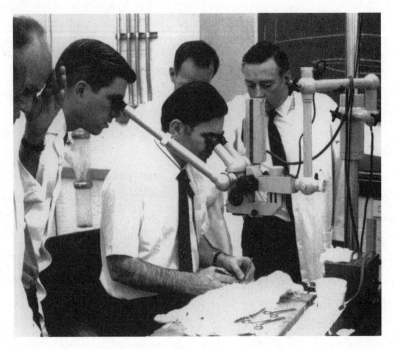

M. Gazi Yaşargil teaching microdissection at the first microneurosurgical course in Zurich, October 1968.

Photograph courtesy of Dianne Yaşargil

Yaşargil recalled that back then even *he* couldn't imagine using the microscope to remove a tumor or clip an aneurysm. Should a rupture occur, he thought the small field of view would be far too limiting.

Yaşargil spent only fourteen months with Donaghy, but in that time he was able to develop the fundamental principles of microneurosurgery that are still in use today. His work led to the publication, in 1969, of his groundbreaking book on the topic, *Microsurgery Applied to Neurosurgery*. According to one of Donaghy's lab assistants, who'd been put in charge of orienting Yaşargil when he first arrived at the training center, "I spent thirty-five minutes showing him how to operate the microscope, and he spent the next thirty-five years showing us what to do with it."

Yaşargil was able to use his newfound appreciation of anatomy—which he could now see in much greater detail—to discover previously undescribed natural planes of dissection. His contribution wasn't incremental; it was tectonic. He completely reconceived *how* neurosurgery should be performed. In the same way Max Planck saw the subatomic world for the first time, forever changing our understanding of atoms, Yaşargil saw the anatomy of the brain in an entirely new way, and he was able to use this fresh perspective to improve the surgical treatment of nearly every neurosurgical ailment. Yaşargil's impact on neurosurgery was an Oppenheimer-like explosion from which there was no turning back.

Yaşargil also designed new instruments to work in this neurosurgical version of the invisible subatomic realm. He then helped the various microscope companies redesign and repurpose their scopes to facilitate the surgeon's ability to manipulate the hefty contraption in a seamless, ergonomic fashion. He designed a mouthpiece that enabled him to bite down and control the location of the microscope, which was carefully counterbalanced with a series of judiciously designed weights. This allowed the microscope to float weightlessly above the patient and move in synchrony with Yaşargil's head.

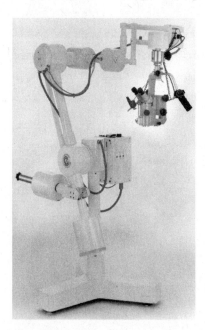

Yaşargil subsequently returned to Zurich, where he created a microneurosurgery mecca to which neurosurgeons from around the world made the pilgrimage to watch the master at work. At times, there were so many visitors in his operating room that he

The Contraves OPMI 6 surgical microscope from 1976.

Carl Zeiss Meditec AG, Germany

feared for the sterility of the environment and the safety of his patients. An authoritarian while operating, he liked to perform surgery in silence, which allowed him to focus his attention on the task before him with no distractions. Rumor has it he once criticized a nurse for breathing too loud.

He never relied on an assistant to retract the brain lest another set of hands introduce a variable he could not control. Rather, he designed a self-retaining retractor system—named the Leyla, after his daughter—that would prop the lobes of the brain aside so he could bloodlessly penetrate their secluded recesses, avoiding any superfluous movements that might detract from his graceful performances. Walter Dandy once said of his mentor Cushing, as a backhanded compliment, "Horsley made the first airplane flight and Cushing improved the plane and flew it better." One of Yaşargil's students added, "Yaşargil has taken us into the space age." Watching Yaşargil operate, this same student recounted, "was the human brain at its best operating on the human brain at its worst."

Yaşargil, like Cushing, was a workaholic. His devotion to both his career and his patients far exceeded his commitment as husband and father. He was not only figuratively married to his profession; he literally married his OR nurse after his first marriage collapsed. One Saturday morning, in the twilight of that first marriage, he sat down to breakfast with his children after spending a week in his apartment near the hospital.

"Did you miss me?" he asked.

To which they responded, "No, not particularly."

GAME OF COILS

Emilia Isobel Euphemia Rose Clarke is a British actress best known for playing Daenerys Targaryen in the HBO epic fantasy television series *Game of Thrones*. In 2011, just after finishing the first season, Clarke, then twenty-four, felt a severe pain in her head while she was working out in a gym near her home in North London. In an article published in *The New Yorker*, she described the sensation: it was, she said, "as though an elastic band were squeezing my brain . . . I made it to the locker room. I reached the toilet, sank to my knees, and proceeded to be violently, voluminously ill. Meanwhile, the pain—shooting, stabbing, constricting pain—was getting worse." She was rushed to the hospital and diagnosed with a subarachnoid hemorrhage, the result of a ruptured aneurysm.

As with Biden, Clarke had a second, smaller aneurysm discovered in a separate location in her brain. Clarke, however, didn't undergo a craniotomy and clipping but rather a minimally invasive alternative to craniotomy called endovascular coiling. During this procedure, a neurosurgeon—or an appropriately trained radiologist or neurologist—places a catheter into an artery in the groin or wrist and threads a wire through the catheter all the way up into the arteries of the brain. Working from within the vessel, using X-ray guidance and a radiopaque contrast material that is continually squirted into the artery for visualization, the surgeon coils the wire into the dome of the aneurysm and then releases it, which causes rapid clotting and obstruction of the aneurysm. Essentially, the wire curls up like a ball of yarn and fills the aneurysm with metal so no blood can enter it. Endovascular coiling provides long-term security against a future rupture, nearly identical in efficacy to that of the craniotomy and clipping but with slightly less risk, no shaved head, and no scars.

Although Clarke briefly had trouble speaking after the hemorrhage, these symptoms quickly resolved, and her coiling procedure was considered a success. After returning to work, however, she battled all the normal fatigue, headaches, and limited concentration so common after suffering from a ruptured aneurysm. Adding insult to aneurysm, she then needed to have the second aneurysm repaired after it was found on subsequent brain scans to be enlarging over time. Another endovascular coiling procedure was recommended; only this time it didn't work. The aneurysm started to bleed, and the procedure was aborted. She underwent an emergency craniotomy to clip the aneurysm and stop the bleeding. Clarke eventually

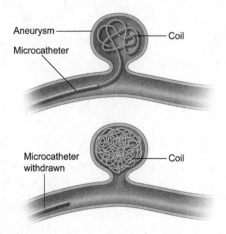

Endovascular coiling of an aneurysm involves threading a wire from a small incision made in the upper thigh or wrist and then passing the wire into the vessels of the brain. There it releases a ball of wire that coils up in the aneurysm and triggers a clot to form that blocks off the aneurysm.

made a full recovery. After going public about her experience, she founded SameYou, a charity that provides therapy and rehabilitation services for people recovering from brain injuries and stroke.

The endovascular treatment of aneurysms is yet another example of more modern, less invasive procedures that have slowly replaced older, more intrusive methods. The craniotomy approach, perfected by Yaşargil into a remarkably safe and elegant procedure, still requires a long, curved incision in the scalp, removal of a sizable piece of bone, and some displacement of the brain to expose and reach the aneurysm. Endovascular therapy, on the other hand, treats the problem from *within* the blood vessel, rather than from the outside; picture the difference between fixing a clogged pipe in your home by ripping open the walls and floors versus snaking a coil down the sink to achieve the same goal.

At first, coiling met with as much skepticism as the microscope had. But progress is inevitable. Only a legend like John Henry could beat the steam-powered drill, but that was a onetime deal. In the 1990s, coiling was reserved only for those aneurysms that were considered unclippable. To-day, the opposite holds true: nearly 80 percent of aneurysms are coiled, with clipping reserved for the small minority of cases where coils cannot reach.

The development of endovascular treatment for neurosurgical diseases was completely dependent on the use of a technology called an angiogram, which was invented in 1927 by Portuguese neurologist Egas Moniz. This was around the same time that Walter Dandy developed the ventriculo-gram, his method for visualizing the brain by injecting air into the ventri-cles and shooting an X-ray. Angiograms, like ventriculograms, rely on the fact that some substances absorb X-rays more readily than others and can therefore be seen more vividly on an X-ray. When you insert these sub-stances into different compartments in the brain, the outline of its struc-ture becomes visible. Whereas Dandy's ventriculogram depended on air injected into the ventricles to visualize their silhouettes, angiograms work through the injection of contrast dye into the patient's blood vessels to highlight the vessels' branching pattern as they course through the brain.

Moniz had originally developed the angiogram to locate brain tumors, a task for which it was not particularly well suited. As a result, the value of the angiogram was not fully appreciated until much later. (Moniz's first patient died soon after their angiogram was performed.) As a side note, Moniz—who suffered from severe gout that left his hands knotted and mis-shapen with arthritis—could not perform the angiograms himself but rather relied on the assistance of a neurosurgeon named Pedro Almeida Lima, whose name we will hear again shortly.

The first successful angiogram was performed on a patient with a large pituitary tumor, which Moniz was able to visualize by seeing how it dis-placed the blood vessels. Like deer tracks in the snow, the distorted vessels provided indirect evidence of the tumor's presence.

Moniz was nominated on three separate occasions for the Nobel Prize, but the first two attempts were rejected by the committee, who felt that the angiogram was not nearly as useful in finding tumors as Dandy's ven-triculogram. Although they may have been correct at the time, the Nobel committee lacked the foresight to appreciate how useful Moniz's invention would one day become. The angiogram remains to this day one of the most frequently performed imaging procedures, whereas the ventriculogram has long since been abandoned.

Ironically, in 1949, Moniz would win his Nobel Prize not for the angiogram but instead for one of the more destructive procedures in the history of neurosurgery: the prefrontal leukotomy, now better known as the frontal lobotomy, which he invented as a treatment for schizophrenia. It's a surgery now considered to be, at best, an unnecessarily aggressive treatment of mental illness and, at worst, a dangerous form of brain mutilation. (This topic, worthy of a deep dive but not relevant to the treatment of aneurysms, we will save for later.)

In 1999, when I finished my neurosurgical training, endovascular treatment for aneurysms was in its infancy. Few doctors already practicing knew how to perform them, and the young neurosurgeons interested in vascular neurosurgery were just beginning to learn the technique. Within a few years, however, endovascular training was incorporated into most neurosurgery residencies, and angiograms and endovascular procedures have now become some of the most common procedures performed by vascular neurosurgeons. We use them to treat not only aneurysms but also arteriovenous malformations and strokes, two other diseases that assault the brain's blood vessels. In fact, today, just a quarter century later, every neurosurgical department has at least two or three full-time staff devoted to endovascular therapy.

This radical shift in neurosurgical methodology has produced a new problem. Given the success of endovascular therapy, most neurosurgery departments end up clipping only a handful of aneurysms each year via craniotomy, and these tend to be the most difficult cases. Since a resident will not usually operate on aneurysms until their final year of training, they may witness and participate in just a few cases—hardly enough repetitions to master the microsurgical techniques required to tackle the more challenging ones.

The solution, of course, is to provide additional training. Today, several high-volume centers do offer post-residency fellowships for trainees who want to become competent at performing open craniotomy–based clipping procedures. In fact, most vascular neurosurgeons will tack on a few extra educational years of training to acquire the necessary skills to both clip and coil aneurysms, and neurosurgical fellowships are becoming increasingly common in not only vascular neurosurgery but also tumor surgery, pediatric neurosurgery, spine surgery, and functional neurosurgery, which involves the treatment of epilepsy and movement disorders such as Parkinson's disease.

How is this information relevant? If ever you find yourself in need of a neurosurgeon, you'd do well to determine if they went through fellowship training specific to whatever problem landed you in their office in the first place. While not always the case, fellowships generally indicate the neurosurgeon's commitment to increasing their expertise and may be a sign of additional experience when compared to non-fellowship-trained neurosurgeons.

CECI N'EST PAS UN ANEURYSM

A few years back, I got a call from the wife of a good friend. She was concerned about her husband. He'd been out for a run, and when he got home, he told her he wasn't feeling well. They had four children of similar ages to mine, and our lives increasingly overlapped, as so often occurs in suburban communities when your kids go to the same school, play on the same teams, and attend the same summer camps. Over the years we'd developed a close friendship, not only on the sidelines of games but also through our frequent dinners and occasional weekends spent together.

I asked her to tell me exactly what her husband had said and what she was currently observing. She told me that as soon he got home from his run, he'd slumped down on the couch and started complaining of a bad headache. Now he was just sitting there unable to—or at least uninterested in—getting up.

As you might imagine, given my profession, I get a lot of calls from friends and neighbors with a variety of general medical and neurological questions, the majority of which require an ice pack, rest, and a few Advil. Real neurosurgical emergencies are rare. Yet something about this story got my attention. This guy had rowed crew in college and was known to bike fifty miles on an average Saturday. He wasn't a complainer. I told her I was on my way over to lay eyes on him before making any decisions. If experience has taught me anything, it's this: there is no substitute for seeing a patient face-to-face.

When I walked into the kitchen, I saw him sitting at the breakfast table, his head slumped forward onto his crossed arms. I called out his name and he slowly looked up as if a more sudden movement might make things worse. "So, what's going on?" I asked.

He told me that he'd been out for a run when all at once he was hit with one of the worst headaches of his life. His eyes were glassy, and I could see that he was not only incredibly uncomfortable but having trouble focusing. My neurosurgical spidey sense immediately started tingling. Within seconds I had formulated my diagnosis: a ruptured aneurysm.

Over the years I've seen plenty of patients suffering from subarachnoid hemorrhages in the emergency room, and that look of helpless incapacitation as the brain is in the process of shutting down is unmistakable. Instantly, I knew exactly how his future was likely to play out: he had about a 50 percent chance of dying within the next twenty-four hours. Should he be lucky enough to survive, he would most likely emerge with some degree of permanent brain damage that would not only end his career but forever change his life and the lives of everyone in his family. I looked over at his wife. She was clearly concerned, but she had no idea of the severity of what I intuited was likely going on inside her husband's skull.

I didn't want to panic his wife, since I needed her to focus and act rationally in the next few minutes, and I also wasn't 100 percent sure of my hunch. Rather than blurt out that I thought he had a ruptured aneurysm or ask her to call an ambulance, which also would have taken too long to arrive, given the nature of his condition, I said that I thought it would be wise for her to put him in their car and take him to the nearest emergency room for a CAT scan. She wondered if he could drive himself, since her son needed to be picked up after hockey practice. Knowing what a bad idea that would be, I offered to pick the boy up myself and drive him home, since my own son was at the same practice. I let her know in no uncertain terms that she ought to take her husband to the ER immediately and then to have the doctor there contact me as soon as the scans were done.

I tried to give her the sense that I thought this might be something serious without letting her know exactly what I was thinking at that moment. Raising his blood pressure could be deadly and I could only imagine her trying to obey the speed limit, waiting at every stoplight, and trying to suppress her road rage, knowing that her husband was on the verge of suffering a fatal brain hemorrhage should his presumed aneurysm rupture again before it could be treated. I also knew we could rapidly transfer him to my hospital if need be. I would have taken him to the ER myself, but I thought it best that she be with him, at least until his scan was completed. Once in my car, I called ahead to the ER to let them know what was coming to make sure there were no delays.

Sure enough, within twenty-five minutes, the call came in: my friend's CAT scan showed a subarachnoid hemorrhage, presumably caused by a ruptured aneurysm. I immediately transferred him by ambulance to my hospital. He was already there, getting his angiogram, when I arrived. Since I'm not an aneurysm specialist, one of my partners was performing the study while I sat in the control room and waited for the images to appear on the monitor. While they were still setting up for the procedure, I began poring over my friend's CAT scans from the first hospital. I had seen this pattern of blood before, the way it was distributed in the subarachnoid space, and I now had a nagging suspicion that maybe something else was going on.

Experience in medicine is one of our most powerful diagnostic tools. Although we learn about the classic ways in which each disease might present itself—the most common symptoms, how the imaging studies look, the clinical course—each instance of a disease plays out differently in every person, unfolding along its own idiosyncratic path, depending on the patient's DNA, the severity of their illness, and their specific anatomy. But doctors form their strongest diagnostic impressions based on previous experience. The more variations of each disease we've seen, the more likely we are to make the correct diagnosis the next time we see it. These skills can't be learned in a book, nor can they be taught. When I saw the CAT scan from the first hospital, it triggered a memory from over a decade earlier, which raised the possibility of another diagnosis that mimicked an aneurysm but was much more benign.

During my residency, I wrote a paper on a condition called perimesencephalic subarachnoid hemorrhage, an uncommon type of subarachnoid hemorrhage caused by a tear in a small vein, not by an aneurysm. The blood from the tear doesn't damage the brain and there is almost no chance of rebleeding. Although the symptoms are identical and the CAT scan nearly indistinguishable from an aneurysmal bleed, it has a slightly different telltale configuration, hence the name "perimesencephalic," which refers to the pattern of blood distribution. An astute, experienced neuroradiologist or neurosurgeon might look at the CAT scan, and when everyone else in the room is thinking aneurysm, they confidently remark that there's nothing to worry about, since this is undoubtedly an example of a more benign condition.

"You think it's a perimesencephalic bleed?" I asked through the microphone wired into the procedure room.

"Yeah, probably," my partner responded. He was already a few steps ahead of me. He *was* the expert after all.

Once the angiogram was complete, it confirmed my hunch: no sign of an aneurysm, meaning the hemorrhage was almost certainly caused by a small tear in a vein. These small leaks generally repair themselves, so nothing needed to be done. I went out to the waiting room to speak with my friend's wife. She was a wreck, having been told by the doctor in the ER at the first hospital that her husband had a life-threatening brain aneurysm and needed emergency surgery. I was able to calm her down and let her know that I thought everything was going to be okay. I was not only thrilled for them but also grateful that the work I had invested in writing that article—published over a decade earlier—was now helping me sort out my friend's situation.

The diagnosis of a perimesencephalic hemorrhage is a diagnosis of exclusion. You can never see the tear in the vein, since it's so small. The best treatment is to repeat another angiogram a few days later and, if there's no sign of an aneurysm, to assume the diagnosis is correct. My friend's next angiogram was clean, and he's never had another problem since.

ELEVEN

TOO CLOSE FOR COMFORT

When I was a senior in high school, circa 1982, I heard a lecture by Robert Jastrow, the noted astronomer, physicist, and futurist, in which he predicted that someday we would all be carrying around briefcase-sized computers to manage the complexities of modern life. Back then, when the iPhone was a mere glimmer in Steve Jobs's eye, I had one or two friends who owned clunky desktops given to them by a parent who advised them that this device would someday become important. But the only use we could find for these clumsy digital typewriters was to create unsophisticated video games with barely recognizable pixelated graphics. Phones were rotary, cash came from a human teller, and only seven channels were available on TV, which in my home was still black-and-white and controlled by walking over to the set and turning a dial. Jastrow's prediction, in other words, was both laughable in its absurdity but also an incredibly exciting vision of what lay ahead.

Now, forty years later, the iPhone is not only a fraction of the size of Jastrow's imagined briefcase computer but also roughly 100,000 times more powerful than the Apollo guidance system that first landed us on the moon. And this multiple increases every year.

This comes to mind when I consider how the founding fathers of neurosurgery might view modern neurosurgery. (I say "fathers" since they were, in fact, all men. This was not yet a field welcoming to women.) Early neurosurgeons struggled to safely open the skull without producing massive infections and often caused more harm than the disease they were treating. The current generation of neurosurgeons—which now thankfully includes women—is reinventing the concept of brain surgery using sophisticated computer-guided procedures performed through tiny entry points: small holes in the skull, needle sticks in the groin, or natural passageways like the nostrils.

One of the best examples of this new way of thinking is typified by the field of interventional neuroradiology, which we described in the prior chapter on aneurysms. Soon it quickly became apparent that other vascular diseases besides aneurysms could be treated using these same techniques. Just as stereotactic radiosurgery, originally designed for pain management, and endonasal endoscopy, originally designed to treat sinusitis, were both repurposed to treat brain tumors, so, too, was the new field of interventional neuroradiology quickly refocused on a disease that has plagued neurologists and neurosurgeons for years: stroke.

THE CASE OF
LESTER SCHWARTZ

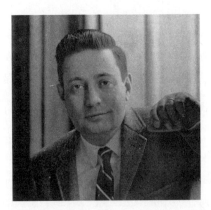

Lester Schwartz was a psychoanalyst who lived and worked on the Upper West Side of Manhattan, which was to late-twentieth-century Freudian psychoanalysis what Texas is to American football. He was born in 1928, in the South Bronx, which at the time was a primarily working-class Jewish neighborhood. Neither of his parents had attended college. Lester, a gifted child, was admitted to the selective Townsend Harris High School. He went on to receive his medical degree from NYU and then trained to be a psychiatrist, first in Cincinnati, then at the Albert Einstein College of Medicine.

On Sept 14, 2000, at the age of seventy-two, Lester underwent a simple operation for a benign fatty tumor in his stomach. He woke up the next morning in the hospital and realized he had lost his ability to speak. He immediately called his son, who happened to be a neurosurgeon.

I was awakened from a deep sleep that Saturday morning by a call from an unidentified number. The voice on the other end of the line was familiar yet also unrecognizable. I thought I could make out a few words, but the staccato phrases were halting and garbled. Each utterance was distorted, requiring enormous effort. Although I couldn't understand what the voice was saying, I had no doubt that it belonged to my father. "I'm on my way" was all I could say as I jumped out of bed. I felt a pit growing in my stomach. I'd heard that type of distorted speech before, and I knew something was terribly wrong inside my father's brain. I also knew that time was not on his side.

When I arrived at his bedside, I noticed that my father looked distressed. I began by asking him a few questions, probing his ability to comprehend and convert thoughts into speech. He tried to speak, but the words wouldn't come. A disconnect seemed to stand between his brain and his mouth. He just stared at me, wide-eyed, his face full of profound helplessness and fear.

My father's stomach surgery had been performed at a different hospital from mine, so I didn't know the staff, and they had no knowledge of my professional training. To them, I was just another concerned family member they had to manage. I ran over to the nurses' station, found my father's nurse, and implored her to contact my dad's doctor and ask him to order a

CAT scan immediately. She tried to calm me down and told me that they had called in a private neurologist to see my father and were waiting for his response. It was Saturday morning. I knew that it was unlikely the neurologist would respond as rapidly as my father's condition demanded. I had no way of ordering a CAT scan myself, so I asked for the neurologist's name and contact information. I was able to reach him by phone and explained that my dad had just developed the acute onset of a Broca's aphasia.

Born in 1824, Paul Broca was a French neurologist who, you will recall, identified one of the key areas of the brain important for language processing. At the time, Paris had become the epicenter of the burgeoning field of neurology, led by the great Jean-Martin Charcot, who worked at the Salpêtrière Hospital. One of the central debates in medicine in the late 1800s concerned the organization of the brain. Two schools of thought prevailed. One held that the brain was arranged into discrete units, each concerned with a different function. The other proposed that the brain was a homogeneous calculating machine with widely distributed processing networks.

Franz Joseph Gall, the main proponent of the first localization theory, believed that the brain was divided into twenty-seven different faculties, each concerned with a unique mental ability. Individuals who were particularly adept at a task, such as having an exceptional memory or fine mechanical skills, were thought to have built up that specific area of the brain, which would, in turn, enlarge and then push into the skull, creating bumps that could be felt externally. Practitioners of this new science, called phrenology, would palpate the skull and interpret the geography of the cranium to draw conclusions about someone's personality and their aptitudes.

Marie-Jean-Pierre Flourens led the other side of the debate. He proposed that mental faculties were widely distributed throughout the brain. Individual areas were not devoted to specific functions. Rather, the whole brain was required to process information and control our behaviors.

Into this debate stepped Paul Broca. Broca had a patient named Louis Victor Leborgne, who had been living for several years in Bicêtre Hospital, in the southern suburbs of Paris. Leborgne had developed an odd speech disturbance and could utter only one short phrase: "Tan." In response to any question or when trying to express an idea, Leborgne would simply parrot the word "Tan" repeatedly. After Leborgne died, Broca performed an autopsy on his body and found a soft area of atrophy in his late patient's brain, likely the result of an old stroke. The damage was in the posterior part of the left frontal lobe. He concluded that this area of the brain, now called Broca's area, was responsible for the production of speech.

As is typical in a case of Broca's aphasia, my father was not only unable to verbalize his thoughts; he was also acutely aware and disturbed by his deficit. The look of fear on his face was haunting, and I could only imagine what was running through the mind of this widely read and erudite student of Freud, now rendered a near mute. The irony and cruelty of his affliction was only exacerbated by the fact that my father's interest in the brain and its organization was one of the primary inspirations for my own career choice.

After reaching my father's neurologist, I convinced him that he needed to order a CAT scan stat. I ran back to the nurses' station and informed the nurse that the scan had been ordered and it was time to go. I knew that if my dad had a stroke, every passing minute meant that more neurons in his speech areas were dying from lack of oxygen. She checked the computer and, sure enough, the order had been placed, but she then informed me that now we had to wait for someone to come transport him to the scanner.

I could feel my blood pressure rising. I asked her, in as calm a voice as I could muster, where exactly the CAT scan was located.

"Fifth floor," she said.

I ran back to the room, packed up all the IVs and unplugged the monitors, as I had done countless times during my training. Then I pushed the bed headfirst out the door toward the elevator with my dad facing me the same way I'd faced him as a toddler when he used to push me around the supermarket in a grocery cart.

"You can't do that!" the nurse was yelling behind me. I was already in

the elevator before anyone could stop me. I was acutely aware of how inef-
ficiently some hospitals run on the weekends and I was not going to let my
dad become some administrator's "areas for improvement" statistic. I located the scanner, let the technician operating the machine know that I
was a doctor (I may have left out that I wasn't a doctor at this *particular*
hospital), and said that the patient on the stretcher was Lester Schwartz,
who was there for his CAT scan. I also offered to help move him out of his
bed and onto the scanner's stretcher.

A few moments later, I found myself sitting in the control room, watching as my father's brain appeared on the viewer, one slice at a time. This
psychoanalyst's brain was so familiar to me, but in such a different way. It
belonged to the man who had raised me, who had held my hand and walked
me to school when I was a boy and taught me how to hold a razor and shave
when I became a young man. He had bequeathed to me not only his love
and his wisdom but also his love *of* wisdom, as well as his passion for books,
movies, science, philosophy, art, and music. How he loved to discuss every
new idea I ran by him, always able to provide a fresh angle or perspective that
I had overlooked. It was no coincidence that I had become a neurosurgeon—
a way to touch the human brain in a way my father never could, a way to
show him up in a defiant Oedipal challenge. Or perhaps just a little boy's
attempt to win his father's affection?

CAT scan images of the head are displayed as horizontal slices emerging one after the other, from the bottom up. Each appears about ten seconds before being replaced by the next. I had viewed and interpreted
hundreds if not thousands of CAT scans in my career, and I knew exactly
what I was hoping not to see.

The first ten slices looked clean. The normal brain appears gray on a
CAT scan. Blood is white, and a stroke looks black. As the frontal lobe came
into view, there it was: a big black spot sitting in the left posterior inferior
frontal lobe, also known as Broca's area.

On slice after slice, the same black hole appeared, so I couldn't pretend
it was an artifact. It was a stroke. A small blood clot must have formed in
an artery that brought blood to that area of my father's brain, which was

now gone forever, as was his ability to speak. Like the black hole in the center of our galaxy from which no light can escape, this black hole in my father's brain could also not be escaped. All his light was being sucked away with the inexorable pull of the gravity of this bleak situation.

Further tests revealed that he'd developed a hypercoagulable state following his stomach surgery, meaning his blood was clotting more rapidly than normal. Another test uncovered a previously undetected lung cancer that was releasing proteins into his blood, which promoted clotting. He was placed on an anticoagulant, started on chemotherapy, and died three weeks later, surrounded by his family, all of us holding hands at his bedside.

Everything happened so quickly. Throughout those three weeks, I struggled to remain positive, trying to convey as best I could a sense of optimism. I wanted him to believe that his situation might improve even as I knew it probably would not. As a result, we never had that final conversation where I could let him know how much he meant to me. I maintained the stalwart veneer of the professional I was becoming at the expense of the son, who needed to let his guard down and bare his soul one last time to his father. My dad's aphasia prevented him from expressing his thoughts at the time. What was my excuse? To this day, my inability to have a heart-to-heart conversation with my dad in the last weeks of his life is one of the regrets I still carry with me.

SHIFTING DULLNESS

Stroke is the second leading cause of death and the number one cause of disability in the United States. A stroke occurs every forty seconds. Someone dies of a stroke every four minutes. The cause of a stroke is straightforward: a blood vessel that brings blood and oxygen to a part of the brain becomes occluded—blocked—and as a result, that part dies. Think of it like a heart attack in the head.

One of the most common symptoms of a stroke is loss of vision in one eye, experienced by the patient as a shade being lowered. This phenomenon is called amaurosis fugax, Greek for "fleeting darkness." Other common symptoms include weakness in an arm or a leg and loss of language.

A stroke is an emergency. There is limited time after symptoms first appear before it is too late to reverse them even if oxygen is eventually restored to that part of the brain. If the patient is lucky, the clot melts away on its own, dissolved by the body's anticlotting enzymes combined with pressure from the inflow of blood that redistributes the clot. When stroke symptoms resolve, we call it a transient ischemic attack, or TIA. More commonly, however, treatment is delayed, and paralysis or aphasia become permanent, resulting in a severe and life-changing disability.

As recently as the mid-twentieth century, there were no treatments for stroke. It was considered a hopeless condition. Few neurologists were willing to devote their careers to taking care of stroke patients, who mostly ended up languishing in remote wings of the hospital. The earliest stroke neurologists were mostly concerned with making the diagnosis, after which nothing could be done. Before CAT scans or MRIs, patients with a stroke were presumed to have sustained some sort of damage to their brains, but the cause remained a mystery. Strokes don't show up on ventriculograms or angiograms, which at the time were the only existing methods for imaging the nervous system.

Early neurologists focused mainly on diagnosing a stroke and connecting the patient's symptoms with the location in the brain where the injury occurred. Charcot, the famous French neurologist working at the Salpêtrière Hospital in the mid-1800s, was particularly renowned for his ability to perform a detailed examination of the nervous system to try to deduce the source of the problem. Like a detective, he would sort through subtle clues to find the culprit, using his well-honed powers of observation combined with a meticulous and systematic method of inspection called the neurologic examination, or the neuro exam. This exercise, in addition to history taking and imaging, remains a fundamental component of any neurologist's or neurosurgeon's interaction with their patient.

Eighty years after Charcot, neurology had still not made much progress understanding the cause of stroke. One of the pioneers at the time was neurologist C. Miller Fisher, who worked at the Massachusetts General Hospital in Boston. Fisher was motivated to pursue a career in neurology by his mentor, the neurosurgeon Wilder Penfield. He was also an expert at performing and interpreting the neuro exam, but his pace was even more painstaking than the average neurologist's. His own students called rounds with him "shifting dullness," an allusion to a phrase used to describe the sound created by surgeons when they tap on the belly to diagnose appendicitis. Fisher famously never wore a watch, as if time itself were irrelevant: a bothersome dimension not worthy of measurement.

In addition to his expertise in neurology, Fisher was also an expert in neuropathology—the science of examining postmortem damaged brains under a microscope—which he applied in his quest to determine the cause of strokes. The only catch was that performing these studies required him to wait until his patients died to obtain his specimens, which could take years. Some of the best neurologists in those early days were known to sneak into funeral homes to snatch the brain just moments before the ceremony began, just as Cushing had done with John Turner, the acromegalic. In the end, Fisher's dedication paid off. Most strokes, he was able to determine, were caused by small clots, or emboli, that would plug up arteries like the balls of hair that clog your drain.

Once neurology had conquered the *diagnosis* of stroke—aided in no small part by the invention of the CAT scan in the 1970s and the MRI scan in the 1980s—the next step was prevention. One of Fisher's greatest contributions to neurology was the understanding that patients with atrial fibrillation—a heart condition in which one chamber of the heart moves irregularly—have an increased risk of stroke. If the walls of the heart don't pump normally, blood can stagnate in motionless areas and form clots. If these clots are dislodged, they can pass into the brain's vessels and obstruct them, thereby causing a stroke.

To prevent this from happening, Fisher championed the idea of treating atrial fibrillation with anticoagulation, using a pill that impairs the blood's clotting abilities. His idea initially met with some resistance. His colleagues were not only skeptical about the hypothesis but feared that the anticoagulation would cause brain hemorrhages. But several randomized trials eventually proved Fisher correct.

Antithrombotic medication—that is, drugs that impair blood from clotting—has now become the standard of care for preventing strokes in patients with atrial fibrillation as well for strokes attributable to their other leading cause: atherosclerosis. Atherosclerosis is a condition in which plaques form in the arteries that bring blood to the brain. It arises from a buildup of fat, cholesterol, and calcium in blood vessels from a combination of bad genetics and poor diet, which can be further exacerbated by hypertension and diabetes. The disease really takes off if you choose to smoke cigarettes and don't exercise. While some degree of atherosclerosis exists in all of us as part of the normal aging process, ignoring your doctor's healthy lifestyle advice is like playing Russian roulette with your arteries. As atherosclerotic plaques enlarge, either they completely block the artery or their irregular borders trigger small clots to form, which dislodge and flow downstream into the brain's arteries. These floating spheres of sludge eventually interrupt the flow of blood and cause a stroke, just like the emboli from atrial fibrillation.

NOT THE FINAL SOLUTION

THE CASE OF
MARA SCHWARTZ

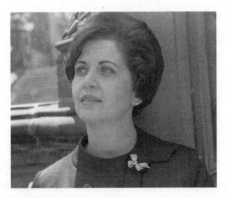

Mara Schwartz was born on December 22, 1925, into a Jewish family in Vienna, Austria. Her father was the successful owner of a dry goods store. She was raised in a comfortable apartment near the center of the city. Her first childhood memory was of the death of her younger sister, who'd contracted meningitis when Mara was five. Her parents' grief, sudden and profound, left Mara feeling twice abandoned: first by her sister, then by her parents. She nevertheless found solace in her many friends, both Jewish and non-Jewish, who filled the aching void.

Mara was twelve when Hitler marched into Austria. The crucifix in her schoolroom was taken down and replaced with a picture of Hitler before she was forced to leave school altogether. To her confusion and dismay, her non-Jewish friends stopped talking to her. She once again felt abandoned, this time by her schoolmates, who now looked away when they passed her on the street.

Mara watched in disbelief and horror as Nazis marched down Vienna's broad tree-lined boulevards, their outstretched arms encircled with red-and-white armbands bearing black swastikas. She also watched in dismay as her neighbors greeted these German soldiers with cheers and applause. On November 9, 1938, she was awakened from a deep slumber and could hear from her bedroom the sounds of windows being shattered. Kristallnacht, the night of shattered glass, had begun. She stumbled onto the sidewalk in front of her home and witnessed firsthand the flames that consumed her family's synagogue down the street.

The next morning her family huddled around the radio and listened to one of Hitler's angry tirades: a voice she would never be able to get out of her head. A lock was placed on her father's store. Soon her apartment and all its contents were confiscated, and she and her family were forced to move out.

When asked about her memories of that time, she recalled feeling an overwhelming sentiment of disbelief. She couldn't stop thinking, *This cannot be true.* The next day she waved goodbye to her grandparents and boarded a train to Belgium with her parents. That was the last time she would ever see her beloved Oma and Opa. They, like 6 million others, would be murdered in the camps.

My mother spent the next five years mostly on her own, evading the Germans and narrowly avoiding capture. She hid in basements and attics throughout the Belgian countryside. She picked up French and refused to speak another word of German. She worked in a weapons factory and lived with a painter who used her as a model. She relied on random acts of kindness by strangers to stay one step ahead of the Nazis.

She was across the border from Dunkirk when the Germans bombed the British soldiers. She was in Antwerp during the Battle of the Bulge. She eventually obtained false papers and changed her name to Simone Mabiét, an identity she would assume for the rest of the war. She was finally relocated by the underground movement to a convent in the village of Banneux Notre-Dame, where she was reunited with her mother, and the two of them lived under the protection of a Catholic priest. Her father was also close by, living in the priest's attic, where he pretended to be both deaf and mute so he wouldn't have to speak with the German soldiers coming and going on the floors below.

In September 1944, a few months after D-Day, Mara saw her first Americans. They were sweeping for mines, waving their metal wands back and forth as they delicately descended the hills adjacent to the convent. This vision marked the end of her nightmare. Desperate for a secure life free from persecution, she married a non-Jewish American soldier whom she'd met in Belgium and moved to Washington, DC, where she embraced the anonymity and security of living as a Christian in America. But she became deeply unhappy and confused by her counterfeit existence. She divorced her first husband, moved to New York City, and got a job as a secretary in the department of psychiatry at the Albert Einstein College of Medicine. There she met my father, Lester, who was working as the chief resident.

My mother's story was recorded on April 9, 1995, by the Survivors of the Shoah Visual History Foundation,* now renamed the USC Shoah Project.

---

*For anyone interested in listening to Mara's story in her own words, the link to the interview is https://www.youtube.com/watch?v=_fKqrfQ3rqc.

Founded in 1994 by Steven Spielberg in the wake of *Schindler's List*, the project documents the testimonies of survivors and other witnesses of the Holocaust as a collection of videotaped interviews. Spielberg realized that the best way to counter a growing Holocaust denial movement was to safeguard the direct testimony of its witnesses, who were aging rapidly and, soon enough, would no longer be alive to provide firsthand accounts.

Four years after the Shoah interview, my mother woke up one morning unable see to out of her left eye and unable to speak, neither in her mother tongue of German, nor in her refugee tongue of French, nor in her liberated tongue of English. Fortunately, these symptoms were transient. The cause was a thick atherosclerotic plaque that had built up in the left carotid artery in her neck, which had temporarily reduced the flow of blood to her brain. Fortunately, the blockage cleared, and she recovered completely without treatment. Had it persisted, she would have suffered a stroke that would have left her not only permanently blind in that eye but also mute. But what was the cause of her atherosclerosis? Although she rarely exercised and even smoked cigarettes for a brief period, she ate a mostly Mediterranean diet and saw her doctors regularly. But what about her past? Could my mother's stressful experiences during the war have put her at higher risk of having a stroke?

———

Hans Selye was born in Vienna a few years before my mother. As a physician, he was best known for characterizing what is now commonly known as the stress response. Though this stress response was originally discovered by Harvard professor Walter B. Cannon, who described the fight-or-flight mechanism, Selye advanced and popularized the notion of stress as a cause for a variety of diseases.

Acute stress, triggered in the brain, is the body's response to danger, whether real or imagined. Not only does it raise the heart rate and sharpen focus, but it also causes the release of hormones, such as cortisol and adrenaline, into the bloodstream, which readies the body for either confrontation or escape. This mechanism was designed to provide primitive humans with a chance to run away from an emergency, such as a predator or a natural disaster. However, stress endured over a sustained period—such as the stress under which my mother was forced to live daily during the Holocaust—is detrimental to one's health, increasing the risk of chronic illnesses like heart disease, diabetes, hypertension, and stroke.

Few historic events rival the stresses of the Nazi persecution of the Jews in the years leading up to World War II. I vividly recall watching with my mother the movie *Au revoir les enfants,* about a group of Jewish children living in France. The film documents the children's feelings of alienation, isolation, and displacement during the war. In one scene, as the German soldiers march into Paris to begin rounding up the Jews, one young non-Jewish boy asks his Jewish friend, "Are you afraid?"

The boy responds, "All the time."

At this point in the film, my mother leaned over and whispered to me, "*That* is exactly how I felt."

Several studies have looked at the incidence of cardiovascular disease in various racial or ethnic groups that have survived equally traumatic events, including earthquakes in Japan and famine in the Netherlands, not to mention car accidents, combat, or domestic violence. These studies have found that, yes, these groups are more prone to strokes than the general population. As for Holocaust survivors, Israel has one of the most comprehensive medical records of any nation. In fact, for the last few decades, 98 percent of Israel's population has had its health statistics meticulously tabulated and made available for research. This was one of the main reasons Pfizer chose to release its COVID-19 vaccine in Israel first, since the infrastructure was already in place to carefully monitor the results.

In 2018, 189,000 Holocaust survivors were living in Israel. In one study, 83,000 of them were compared to a group of similarly aged immigrants who had not lived under Nazi occupation. The conclusions of the paper demonstrated that survivors exhibited higher rates of diabetes, hypertension, heart attack, and stroke. So it's likely, then, that my mother's traumatic childhood was a key contributor to her carotid artery disease—in addition to genetic factors, her lack of steady exercise, and years of smoking.

The goal, now that my mother had averted a stroke for the time being, was to prevent the next stroke, which might leave her with a permanent disability. She was therefore immediately placed on anticoagulation and told she needed to have a surgery called a carotid endarterectomy. I was still a resident in neurosurgery at the time, but I knew that the chair of the department, Dr. Robert A. Solomon, performed this type of surgery frequently. He was my first choice to do my mom's procedure, not only because of his ability but also because I could be nearby in the hospital to see her before and after the operation and make sure she received the best care.

To clarify, a carotid endarterectomy is not a treatment for a stroke. Rather it's a defense against the *next* stroke.

In this procedure the surgeon makes an incision in the patient's neck and exposes the carotid artery, one of the four primary blood vessels that shuttles blood to the brain. They then clamp the carotid for as short a time as possible and make a lengthwise incision in the artery. This allows access to and removal of the atherosclerotic plaque gluing up the works. The plaque looks like a thick, rubbery, yellow inner tube caked with irregular bumps, and this corrugated mess lines what would otherwise be the smooth wall of the blood vessel—like a season's worth of crusted dried leaves plugging up a rain gutter. A skilled surgeon can find the plane of dissection between the plaque and the blood vessel wall and strip away the entire thing in one continuous lump.

Although the surgery is very satisfying to perform, since blood flow to the brain immediately improves, the risk that a small piece of plaque can flick off during surgery and flow downstream and *cause* a stroke—the very problem the surgeon is poking around in there to prevent—is real. Likewise, because the artery must be closed off during surgery, the risk of stroke increases if the clamps are left in place too long.

And while the surgery is safe and effective in skilled hands, I had witnessed, on more than one occasion, what had seemed to be a flawlessly performed operation result in a devastating stroke that left the patient with permanent paralysis and an inability to speak. In other words, I was acutely aware of the risks and what my mother stood to lose.

While my mother was undergoing her procedure, I was in the next room, assisting with a different operation and trying to stay focused on the patient in front of me and the task at hand. By the time the operation I was performing ended, my mother was already in the recovery room. I ran over and reflexively began to examine her. Both of her eyes were open. Check. Her pupils were round and symmetrical. Check. Her face was not drooping. Check. I stood in front of her and smiled. "How's it going, Mom?"

She didn't respond right away, but she seemed to be looking at me as if she were trying to recognize my face. Then she started gazing past me. Uh-oh. I could see her trying to focus, as if she were in the process of rebooting her CPU. Was she in there? Was she gone?

"Good," she finally said, with a little smile.

Phew! I sometimes forget how long it takes for anesthesia to wear off.

My mother made a full recovery. She was a survivor after all, now in every sense of the word. She had survived hiding from Nazis and fear of discovery and displacement from home and the death of relatives and false identities and marriage to the wrong man and stress-induced illness and now even a carotid endarterectomy. This surgery was just another way for her to stay alive, a chance for her to meet her as-yet-unborn Jewish grandchildren and seal her final victory over Hitler. Her way of ensuring the failure of his final solution.

TIME IS BRAIN

The history of stroke therapy can be separated into three distinct stages. The first was diagnosis, which required astute neurologists correlating detailed bedside examinations with autopsies. The second stage was prevention, which relied on anticoagulation and carotid artery surgery. This brings us to the third stage: treatment. When a patient has a stroke and the blood supply to the brain is interrupted, how do you prevent that part of the brain from dying? Is it possible to reverse the process, or is the damage inevitable? For many years, one strategy was to administer medications that might either slow down the brain's metabolism or block the chemicals released by dying neurons that can be toxic to the surrounding healthy neurons. At best, these attempts reduced the size of a stroke by only a small amount. It took fifty years, but eventually, modern medicine developed a substance that rapidly dissolves clots. It's the medical version of Drano—I jokingly call it Braino—since it cleans out the pipes and dissolves the accumulated crud.

Braino's real name is tissue plasminogen activator, or tPA. In 1996, the FDA approved tPA as the first-ever treatment for acute stroke. It could be administered intravenously, after which it would travel through the bloodstream to liquify any clot in its path. Like Drano, which anyone can buy at the hardware store and pour into their pipes, Braino could be administered via an IV by any ER doctor or even a paramedic absent years of advanced training. This is critical, as Braino must be given quickly—ideally within the first ninety minutes after a stroke but at most within four to five hours—so it can do its work before the brain is irrevocably damaged. Once tPA was approved, emergency rooms around the country raced to create protocols for identifying stroke victims as early as possible to take advantage of this first-of-its-kind treatment. The mantra of this new stroke treatment era? Time is brain. Every minute of delay equals 2 million dead neurons.

But Braino turned out not to be the miracle drug it was advertised to be. Many clots were too large or too thick to be dissolved. Another problem was that many strokes also cause small hemorrhages in the brain, since a lack of oxygen weakens blood vessels, which can then rupture. Giving a clot-busting drug to a patient with a brain hemorrhage is just about the worst thing you can do, since it risks transforming a small hemorrhage into a bigger one. Once this contraindication was understood, stroke patients were first required to get a CAT scan showing that there were no brain hemorrhages before Braino could be administered—a waste of precious time even for the subset of patients who seemed to be good candidates for the drug.

With all these restrictions, only about 10 percent of acute stroke patients ever received Braino. Even when it was administered, it was successful at most only half the time, and in about a third of the cases in which it did its pipe-cleaning magic, the clots quickly reappeared.

A new strategy was desperately needed. The answer came, once again, from our friend the plumber. The idea was to retool the same endovascular techniques that were being used for aneurysms and apply them to treat a stroke as it was occurring. Endovascular therapy—threading a catheter into the blocked blood vessel—offered an opportunity to reach in, grab the clot, and pull it out the same way the plumber threads a metal snake down a drain in search of hairballs. Roto-Rooter to the rescue! As anyone who has ever had to call the plumber knows, it's more expensive than a can of Drano, but it's also way more effective.

The first device for removing clots from within brain blood vessels was called the MERCI retriever, an acronym for "mechanical embolus removal in cerebral ischemia." Approved by the FDA in 2004, the MERCI was basically a corkscrew concealed inside a catheter that could be threaded up into an occluded blood vessel and snaked past the clot, after which it would be deployed to hook the clot and pull it back out of the blood vessel. The concept is not unlike removing a cork from the neck of a wine bottle.

The name's French origin—*merci* means "thank you" in French—may not be a coincidence. The inventor of the MERCI is Dr. Yves Pierre Gobin, one

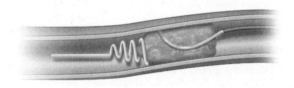

The MERCI device is passed beyond the clot and then snags it.
The neurosurgeon or neuroradiologist performing the procedure
can then withdraw the catheter to clear the clot from the artery.

of my partners at Weill Cornell. Pierre is not a neurosurgeon; he's a radiologist with advanced training in interventional neuroradiology, the specialty that passes catheters into the brain to treat aneurysms and strokes. I always wondered if his love of fine French wines inspired his corkscrew design. (Or perhaps the name echoes the thanks expressed by his patients when the symptoms of their strokes were reversed?) Either way, Dr. Gobin deserves a *merci* from all of us for advancing stroke care.

Since the release of the MERCI, dozens of other catheter designs have been developed to allow a surgeon to either grab or aspirate stroke-causing blood clots. The window of opportunity to use one of these devices is longer than for tPA anywhere from six to twenty-four hours, and, when used correctly, their success rates are almost 80 percent. Although it took seventy years, the field of stroke care has finally arrived at the third stage in its evolution, progressing from diagnosis to prevention to, at long last, an effective treatment.

JUST ANOTHER SUNDAY AFTERNOON

A few months ago I received a call from one of my oldest and closest friends. He sounded panicked, his voice trembling. He had brought his mother, who was exhibiting signs of lightheadedness, to the emergency room at Cornell earlier that day, and things had taken a turn for the worse. He wasn't sure what was going on, but he was on his way back in to see her. As is often the case when I get calls like this, it was a weekend: a Sunday afternoon, and I was out of town. I told him I would make a few phone calls and figure out what was going on. I managed to reach the doctor in the emergency room, who confirmed that one moment my friend's mom was awake and conversing, her vital signs stable, but the next she had lost the ability to move her right arm and couldn't speak. The leading diagnosis was that she had suffered a stroke on the left side of her brain.

I called my friend to let him know what I'd learned, but he was already at her bedside and could see for himself. When we finally spoke, he used the name I went by in high school: "Teddy," he said, faltering, "she can't say anything. It's a stroke, right? That's what they are saying. Is she going to be okay? It's bad, right?"

I know my friend's mom well. She's a lovely woman, as kind as she is smart. She's been a part of my life for over forty years. She watched me grow up. She attended my college graduation. I've been in her home countless times for dinners and holidays, and I've seen her at dozens of family events, from birthday parties to funerals. She is one of those childhood friend's parents who feels more like a second parent. Fifteen years prior, my father had died of a stroke, and nothing could be done for him. Picturing him lying in that hospital bed, unable to move, unable to speak, I couldn't bear to watch the same scenario play out all over again.

I picked up the phone and called the operator at the hospital. "Who's on call for endovascular?' One of my partners, she told me, a neurosurgeon who'd spent an extra two years learning to perform catheter-based endovascular treatments. I called him on his cell. He picked up right away and I filled him in. Although I was interrupting his weekend, he was happy to help and responded casually. Just business as usual. "I'll be in to see her in about twenty minutes. I'll let you know how it goes."

I reached out to my friend to let him know they were taking his mom up for a cerebral angiogram and, if a clot were found, my partner would try to remove it. Approximately forty-five minutes from the time she hit the ER—maybe minutes from the onset of her stroke—she was in the angiogram suite, and the procedure was underway. Sure enough, a small clot had passed into her middle cerebral artery and was stuck there, obstructing the flow of blood to a part of her brain. My partner snaked the catheter up to the clot and fished it out. The whole thing took about fifteen minutes.

Not only was the blockage cleared and her blood flow restored, but by the time my friend saw his mother again, she was already starting to move her arm. A day later she began to speak—first just a few words, but soon in whole sentences.

My friend was eternally grateful, but his mom was also incredibly lucky. If her stroke had happened a few years earlier, she most likely would have been left completely paralyzed in her right arm and unable to communicate with the outside world. At her age, she wouldn't have lived much longer. Moreover, she was extraordinarily fortunate to have been only a few blocks down the street from the hospital when her symptoms began and in the ER by the time they worsened. The timing of it all could not have been more fortuitous.

As for my partner, the guy who had saved my friend's mother's life, to him it was just another Sunday afternoon. For me, the whole experience was bittersweet: sweet because I had a chance to help my friend and his mom; bitter because I couldn't help but remember my father's outcome. If only medical innovation had moved at a slightly faster pace, I thought to myself, maybe it wouldn't have saved his life or cured his cancer, but at least it might have given me the chance to say goodbye.

III

WHO'S IN CHARGE?

TWELVE

PSYCHOSURGERY OR PSYCHO SURGEON?

Rose Marie Kennedy—better known as Rosemary—was born on September 13, 1918, the third child but first daughter of Rose and Joseph Patrick Kennedy. Joe, the first chair of the Securities and Exchange Commission and ambassador to the United Kingdom from 1938 to 1940, had high ambitions for his children, three of whom went on to successful political careers, each of which was abruptly derailed under the care of a neurosurgeon. Rosemary's older brother John served as the thirty-fifth president of the United States; her younger brother Robert served as the U.S. attorney general and senator from New York, and her youngest brother, Teddy, was a senator from Massachusetts. Had he been clairvoyant, Joe might have encouraged one of his children to become a brain surgeon, given the impact our field had on his offspring.

Rosemary, like her brothers, would also be touched by neurosurgery; although in most other regards, she was very unlike her influential siblings. At an early age, she began having trouble in school. Her parents claimed that she'd suffered some sort of brain trauma that had left her mentally handicapped. Most of the evidence, however, points to developmental delays with a significant behavioral component. Because of the social stigma associated with mental illness at the time, she was sent off to a series of boarding schools for children with learning disabilities. As she grew older, she became more aggressive and difficult to control. Although her family stated publicly that she was "mentally retarded"—a term used more commonly back then—it is likely that she also suffered from severe depression.

By her early twenties, Rosemary's psychological state had further deteriorated into florid mental illness. At the time, no treatments were available for her aside from institutionalization, isolation, and a variety of barbaric therapies based on an inadequate understanding of the genetic, neuronal, and chemical causes of psychiatric disease. Turning to his only available treatment option, in 1941, Joe arranged for Rosemary, then twenty-three, to undergo a frontal lobotomy. According to several accounts, the surgery was performed without her mother's knowledge. Joe took Rosemary to two of the top experts in the field, Dr. James W. Watts, a neurosurgeon, and Dr. Walter Jackson Freeman II, a neurologist.

As was customary, Rosemary would have been awake but partially sedated for the procedure. Two small holes were drilled on either side at the top of her head. A dull blade akin to a butter knife was passed through these holes and down through the gray and white matter of her cerebral cortex, where they were gently twisted and cantilevered back and forth, disconnecting the most anterior parts of her frontal lobes from the rest of her brain. During the procedure, Freeman and Watts likely asked Rosemary to speak or to sing. The cutting continued until her talking ceased. The termination of spontaneous speech was believed to be the point at which the frontal lobes were adequately disconnected, and the surgery was declared a success.

While Joe's actions may seem cruel and overbearing from our current perspective, he was likely told that the procedure was not only quick and painless but had a high probability of transforming Rosemary back into the sweet and amiable girl he remembered. Alas, that did not occur. Rosemary emerged from her lobotomy severely damaged. Her personality was erased.

She had trouble with tasks as simple as walking, and her intellect was reduced to that of an infant. Unable to care for herself, she was eventually sent to St. Colleta School for Exceptional Children in Jefferson, Wisconsin, where she spent the rest of her life under custodial care.

For many years, the Kennedy family refused to speak about Rosemary. Indeed, they apparently didn't really know what had happened to her. Joe seemed to have covered up the whole episode. Many of the facts emerged only after his stroke in 1961. Rosemary's sister, Eunice Kennedy Shriver, began visiting Rosie—as she was known to her family—and in 1968 Shriver founded the Special Olympics, a loving tribute to her sister in which people with disabilities could participate in athletic competitions. The full story of Rosemary's condition and her lobotomy were not made public until two decades later when it was put on display as an example of paternalistic power run amok, yet another sin perpetrated by an autocratic, arrogant medical establishment controlled mostly by White men who—not coincidentally—performed a disproportionate number of lobotomies on the opposite sex.

The damage done to psychiatric patients at the time—not just its most famous victim but the tens of thousands of mentally ill patients in the United States who underwent this misguided and ill-conceived operation—was a large-scale tragedy and a dark stain on our field. The frontal lobotomy also became a kind of symbol of the irrational exuberance that often heralds the adoption of new medical procedures before their appropriate indications and potential complications are fully understood.

The macabre tale I'm about to tell involves a mad scientist of sorts, a charismatic and egomaniacal man who abused his medical degree and the trust of his patients to the detriment of our profession. However, this person was not a neurosurgeon but rather a neurologist. And for those who think that the psychosurgery chapter has been definitively closed in the post-lobotomy era, it may surprise you to learn that the idea behind the frontal lobotomy lives on, albeit dramatically transformed into a much more elegant and refined operation.

THE IGNOBEL PRIZE

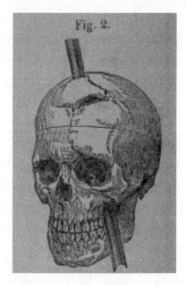

The crown jewel of Harvard Medical School's Warren Anatomical Museum is the skull and tamping rod of Phineas Gage, the most famous case in all of neurology. In 1848, Gage suffered an accident while laying railroad tracks in rural Vermont. He was hammering blasting powder with a tamping rod when a spark prematurely ignited an explosion that sent the three-foot-long iron rod—roughly one inch in diameter—shooting up like a javelin through his left jawbone. The bar pierced his left frontal lobe and exited out the top of his skull. The force was so great that the projectile landed some eighty feet away.

Figure from the 1868 publication by Dr. John Harlow showing the trajectory of the tamping rod though Gage's skull.

Massachusetts Medical Society

To everyone's surprise, despite extensive damage to his forehead, Gage ultimately survived and lived another twelve years. While his left frontal lobe was severely injured, the remainder of his brain remained intact, which permitted the physicians of his day a glimpse into the functions of the frontal lobe based on how its absence impacted Gage's character. According to John Martyn Harlow, the local doctor who followed Gage throughout his recovery, Gage's personality had completely changed. Whereas before the injury he had been shrewd and fastidious, he was now capricious, unkempt, irreverent, and irresponsible. Gage had been so altered by his injury that his friends remarked that he was "no longer Gage." If you recall from chapter 3, Jim Brady suffered a similar personality-altering injury to his frontal lobes.

Although Phineas Gage may have provided some of the earliest evidence that the frontal lobes play a critical role in behavior, early neurosurgeons were also aware of this fact. Cushing, Dandy, and Penfield each noted that patients who had large tumors compressing their frontal lobes displayed alterations in mood and behavior. However, none of these physicians ever considered purposefully damaging the brain to alter its function. Avoiding brain injury was so fundamental to their surgical aesthetic that the idea of willfully desecrating it was sacrilegious.

The first doctor to make the suggestion that destroying part of the brain could be therapeutic was the Swiss psychiatrist Johann Gottlieb Burckhardt. Burckhardt wins my first Hannibal Lecter prize for experimental and egregious brain mutilation. In 1888, based on misguided theories about the location of aggression centers in the brain, Burckhardt decided to remove small chunks of the cerebral cortex in six of his patients with severe mental illness. He described his decision to proceed with the following rationalization: "Doctors are different by nature. One kind adheres to the old principle: first, do no harm (primum non nocere); the other one says: it is better to do something than do nothing (melius anceps remedium quam nullum). I certainly belong to the second category." Although his patients were calmer after the intervention, several lost the ability to speak, most had seizures, and two died.

From the start, treating mental illness with psychosurgery lacked any rigorous scientific foundation. The genesis of the frontal lobotomy can be traced back to a lecture by Yale physiologist John Farquhar Fulton, which he gave at the Second International Neurological Congress in London in 1935. Fulton had trained with Cushing in neurosurgery and was so inspired by his mentor that he wrote the first of Cushing's many biographies, published in 1947. Turning away from clinical medicine, Fulton instead focused his efforts on research. At the congress, Fulton presented the results of a small series of experiments he had performed on two chimpanzees, Lucy and Becky. Lucy was described as independent, calm, and unexcitable. Becky, on the other hand, was more volatile, although also very loving and affectionate. One of Fulton's students subsequently wrote a detailed report about what was done to Lucy and Becky, so we know exactly what was presented to the audience that day.

In one experiment, the animals were asked to solve increasingly complex tasks that involved choosing between sticks of different lengths and then using them to obtain food. Here, both chimps performed well. In another experiment, they had to remember the location of a small nugget of food placed under one of two cups, which were then hidden from view. Once the time was up, the two cups reappeared, and if the chimps could remember where the food was hidden, the reward was theirs. While Lucy was pretty good at playing this simian version of three-card monte, it made Becky anxious, mostly because she was horrible at it. She would become irritable and throw temper tantrums, not only if she made the wrong choice but merely at the thought of performing the test.

Fulton then completely removed Lucy's and Becky's frontal lobes, after which he retested them. The surgery, according to a public report, virtually eliminated Becky's anxiety and her tantrums. What is not as broadly recognized but clearly stated was that the lobotomized Lucy and Becky were also no longer able to use sticks as before to get food, particularly if any sort of complexity was introduced into the task. Their newly fractured brains couldn't unravel what previously had been a simple chore. Post-lobotomy, they were easily distracted, and even Lucy, who had been beating the house and winning fistfuls of food pellets in the cup game before Fulton lobotomized her, was now just guessing—and losing—most of the time. Even worse, she was becoming increasingly frustrated over her lost skills. She began throwing tantrums and acting out *after* her lobotomy—*behaviors she had not previously demonstrated*. Becky, who had been the more affable and affectionate of the two, although admittedly less anxious, became indifferent to human contact, as if she no longer cared about emotional connections. Basically, the frontal lobotomy had robbed these poor animals not only of their IQ but of their EQ—their emotional quotient—and it was just as likely to make them more anxious as less.

Fulton's report caught the attention of one of the conference attendees, a Portuguese neurologist named Egas Moniz (the same Moniz who invented the angiogram). Moniz noted that the surgery virtually eliminated Becky's anxiety and her tantrums. He apparently ignored the other results— the negative impact on cognition, the loss of emotional connectedness— and based on this result (in only one of two chimps, mind you), he returned to Portugal and persuaded a neurosurgeon named Almeida Lima to attempt a similar operation in human beings as a treatment for patients suffering with mental illnesses.

To bring their new surgery from bench to bedside, Moniz and Lima developed a dedicated tool: basically, a wire loop that they called a "leukotome," which could be passed into the brain through two separate burr holes and then rotated and swept from side to side to disconnect the frontal lobes. Moniz called this new procedure a "frontal leukotomy" and went on to perform it, with Lima's help, on some one hundred patients. None of these patients gave their consent for the operation. Permission was obtained solely from family members.

The outcomes from Moniz's leukotomies were reported as follows: "35% healed, 35% improved, 30% unchanged, no worsening, no cases of death." That's it. No other results were provided. Whether patients were rendered catatonic; whether their personalities were irrevocably damaged; how the surgery had impacted their IQs—none of this was recorded nor communicated. This premature application of cherry-picked data from a single chimp makes Moniz the perfect candidate for my second Hannibal Lecter prize for experimental and egregious brain mutilation.

But, as they say, hindsight is twenty-twenty, because in 1949, for his contribution to psychosurgery and psychiatry, Moniz was myopically awarded the Nobel Prize in Physiology or Medicine. This official imprimatur from the Swedish committee not only catapulted the lobotomy into mainstream medical practice but also alerted the general public to the existence of a "groundbreaking" new treatment for mental illness that, as we now know, was not quite as billed.

Years later, relatives of patients whose family members were victims of lobotomies petitioned the Nobel Foundation to revoke the award. I'm sure, in retrospect, the committee wished they could take this one back—although they didn't. But viewed from a different historical perspective, the decision was understandable. At the time, not only were psychiatric illnesses widely prevalent, but no worthwhile medications or treatments were available. Almost half of all hospital beds in the United States were filled with institutionalized, mentally ill patients who were not only isolated from their loved ones but also treated with therapies that were more like punishment than care. These included infecting them with malaria, shocking them with electricity, plunging them in freezing cold baths, and even injecting them with insulin to lower their blood sugar. Overcrowded wards led to neglect and blatant abuse by undertrained staff.

It's also important to bear in mind that history has shown that Moniz was not as crazy as he might appear to our modern eyes. We now know that the selective modifications of specific fibers in the frontal lobe—if done safely, in well-chosen, appropriately informed, and consenting patients—can be quite effective at modifying certain symptoms of some mental illnesses *without destroying the essential elements of personality*. In fact, a shocking number of success stories emerged during the early psychosurgery era. One study, published in 1961, reported that as many as 70 percent of the 10,000 subjects studied were improved by the surgery. Although the procedure seems barbaric to our modern sensibilities, the fact remains that many patients were indeed better off *after* the procedure than they were before.

Moreover, Moniz, together with his neurosurgeon collaborator, Lima, were among the first scientists to adapt findings from animal studies to modulate human behavior. Although clearly in violation of modern ethical principles, Moniz's leukotomy laid the groundwork for the development of a new branch of neurosurgery now called functional neurosurgery, which treats diseases such as epilepsy, Parkinson's disease, depression, obsessive-compulsive disorder, drug addiction, and Tourette's syndrome.

Up to this point, I've described neurosurgery in its most mechanical form: head trauma, brain tumors, and aneurysms are essentially plumbing problems. If the pressure inside the skull is too high, you lower the pressure. If a tumor is pushing on the brain, you remove it. If an aneurysm is about to rupture, you plug the hole. And if a clot is blocking an artery, you suck it out. These treatments tend to overlook the fact that neurosurgeons are operating on the human brain, an organ made up of billions of neurons that together form the basis of human consciousness, thought, and emotion.

The subspecialty of functional neurosurgery, on the other hand, faces these issues head-on, treating the brain's purpose, not its plumbing. In other words, we operate on the brain *with the intention of altering the mind.* In so doing, we expose the fundamental fact that the mind and brain are two sides of the same coin.

And to whom do we owe this modern field, its miraculous cures, and the insights it has provided about humanity? Yes, that's right: Moniz and his frontal lobotomies.

In fact, nearly every field of neurosurgery has benefited. Both stereotaxis and radiosurgery were originally conceived as ways to make lobotomies safer. While we cannot absolve Moniz of the vulgarity of his leukotomy, it's important to understand how it sparked revolutions in other areas of neurosurgery.

Moniz released the frontal lobotomy into the world and, like the scientist who first split the atom, was unable to control the downstream misappropriation of his idea. But the damage done to neurosurgery's reputation—and more broadly to all fields of medicine—cannot be placed entirely on Moniz's shoulders. Had his work led to slow, steady, and thoughtful scientific progress to further understand the circuitry of the frontal lobe—and had safer and more refined techniques been developed to selectively modify this circuitry in well-designed and ethical trials—Moniz would have been viewed, from our vantage point, in a very different way. But history, as we shall see, did not play out this way.

THE ICE PICK LOBOTOMY

In 1840, Thomas Carlyle wrote, "The history of the world is but the biography of great men." Although this "great man theory" has been mostly discredited, and I don't subscribe to its sexism, the opposite scenario—the impact of charismatic, selfish, egotistical men, obsessed with power, who move history in the wrong direction (think Hitler, Stalin, Pol Pot, Bin Laden, Mussolini, etc.)—may be more accurate. If such a theory were applied to the history of medicine, the neurologist Dr. Walter Freeman—the third winner of my Hannibal Lecter prize—would undoubtedly make the list.

Walter Jackson Freeman II grew up around the turn of the century in an upper-middle-class home. He was educated at Yale College before entering medical school at the University of Pennsylvania. Freeman had always been fascinated by neurosurgery. His maternal grandfather, William Williams Keen, was one of the foremost American neurosurgeons. In 1897, Keen performed the first resection of a brain tumor in the United States. However, his grandson Freeman chose to pursue a career in neurology.

Freeman's early career was marked by disappointments. Unable to obtain the job of his dreams working for Dr. Walter Spiller, the leading neurologist in Philadelphia, Freeman instead obtained a position at St. Elizabeths Hospital in Washington, DC, which he secured only with his grandfather's help. There, he was put in charge of the psychiatric unit.

Although bright, hardworking, and insightful, Freeman was also ambitious and narcissistic. Attracted more to fame than to the plodding pace of scientific research, he was less focused on delivering proper patient care than he was on leaving his mark on the field. He dressed flamboyantly and developed an addiction to barbiturates to help himself sleep. In time, he rose to become the chair of the department of neurology at George Washington University and was one of the founders of the American Board of Psychiatry and Neurology. Back then, the fields of neurology and psychiatry were essentially one and the same. Because of the clientele available to him at St. Elizabeths, Freeman turned his attention to psychiatry.

Surrounded by mentally ill patients and frustrated by the lack of effective therapies to treat them, Freeman became intrigued by Moniz's leukotomy procedure. On September 4, 1936, he and neurosurgeon James Watts performed the first frontal leukotomy in the United States. Their first patient, Alice Hood Hammatt, had been diagnosed with "nervousness, insomnia, depression of spirits, anxiety and insecurity." When they tried to obtain her consent for the procedure, Hammatt, who was already concerned about her thinning hair, initially refused when she learned that her head needed to be shaved. Freeman reassured her that her hair would remain untouched. Once his patient was under general anesthesia, however, he shaved Hammatt's scalp bare.

Watts sterilized Hammatt's skin and drilled four burr holes through her skull at the top of her head, two on either side. Using a leukotome that they had purchased from Moniz's supplier, the two men together performed the first psychosurgical procedure in the United States. A few hours after her surgery, Hammatt was asked if she still had any of her old fears. She said no, but upon further questioning, it became clear that she could no longer recollect what problems had brought her there in the first place. Her surgery was declared a success, in part because Freeman noted that she no longer complained about losing her hair. Indeed, she had become apathetic in regard to a great many of her former anxieties.

Freeman quickly became not only a convert but a crusader, promoting and performing the frontal leukotomy with alarming frequency. He modified Moniz's technique, developing new instruments to make the frontal lobe transections more complete, and then he changed the name of the procedure from "leukotomy" to "lobotomy," emphasizing that his procedure did more than just interrupt the white matter (*leukos*, meaning "white" in Greek).*

But the truth is that Watts and Freeman never really knew how much of the frontal lobe they were transecting. CAT scans and MRIs had yet to be invented. Unless an autopsy was obtained after one of their patients

---

*The word "lobotomy" should not be confused with the word "lobectomy." A lobectomy is the removal of an entire lobe of the brain and can be an effective treatment for certain forms of epilepsy and some tumors, particularly those in either the right frontal or temporal lobe.

died, they remained oblivious to the damage they were inflicting. Without any real-time feedback, there was no way to standardize the operation. And with such variability, if one patient improved while another deteriorated, they had no idea if the two patients had had different illnesses or different surgeries. While such uncertainty might have rendered some surgeons more tentative, for Freeman it was liberating.

Freeman's excitement over his few successes essentially blinded him to both the mounting complications and the outright failures. Although the patients who improved did seem less violent and agitated, this came at the expense of their personalities, which were dulled or, in many cases, completely altered.

Sadly, economics also played a decisive role in Freeman's lobotomy zeal. He approached his new procedure not as an analytical scientist using empirical data to advance knowledge but rather as an entrepreneur hoping to maximize economies of scale. He grew frustrated by the tedious pace of the procedure in the hands of his neurosurgeon partner. In Freeman's opinion, Watts was just too meticulous and overly concerned with sterility and avoiding complications. Freeman lamented his dependence on a neurosurgeon to perform what he considered *his* trademarked operation.

When Watts failed to show up for work one day, sidelined by a cold, Freeman decided to attempt the procedure on his own. Although not a disaster, Freeman's renegade operation was strongly censured by the hospital, which forbade him from operating solo, as he had neither formal training nor a license to perform neurosurgery. This restriction only further motivated Freeman to find a way to liberate himself from his neurosurgeon partner.

He found his answer in an obscure article he dug up, written by an Italian psychiatrist, Amarro Fiamberti, who had concocted another method of performing frontal lobotomies. Rather than pass the instruments downward through holes drilled at the top of the skull, as Moniz and Lima had done, Fiamberti realized that the same result could be achieved from the bottom up, by passing a sharp instrument above the eye and under the eyelid—through the thin bone at the base of the skull—and then plunging it upward into the brain. Fiamberti essentially turned Moniz's operation upside down. Once in the brain, the instrument could then be swiped back and forth like a windshield wiper to disconnect the frontal lobe. Of course, this had to be done on both sides, above both eyes, to isolate both lobes.

Freeman customized the transorbital approach by modifying Fiamberti's tool, first trying an ice pick from his kitchen, then designing a dedicated lobotomy blade. Since this new technique could be performed quickly in an outpatient setting, he was finally freed of the hospital oversight he so resented and was no longer shackled to his neurosurgeon.

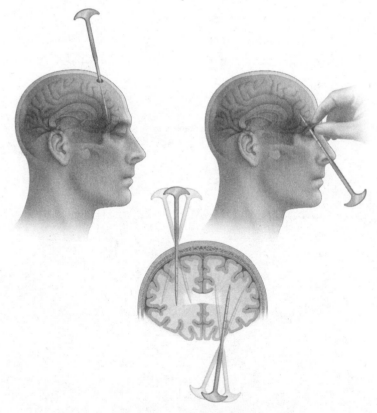

Moniz's leukotomy (top left) accessed the frontal lobe through the top of the head. Fiamberti's and Freeman's transorbital lobotomy (top right) accessed the frontal lobe from below, just above the eye and below the eyelid. The bottom image shows the trajectories of each approach, Moniz's on the left and Fiamberti's and Freeman's on the right.

Rather than anesthetizing his patients, he gave them electroshock therapy, which stunned them into a stupor—a procedure he was licensed to perform on his own, as it was an accepted psychiatric treatment for depression. Not a trained neurosurgeon, he never bothered to sterilize his instruments and wore neither gloves nor mask.

Freeman quickly became so facile at performing the transorbital lobotomy that he could complete as many as twenty-five in a day, each lasting no more than fifteen or twenty minutes. The first time Watts witnessed a gloveless and maskless Freeman in action, performing his new procedure, he was so dismayed that he immediately turned around and walked right out of the room, permanently terminating their working relationship. Freeman's neurosurgeon wanted no part in the transorbital lobotomy. But despite his fractured relationship with Freeman, Watts still offered the more

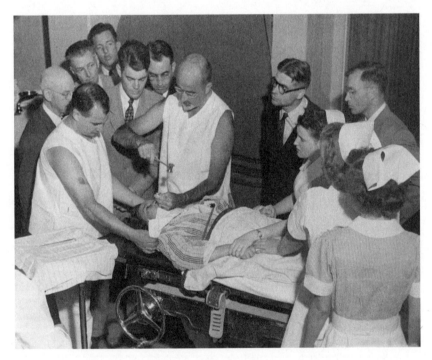

Freeman was a showman and enjoyed performing his "ice pick" lobotomy in front of an audience.

Bettman, Getty Images, July 11, 1949

traditional lobotomies to his patients from time to time and sheepishly even adopted Freeman's transorbital technique.

Thus began the darkest chapter in the history of neurosurgery, though neurosurgery played only the slightest role in its inception and proliferation. Freeman publicized his new cure for mental illness directly with the media. Early public acceptance and acclaim was overwhelming, both for the procedure and for its biggest proponent, Freeman. In pioneering this "miraculous" new therapy—the lobotomy—Freeman finally achieved his life's ambition and stepped into the spotlight.

Freeman's reputation with his scientific and medical colleagues, however, was less exalted. Although the lobotomy was initially embraced by hospital administrators, eager to decongest overcrowded psychiatric wards throughout the country, many of the leading neurosurgery, neurology, and psychiatry luminaries of the time remained skeptical.

Nevertheless, the lobotomy—absent any sanctioned oversight, and with no viable competing alternatives—flourished. Between 1935 and 1955, over 60,000 frontal lobotomies were performed in the United States. Freeman, who charged $25 a pop, did 4,000 of them. He even published before and after photos of his patients in medical journals and textbooks as if he were marketing diet pills.

Eventually it became clear that the lobotomy, like an overprescribed antidepressant, was being abused. Psychiatrists would fall back on the lobotomy as a crutch to help control difficult patients, often without informed consent. Frustrated husbands authorized lobotomies for their disobedient spouses to make them more deferential. Teenagers and even children as young as four were forced to undergo the procedure as a remedy for disrespectful behavior.

As evidence mounted of the operation's lack of sustained efficacy, its dulling effect on patients' personalities, and the high rate of complications, public opinion pivoted from embracing the lobotomy as a panacea to condemning it as an atrocity. Of course, it didn't help matters much when, during one of Freeman's surgeries—while he was posing for a picture—the instrument in the patient's brain inadvertently slipped from Freeman's grasp, instantly killing the patient.

It didn't take long for Hollywood to capitalize on the flip in public sentiment. Movies such as *One Flew Over the Cuckoo's Nest* and *Frances* depicted the barbarity and indiscriminate administration of the lobotomy. Mounting negative press eventually led to the passage of laws that restricted its use. Soon new drugs emerged that effectively treated mental illness without inflicting irreversible brain injury. Then, just as fervently as the frontal lobotomy was embraced, it was promptly abandoned, leaving in its place the caricature of the malevolent neurosurgeon who compels helpless patients to submit to mind-altering experimental brain surgeries to feed their own selfish desire for power and career advancement.

UNPACKING THE MYTH

If we unpack this neurosurgeon-as-mad-scientist myth, several fallacies and distortions bear discussing. First, Freeman was not really an evil man. He truly believed that he was helping his patients more than he was hurting them. At the time, mental illness had no other viable treatment options. Most patients were permanently institutionalized with little hope of recovering. The alternative therapies back then were almost as cruel as the lobotomy. Moreover, Freeman's ego—and his yearning for his procedure to be more effective than it was—blinded him from objectively appreciating both the harm he was causing and the countless patients who gained no benefit from the intervention. But I think it's important not to demonize him through our present-day lens. This man was not forsaking his Hippocratic oath; he had no intention to do harm.

The second element of the specious myth of the malevolent brain surgeon was that the frontal lobotomy was never really embraced by the neurosurgical community. It was the public who were initially enamored of the operation, which was sold to them by the media as a miraculous cure for mental illness. Freeman bypassed the scientific publication process and went straight to the press—after which, neurosurgeons were suddenly inundated with requests for frontal lobotomies, both by psychiatrists as well as by patients' families. At first, these mid-twentieth-century neurosurgeons complied, but their adoption of the technique was circumspect and analytical. If the procedure was going to be performed, they thought, they wanted to be sure it was done safely, using sterile techniques, in the hands of trained professionals.

Wilder Penfield, an early critic of the lobotomy, famously said, "It may be urged that to destroy a delicate instrument is not the best way to study its function." Although Penfield felt that the lobotomy was a grotesque and uncontrolled defilement of the brain, he couldn't completely discount the widespread reports of successful outcomes. To determine if a more refined procedure might be more effective, he collaborated with his psychiatric colleagues at McGill University in Montreal and developed a modified version where he removed only a small portion of the frontal lobe.

Whereas Freeman's procedures were performed haphazardly, without the benefit of directly seeing the transected tissue, Penfield's surgeries targeted specific parts of the brain and were performed under direct vision. Still, the complications were high, particularly when it came to postoperative seizures, and Penfield could see no clear benefit derived from the procedure. After trying the operation on seven patients, he abandoned it.

This brings us to the third fallacious element of the psychosurgery myth, which was that patients were uniformly harmed by the procedure. J. Lawrence Pool—the Renaissance man, chair of the Neurological Institute of New York, and pioneer of the operating microscope—launched a research study in 1947 using a variation of Penfield's surgery in collaboration with the psychiatrists at nearby Greystone Park Psychiatric Hospital in New Jersey. He relied on a team of psychiatrists and social workers who carefully selected suitable patients, performed baseline psychological tests on them, and then divided them into two groups.

One group underwent a limited frontal lobe removal under general anesthesia, which Pool called a topectomy—from the Greek *topos,* meaning

"place," as in "removal of a place in the brain." Pool's technique, unlike Freeman's, was a meticulous, sterile, and well-choreographed neurosurgical
intervention that relied on direct visualization of the tissue he cut out. His
other group of patients didn't undergo any sort of surgery. These were examined for comparison and used as a control group.

One year later, all the patients were again tested by the same evaluators,
who didn't know which patients were in which group. The results were
clear: roughly half of the operated patients got better. Twenty of them were
even deemed suitable for discharge from the hospital. In comparison, only
four from the non-operated group saw similar improvement. As for long-
term cognitive changes, the tests showed that the lobotomized group
hadn't lost many IQ points. One patient commented after the procedure,
"I'm well. The torment is gone. The voices are quiet." Another felt that the
doctor didn't take out quite enough brain, since "most of the trouble was
gone, but not all."

Pool admitted that he had no idea why the operation worked, but his
high success rate was impressive, given the low risk of the operation. Pool
described a few of his patients:

> One man, who had been unable to work for eight years, was re-
> cently kept at his job as a skilled electrician, though several others
> in the shop were discharged because business had slackened. An-
> other, a government tax expert, has been promoted since his to-
> pectomy. One woman has been paid handsomely for a magazine
> article she wrote after her topectomy; another has been retained
> as a secretary despite two attacks of convulsions; and so on. Mu-
> sical and artistic skills are preserved, and businessmen have re-
> turned to their usual office work. One family wrote that, since
> topectomy, their mother had become "100% perfect, with interest
> in and love for her family, the capacity to act as hostess at dinners,
> etc., whereas she had never spoken a single word to her family for
> ten years."

James L. Poppen, one of the foremost American neurosurgeons in the middle of the last century, did a similar study from 1943 to 1947 at the Lahey Clinic in Boston, in collaboration with the psychiatrists at the Boston Psychopathic Hospital. They enrolled 147 patients with severe mental illnesses. Their conclusions? "The operation was worth doing in 88 cases; gratifying results were achieved in 36; and stellar results were achieved in a dozen." While their grading scale of "worthwhile," "gratifying," and "stellar" would not hold up to modern scrutiny, the authors were clearly boasting about the operation's success.

A year later, in 1948, Poppen published a larger series of cases in the *Journal of Neurosurgery* in which he described his own method for performing lobotomies, one he had developed to improve the safety of the procedure. At the time, Poppen had performed 470 lobotomies, not just for his patients with mental illnesses but also for those with uncontrolled pain, since the lobotomy had the additional effect of rendering chronic pain more tolerable. His description of the technique was clear, thoughtful, and well-illustrated. There was no shame in it. If anything, Poppen was proud of his safety record, almost boasting about his expertise.

However, he was very clear on the role of the neurosurgeon in selecting suitable candidates for surgery:

> *I feel strongly that it is the neurosurgeon's duty to perform the operation as safely and accurately as possible, but that the burden of deciding whether a mental patient should be subjected to the procedure falls on the shoulders of competent neuropsychiatrists who have had an opportunity to study many patients before and after the operation. No neurosurgeon wishes to be a technician only. In most instances, however, the neurosurgeon has not had the proper training nor has he the time to devote the many weeks and perhaps months of intimate contact with the patient and his relatives to reach a just decision. Therefore, he is not in a position to weigh justly the merits for or against operative interference.*

Poppen shows humility here and summarizes neurosurgery's role in the frontal lobotomy at the time. We were the technicians performing the surgery. The decision whether to operate and whom to operate on was not in our hands, nor should it be. Like Moniz's neurosurgeon Almeida Lima, we were performing a service for the psychiatrists. Very few neurosurgeons made psychosurgery the primary focus of their practice. Even for those neurosurgeons who embraced the procedure, the lobotomy might represent some 10 percent of their total caseload, the majority of which were traumas, tumors, aneurysms, and spine surgeries.

The rise and popularity of psychosurgery, in other words, was not driven by neurosurgeons but rather by both the public, hyped up by media reports of its efficacy, as well as psychiatrists in an era before antidepressants, antipsychotics, or any other effective medical interventions for severe mental illness.

Now, looking back nearly a century later, we are left with several pressing questions: What is to be made of the reasonably good results reported in these and many other studies published around the same time? Did the lobotomy really work? Is the world now being deprived of an effective treatment option? My point in asking these questions is not to propose that the frontal lobotomy be revived. Rather, I believe that the *concept* of modifying the circuitry of the frontal lobe to alter behavior in a way that benefits patients is not, perhaps, so far-fetched.

The lobotomy was an idea ahead of its time. Scientists in the 1950s simply didn't understand enough about how the brain works to justify such an aggressive intervention. Which raises two additional questions: Do we now know enough to develop a more modern and sophisticated version of the lobotomy? Can a targeted and scientifically based neurosurgical intervention be developed that might uniquely treat the symptoms of mental illness while preserving personality and intelligence? In short, yes to both. The failure of psychosurgery provided neurosurgery with the motivation it needed to make dramatic advances. But before we jump forward to modern versions of psychosurgery, there is one last chapter in this saga that is worth a visit.

EVITA

THE CASE OF
EVA PERÓN

María Eva Duarte de Perón, better known as Eva Perón, or Evita, was raised in poverty in a small town in Argentina. She moved to Buenos Aires to find work as an actress, where she met and fell in love with her future husband, Colonel Juan Perón. When he was elected president of Argentina, she began her political career, advocating for labor rights and women's suffrage, and even starting her own political party. She also created a foundation that donated clothes to the poor, built hospitals, and promoted a system of equitable healthcare. She was beloved by the country and treated like a saint by the working class. Over time she increasingly expressed her fanatical outrage over the poor living conditions in her country.

In January of 1950, when she was only thirty years old, Eva Perón was diagnosed with advanced cervical cancer. She secretly underwent a hysterectomy performed by the American surgeon Dr. George Pack. The participation of an American doctor was kept secret, not only from her, since she was vehemently anti-American, but also from the public. Perón experienced horrible pain from widespread metastases and suffered unrelenting anxiety over her diagnosis. Her health continued to deteriorate until sadly, on July 26, 1952, she passed away. The country mourned as if she had been the president and not the first lady. After her death, her body was embalmed for display, but before a monument could be constructed, her husband was overthrown in a military coup and her body disappeared. In 1971, Evita's remains were eventually tracked down to a crypt in Milan, after which the coffin containing her remains was moved to Spain, where her husband installed it in the living room of his apartment, like a morbid memento mori coffee table. It was eventually returned to Argentina, where her body was finally laid to rest.

Eva Perón's health and her treatments were kept hidden like state secrets, never fully revealed to the public. Then, in 2005, George Udvar-helyi, a neurosurgeon working at Johns Hopkins Hospital, released a startling bit of previously undisclosed information in an interview with *The Baltimore Sun*. According to Udvarhelyi, Eva Perón had allegedly undergone a frontal lobotomy just prior to her death as a treatment for the intractable and unremitting pain caused by her cancer. Udvarhelyi, originally from Hungary, had trained in Argentina, where he met Perón. He learned of her lobotomy while working at the Institute for Neurosurgery in Buenos Aires, several decades before immigrating to the U.S.*

Even after Udvarhelyi's shocking revelation, doubt remained over Evita's lobotomy, since there was still no solid evidence, just hearsay. It took another neurosurgeon, Daniel Nijensohn, to complete the investigation. The Argentinian-born, Mayo Clinic–trained Nijensohn spent several years trying to track down and interview Evita's remaining caregivers. Few were still alive. Eventually, while watching a documentary on Evita, Nijensohn saw her picture flash by. Above her head, in the background, he spied a light box on which were hanging X-rays of Evita's skull.

Nijensohn captured the image and zoomed in. There, in just the right location, he saw two small lucencies—areas of low density indicating missing bone—precisely in the part of the skull where the burr holes would have been drilled if she'd had a lobotomy. Digging even deeper, Nijensohn found another photograph of Perón taken just before her death, in which he discovered two slight indentations in her scalp in exactly this same area. Such circumstantial evidence, however, was hardly definitive.

One piece of the puzzle remained. Nijensohn needed to identify the neurosurgeon who performed the procedure. His only hope was that somehow, by accident, the surgeon had inadvertently divulged his involvement in the clandestine operation. The most likely candidate was Dr. James Poppen, the expert lobotomist from the Lahey Clinic. Nijensohn dug up a

---

*While in Hungary during the Second World War, Udvarhelyi risked his life providing Swiss passports to Hungarian Jews alongside Raoul Wallenberg.

Lahey Clinic newsletter published around the time of Perón's rumored lobotomy and almost fell off his chair when he read the following announcement: "Neurosurgeon James Poppen, MD, was summoned to Buenos Aires to operate on Evita Perón."

Poppen had been well known to the Peróns. The Argentine government had awarded Poppen merit decorations and made him an honorary member of the Argentine Society of Neurology, Psychiatry, and Neurosurgery. But what procedure had Poppen performed on her? Nijensohn still could not eliminate the possibility that Poppen had done another type of neurosurgical operation, a hypophysectomy, in which the pituitary gland is removed to treat cancer-related pain.

Finally, Nijensohn tracked down Poppen's nurse assistant, Manena Riquelme, and asked her point-blank if Poppen had done Evita's lobotomy. Riquleme not only confirmed the story but revealed an even more shocking detail. Apparently, before being allowed to lay a gloved hand on Evita, Poppen was told he first needed to practice the surgery on a few of the prisoners held in a Buenos Aires prison. And not just any prisoners: ones specifically selected by Juan Perón.

Poppen didn't know anything about these prisoners, their lives, or their mental states. He didn't know the indication for their surgeries. I think it's also safe to assume that he did not get their consent for their lobotomies before proceeding. He simply trusted Juan Perón's judgment that these surgeries were necessary and then blithely lobotomized a few of the inmates just for practice, *to work out the kinks!* According to Riquelme, Poppen later expressed remorse about the events surrounding Evita's lobotomy, also likely done without her full consent. Once again, Poppen was used as a puppet, though this time not at the hands of American psychiatrists but rather at the behest of a foreign dictator.

Nijensohn also suggested that the surgery might not have been performed only to alleviate Evita's intractable pain. Political motivations might have played a role. Near the end of her life, Evita was becoming increasingly aggressive, threatening her enemies. She began encouraging her followers to rebel. She even purchased weapons and ammunition to arm her own militia, who had begun training in the mountains of Argentina. Did Juan Perón want Poppen to perform a lobotomy on his wife to eliminate a political opponent and squash a nascent rebellion? The hypothesis is not so far-fetched.

———

Perón's story highlights the unfortunate politicization of psychosurgery. Its critics raised fears that the lobotomy could be used as a weapon by an authoritarian regime to enforce its political power. In the United States it was suggested that perhaps violent criminals could be forced to undergo lobotomies to treat uncontrolled aggression. One of the more famous proponents of this line of thinking was a neurophysiologist named José Manuel Rodríguez Delgado. Delgado had begun his career at Yale in John Fulton's lab, where the idea of the frontal lobotomy was spawned. However, unlike Moniz and Freeman, Delgado found the lobotomy distasteful. It was, he thought, inelegant and destructive of healthy brain tissue. He imagined a more refined method for modulating brain function that involved electrodes, which could be inserted into the brain and then stimulated to alter neuronal function—a precursor of the deep-brain-stimulating electrodes we now use to treat Parkinson's disease. Delgado's apparatus, which he called a "stimoceiver," consisted of an electrode implanted in the brain that could be activated at a distance using a radiofrequency transmitter.

In 1964, in one famous demonstration, Delgado implanted his stimoceiver in the brain of a bull. He then entered a bullring in Córdoba, Spain, armed only with a red cape and a remote control. With dramatic flair (and video cameras running), Delgado, by simply flicking a switch, was able to halt the animal's charge, demonstrating not only the power of his high-tech cow prod but also the behavior-controlling potential for implanted brain electrodes. When the public got wind of his work, he was quickly stereotyped and labeled a mad scientist keen on world domination. In Delgado's case, it must be said, this description was not too far off the mark. In 1970 he published a book, *Physical Control of the Mind: Toward a*

Psychocivilized Society, in which he hypothesized that his electrodes could, and in some circumstances *should,* be used to control human behaviors, including aggression, anxiety, sleep, feeding, and even sexual function.

Delgado was yet another non-neurosurgeon, in this case a neurophysiologist, whose reckless pseudoscientific recommendations served to compound the myth that the patient's well-being might not be the primary goal of most brain surgeries. In 1972, the California prison system began discussing the possible use of psychosurgery to control their incarcerated inmates, many of whom were Black or other minorities. Suddenly the lobotomy was portrayed as yet another tool for society's systemic racist oppression, like the broken prison system itself.

In response, the federal government finally stepped in in 1974 and convened a conference on psychosurgery that published guidelines prohibiting the use of such procedures unless performed in a research protocol approved by an institutional review board, or IRB, and then only on adult patients. An IRB is a committee of objective individuals, including both experts and laypeople, who assess whether a medical research study involving humans is safe, appropriately designed, and performed with informed consent.

The government's recommendations did leave open the possibility of permitting psychosurgery under certain circumstances, such as when the procedure had "a demonstrable benefit for the treatment of an individual with a specific psychiatric symptom or disorder." Although the commission was formed in response to the public's desire to completely outlaw psychosurgery, following its report, psychosurgery found new life in the hands of responsible psychiatrists and neurosurgeons at academic institutions in compliance with appropriate safety and ethical guidelines.

PSYCHOSURGERY 2.0

In retrospect, although the psychosurgery debacle was not helpful to neurosurgery's reputation, ironically it helped propel neurosurgery into the modern era. First, as motivation for the development of new technologies, such as stereotaxis and radiosurgery, but also as a precursor to the modern field of functional neurosurgery, in which electrodes rather than ice picks alter the circuitry underlying human emotion. This technique, called deep brain stimulation, or DBS, is now used to treat a variety of behavioral disorders, including depression, anorexia, substance abuse, drug addiction, and obsessive-compulsive disorder.

THE CASE OF
AMANDA AND SARA ELDRITCH

Amanda and Sara Eldritch were identical twins diagnosed at age sixteen with severe OCD. Their obsession was with order and cleanliness, and they spent their days compulsively self-washing to avoid dirt. The slightest wrinkle in their socks would bring on unbearable and paralyzing anxiety. Just the act of putting on their shoes could take hours: each step had to be done perfectly. They were also hypochondriacs, fearing that they might be penalized for any sort of deviation with some deadly disease or, worse, eternal damnation.

The twins would stay in the shower for hours each day, dissolving entire bars of soap during a single hand wash. They would scrub their skin with alcohol or hydrogen peroxide until it burned. One of the girls described it as if she were being held hostage by her disease. "The OCD is saying, 'Do this, do this,' and I'm like, 'OK, OK, I'm doing it.'" They were terrified to leave their house, for fear that they might need to use a public restroom. If they absolutely had to go out, they would avoid drinking water for days beforehand. Eventually they lost all connections with their friends and fell into a deep depression, even attempting suicide on several occasions. After twenty different medications and hypnosis failed, at age thirty-three they turned to the procedure of last resort and agreed to have deep-brain-stimulating electrodes implanted in their frontal lobes.

In February 2015, neurosurgeon David VanSickle operated on the twins in a small private hospital in Littleton, Colorado. Each operation began with two tiny incisions made just behind the hairline. Then two holes no bigger than the diameter of a pencil were drilled into their skulls. Through each of these openings, VanSickle slid two wire-thin electrodes, one on each side, using computer-guided navigation—a stereotactic system based on the same ideas introduced by Horsley, Spiegel, and Wycis. To be clear, this surgery was nothing like the lobotomy. There was no damage done to the brain, and the electrodes were not advanced blindly but rather placed precisely in specific brain areas.

The target was the nucleus accumbens, a part of the brain that has been called its pleasure center. When rats are given the choice between having this area electrically activated or eating food, they choose the electrical activation to the point of starvation. In humans, the nucleus accumbens is a hub in the circuit of the brain that neuroscientists call its reward system, which provides positive feedback for good behavior. Think of it like your mom saying, "Great job!" when you made your bed or cleared the dinner table.

VanSickle then connected the electrodes to two small battery-powered generators that he placed in two small subcutaneous pockets created under the skin in the front of the chest, just below the clavicles.

Once the electrodes were activated, their effect was immediate. Each sister had a similar reaction, stating that they unambiguously felt "like a different person." They no longer needed their medications and began cognitive behavioral therapy. For the first time, they understood the oddities of their obsessions and could examine them through more rational eyes. They began taking control of their lives. They could leave the house and even separate from each other, a behavior that seemed impossible to consider before the surgery. They hugged their mother, Kathy, for the first time in years, taking the risk that they might contaminate themselves with her germs. Kathy was quoted as saying, "This surgery has changed their lives— and saved their lives."

Only a few years after their surgery, despite this brief respite from their debilitating symptoms, the twins were both found dead in a car, victims of a suicide pact. What is perhaps most upsetting about this surprising turn of events is that each woman had tasted what life could be like without her disease, making the return of their symptoms, we must conjecture, that much more devastating.

Several aspects of the Eldritch twins' tragic case bear further discussion. Foremost is the fact that they were twins, which provides an important window into the relationship between our genes and our personalities. Identical twins look alike and they sometimes have similar personality traits, but we tend to think of mannerisms and expressions as being environmental: acquired from growing up in the same household. We all know twins who, despite looking alike, don't behave alike. In some sets of twins, the longer they're apart, the more different they become.

Here, however, we have two women with the same DNA who both developed a severe form of OCD, and their symptoms and behaviors were indistinguishable. Sure, it may be eerie to think that our personalities are, to a large degree, determined by our DNA. But what's even more uncanny here is the parallel effect that their brain surgeries had on them.

This parallel effect provokes several important questions: What does it mean that both girls felt like different people when the device was turned on? Is it possible to change one's identity so drastically merely by stimulating one small area of the brain with an electrode? And what does this transformation say about our commonsense notion that who we are, our identities, is constant? Did the procedure turn them into different people, like a complete home makeover, or were they living in the same home with a few new decorations and a slightly adjusted thermostat?

Obsessive-compulsive disorder is characterized by obsessions, such as fear of contamination, and compulsions, such as excessive washing or hoarding. While many of us are somewhat compulsive and jokingly label ourselves OCD, the actual disease provokes a completely different level of obsessiveness than just trying to keep your kitchen clean and your sock drawer neat. Patients with OCD are unable to hold down jobs and they get very little joy out of life. Although symptoms wax and wane, they are a constant burden, always waiting in the wings, frequently pushing themselves onto center stage. After years of inadequately treated OCD, patients often become depressed and even suicidal.

The deep brain stimulation done by VanSickle is not a common treatment for OCD. For a doctor to even consider it, the patient must have already failed multiple forms of behavioral therapy. Most important, a committee of psychiatrists *not associated with the care of the patient* must review the case and decide if brain stimulation should be offered. This last bit is critical. One of the main issues with Freeman's psychosurgeries was that he served as judge, jury, and executioner in the treatment of his patients. In other words, he diagnosed their disease, determined the need for treatment, and then performed the operation himself. He was biased and *not* a disinterested party, since he also benefited from the procedure, both financially and as food for his ego.

In 2009, deep brain stimulation received a humanitarian use designation from the U.S. Food and Drug Administration for the treatment of OCD. Placing DBS electrodes is not considered a technically difficult operation for a neurosurgeon. Unlike clipping an aneurysm or removing a tumor from the third ventricle, DBS placement does not require supreme dexterity. The surgery doesn't involve watchmaker-like precision or 10,000 hours of practice to master. Drilling holes in the skull is a procedure so basic that sometimes it's turned over to medical students to kindle their interest in neurosurgery. Moreover, a computer decides the trajectories of the electrodes and the surgeon complies, leaving little to no room for either error or artistic license.

But placing the electrodes in the brain is only the first half of the battle. The next step—the programming—is even more time-consuming and challenging. Each DBS electrode has four contacts at its tip, each of which can act as either an anode or a cathode. In other words, one is positive and the other negative, and current can be passed through them in a variety of different ways. Electricity is not just an on-or-off phenomenon. Think of a dimmer switch: it can be fully on, fully off, or somewhere in between. Similarly, currents in the DBS can vary in amplitude, or strength, as well as frequency, pulse width, and duration. Imagine current as a wave rolling into shore. As any surfer knows, each wave rises to a different height and they arrive at uneven intervals. Likewise, electrodes can have dramatically different effects on the brain's neurons and circuitry, depending on how the waves of electricity are set.

What is perhaps most remarkable about the programming process of DBS electrodes is the dramatic effect that very minute changes in current can induce on a person's mood, sensations, or experiences. For example, as soon as the device is turned on, it is common for people to report an immediate and overwhelming sense of joy. Such giddiness can occur within seconds to minutes of the adjustment. Sometimes these feelings persist, and sometimes they subside as the brain accommodates. However, if the current is extinguished, these feelings are snuffed out just as rapidly as they were ignited. With another set of stimulation parameters, a patient might suddenly experience a panic attack or a deep sense of foreboding. Anger or irritability can similarly be titrated up or down with the flip of a switch.

Even cognition can be manipulated. Brain stimulation can create a sense of cloudiness or difficulty concentrating, otherwise known as brain fog. In some instances, distant memories can be triggered. As quickly as these flashbacks are re-illuminated via the prodding of electrodes, they fade into the haze of distant memory in lockstep with changes in the stimulation current.

Let's think about this for a second. The fact that our personalities and emotions can be manipulated so readily with brain stimulation also reveals how ephemeral the self really is and how little control we may have over our behavior. In one reported case, activating a brain electrode triggered a love for the music of Johnny Cash. Once the electrode was turned off, the patient no longer enjoyed his music. If love of one type of music can be controlled, what about one's taste in food, art, or even sexual partners? Indeed, the fact that the Eldritch twins shared the same DNA and both suffered from severe OCD implies that a significant chunk of our personality is determined by our genetic codes, which is fixed before we're even born.

Several studies have shown that OCD is inherited in almost 50 percent of cases. The twins did not choose to have OCD, just as they did not choose to get better once VanSickle activated their DBS electrodes.

So, what went wrong? Why did the sisters kill themselves? Many patients with severe OCD, like the Eldritch twins, have not only contemplated suicide but have made prior attempts. Since DBS doesn't provide 100 percent improvement in all symptoms, and its effects wax and wane, a complete and durable cure was neither implicit nor promised. Based on their television appearance on *The Doctors* and their mother's interviews, the twins' procedure clearly provided them with temporary relief, a furlough from the prison of their disease. Who can say whether these transient moments of freedom were worth the risk of relapse? We'll never know whether they might have ended their lives years earlier had they *not* undergone the procedure.

Another possibility is that the battery powering their DBS may have simply run out of power. Dramatic mood swings and increases in depression are known to occur as the device's energy source is depleted. Such a sudden relapse in symptoms and crash in their moods—not to mention their disappointment at the seeming failure of their operation—might have been a sufficient trigger to plan and enact a suicide pact.

Battery life lasts roughly three to five years, depending on how the stimulation amplitude and frequency are set. Changing out the power supply is a simple procedure that can be done under local anesthesia. It takes about twenty minutes. But sometimes the surgery to swap out the battery can get delayed for mundane reasons. The loss of power might not be recognized at first, or the insurance company might not immediately approve the surgery. Is it conceivable that something as trivial as bureaucratic red tape might have caused the twins' deaths?

I—and probably every other surgeon in our healthcare system—can attest to the fact that insurance companies are loath to approve surgeries for novel or unusual indications. These approvals often require that the surgeon submit supporting paperwork, which the insurance company must review, after which we are usually forced to schedule a peer-to-peer conversation with a doctor who works for the insurance company. These doctors rarely specialize in neurosurgery and generally know little about our procedures. One day I might speak to a gynecologist to get approval for a new way to remove brain tumors; the next day a pediatrician will question why I need a new specialized MRI to plan robotic surgery. Insurance company approvals for nonemergency operations often take weeks, if not months, and then, after all the paperwork and conversations, our requests are often denied anyway as a matter of course.

Did the insurance company drag its feet? Let's hope not. But given the timeline of the suicide, the half-life of the battery, and my experience with insurance companies, I would not be surprised at all if this was the case. Although it would be easy enough to ask their neurosurgeon, Dr. VanSickle, this would be a violation of the Health Insurance Portability and Accountability Act of 1996 (HIPAA), which protects patient information for a good fifty years after death. So we may have to wait a few more decades to know the answer.

PANDORA'S SKULL

When I look back on the history of psychosurgery, I try to place myself in the shoes of my predecessors. I imagine a reputable psychiatrist who, let's say, refers a severely depressed patient to me for a frontal lobotomy. Perhaps this man was in an asylum for over a decade and failed all medical therapy, including the state-of-the-art treatments of the time. After I agree to consider it, I speak with the man's family, who, desperate for help, beg me to perform an operation that might pull their loved one out of his misery and back into the real world.

I explain to the family that he has a 60 percent chance of improvement but little chance of cure. We then review the risks: a 3 percent chance of stroke, hemorrhage, or death. I tell them that he might be somewhat altered after the surgery, maybe a bit quieter, more distant; he might even lose a few IQ points. What if both he and his family were so desperate, so miserable, that they were willing to take that risk? Would I proceed?

Knowing I could perform the procedure safely and wanting to help this family and their loved one, I have to believe that, yes, I would.

But now imagine the following scenario, one that holds much more promise as a treatment for mental illness: a patient with severe depression, unresponsive to all medical and psychiatric therapy, enters the hospital for a surgery. A group of neurosurgeons and psychiatrists don virtual reality goggles and together rotate a holographic 3D model of this patient's brain, calculating the entry point and target for each of the sixteen electrodes they plan to place in his brain. They then bring the patient into the operating room and insert them under general anesthesia.

First, the surgeons place four *stimulating* electrodes, each with eight contacts, into the spots in the patient's brain that are most critical for controlling mood. Call these regions master mood nodes. Then the surgeons implant a dozen more *recording* electrodes throughout the extended mood network: areas downstream from the nodes, where the electrical activity of the mood network can be sampled. The surgeons place each electrode using a robotic arm, since the trajectories have already been calculated from the virtual reality planning session.

The next day, the psychiatrists show the patient images, play music, or tell them stories that create different mood states—happiness, sadness, optimism, pessimism, anxiety, lethargy, exuberance, jealousy, etc.—and record the electrical impulses from the mood network during each of these emotions. This is essentially a way to map the state of the brain when the patient feels different emotions—like taking a picture of a smiling face and a frowning face captures the expression of those moods.

The doctors then sequentially activate each of the eight contacts of the four stimulating electrodes sitting in the master mood nodes, quickly shuffling through each of the roughly 4 billion different possible stimulation combinations while measuring the effect of each stimulation paradigm with the recording electrodes that were placed in the extended mood network. The goal is to find just the right stimulation parameters to recapitulate the state of the brain when the patient was experiencing happiness or optimism. The surgeon then removes the recording electrodes and sets the stimulating electrodes to their most effective joy-producing settings.

Continuing with the face analogy, imagine if you could record and capture, via all the muscles in the face, the physical state of smiling. Anytime you wanted to reproduce a smile, all you would need to do is to stimulate the muscles in the face to create a smile. Now imagine doing the same thing directly in the brain, but to create the feeling of pure ecstasy. To put the brain in a state of bliss becomes as simple as pushing a button, passing a small current through the electrodes, and voilà! Instant rapture. Bye-bye, depression. It's like a shot of heroin without the needles and track marks. But would this be addictive, absent the narcotics? You bet.

Sounds like a fantasy, right? Well, it's not. In fact, a collaborative team led by neurosurgeons Sameer Sheth and Nader Pouratian implemented a version of this remarkable surgery at Baylor College of Medicine and UT Southwestern to treat a patient with severe and unrelenting depression. Not only did the patient achieve a complete remission from their depression, but once the device was turned off, all their symptoms returned. When it was turned on again, the depression lifted. Just like Delgado's electrically pacified bull.

If such results can be verified and reproduced, the implications are staggering. It means we can create literally any imaginable brain state and its corresponding mood simply by stimulating the brain with electrodes— not just joy, but jealousy, affection, hope, fear, and even desires and beliefs.

Sheth and Pouratian's highly personalized brain stimulation technique could help patients with countless other psychological illnesses, including addiction, schizophrenia, severe anxiety, paralyzing phobias, eating disorders, and post-traumatic stress disorder. In the wrong hands, however, it could be used to achieve a degree of mind control that puts *The Manchurian Candidate* to shame. With the push of a button, we could make soldiers fearless. We could implant false attractions between two strangers to create unwanted desires. We could render prisoners less aggressive. Powerful governments could falsely diagnose dissidents with bogus disorders and alter their personalities to make them more compliant. The possibilities for controlling brain function are unlimited, but the ethical and legal issues pertaining to the patient's civil rights, their ability to consent, and their right to self-determination remain pressing and yet unanswered concerns.

We are on the cusp of a revolution in our ability to control the brain and the mind. But how—and who—will regulate this power must be clearly addressed by those who understand the implications of unleashing it on the world before we surgically crack open Pandora's skull.

THIRTEEN

LUCK FAVORS THE PREPARED MIND

Once my residency and fellowship were completed, it was finally time for me to find a real job. I wanted to work at an academic medical center where I could both perform surgery and pursue a research career. Just over a hundred such programs exist, and they are scattered throughout the United States. Since my goal was to stay in New York City, that left me with only five hospitals to choose from. Just one, Cornell, was looking for someone with my interest in tumor and epilepsy surgery. After a few interviews, I was offered the job. So eager was I for the position that I may have missed some of the fine print in the contract. On my first day the chair called me into his office and informed me that my duties would include taking call at some of Cornell's surrounding network hospitals. Before I knew it, I was made the chief of neurosurgery at St. Barnabas Hospital in the Bronx, one of the busiest Level I trauma centers in the metropolitan area.

The work was important and satisfied my aspirations to care for an underserved population. But for a time, I was practically the only neurosurgeon on call, which meant I spent most of my nights and weekends dashing in and out of the hospital tending to the many gunshot wounds and traumatic head injuries that flooded the hospital on a nightly basis.

On many days I felt as if I were drowning. I had no time to write the papers and grants required to jump-start my academic career. I had no time for my family. I had no time to get my lab up and running or fully develop my other clinical skills.

One evening, while I was waiting for the next patient to roll into the operating room, one of the nurses, sensing my frustration, tried to cheer me up. "Did you know that, back in the day, St. Barnabas Hospital was one of the most famous neurosurgery hospitals in the world?" she said. I tried to determine from the expression on her face if she was playing me. The original name for St. Barnabas was—no joke—the Home for Incurables. Founded in 1866, it was essentially a charity hospital for the chronically ill, supported mostly by the nearby Grace Episcopal Church and a few generous families. The name was changed to St. Barnabas in 1947, and few if any neurosurgery cases were done back then, other than the occasional ones that slipped in through the emergency room.

Raising an eyebrow, I replied, "You're kidding, right?"

She looked me in the eye and began to reprimand me. "Do you mean to tell me that you've never heard of Irving Cooper?"

Admittedly, I had not.

"Irving Cooper," she went on to say, "was one of the most famous neurosurgeons in the world. He invented surgery for Parkinson's disease, and he did it right here at St. Barnabas. In fact, he operated in the very same operating room where you're standing right now. People came from all over the world to see him. He put St. Barnabas on the map!"

Now I was completely baffled. Was it possible that right here, in the middle of the Bronx, in one of the most underserved neighborhoods in the city, a world-famous neurosurgeon invented a surgery for Parkinson's disease? Who was Irving Cooper and how had I never heard of him? What had happened to him and his legacy?

To fully understand Cooper's story and the impact of his discovery, we must first take a brief detour into the disease that he treated.

BACK TO THE SUTURE

In 1817, Dr. James Parkinson published *An Essay on the Shaking Palsy*, a short monograph in which he described a few of his patients who all displayed the same symptoms: tremors, a tendency to hunch forward, and difficulty initiating movements. He also observed that once these patients began moving, they had trouble stopping.

Jean-Martin Charcot, the famous French neurologist working at the Salpêtrière, further refined Parkinson's description. Charcot described not only the muscular rigidity of what we now call Parkinson's disease but the associated hesitancy called bradykinesia, which translated from Greek means "slow movements."

Since the symptoms of Parkinson's disease mostly affect movement, early treatments tried to counterbalance one motion with another. Thus, doctors created vibrating chairs or oscillating helmets to retrain the body, as if to realign an imagined internal pendulum. We now understand that Parkinson's disease is caused by the degeneration of a small group of neurons that produce a chemical called dopamine, one of the several neurotransmitters that neurons use to communicate with each other.

This degeneration occurs in a specific part of the brain, an island of neurons known as the substantia nigra (Latin for "black substance"), named for its dark appearance when viewed under the microscope. The dopamine secreted by the neurons of the substantia nigra modulate yet another group of neurons in a separate location called the basal ganglia. Together this circuitry regulates the smooth coordinated execution of movement.

In Parkinson's disease, the problem lies deep within the brain's very core, underneath layers of gray and white matter in areas known as the caudate, putamen, globus pallidus, thalamus, subthalamic nucleus, and the abovementioned substantia nigra. Together these regions are also called the basal ganglia, and they ensure that your arms and legs don't flail about wildly as you try to move from point A to point B. They regulate the motor system without controlling it, like the gyroscopes that balance a missile or a Segway.

While the incidence of Parkinson's disease has remained relatively stable, our awareness about it has been raised by a few notable celebrities who've publicized their struggles dealing with the often relentless progression of their symptoms.

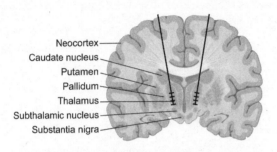

Neocortex
Caudate nucleus
Putamen
Pallidum
Thalamus
Subthalamic nucleus
Substantia nigra

Two deep-brain-stimulating electrodes are placed in the basal ganglia, the structures deep in the brain that coordinate the movements initiated in the neocortex.

THE CASE OF
MICHAEL J. FOX

Michael Andrew Fox, born in Canada on June 9, 1961, changed his middle initial to create a more appealing stage name. As Michael J. Fox, he became one of the most popular comedic actors of his generation. After starring in the popular TV sitcom *Family Ties*, Fox was propelled to mega-stardom after appearing in Robert Zemeckis's *Back to the Future* film trilogy.

In 1988, he married co-actor Tracy Pollan. The two are still married today, having raised their four children to adulthood. Ten years after his wedding, Fox stunned the world when he announced that he had been diagnosed with early onset Parkinson's disease.

Fox's symptoms—chronicled with wit and honesty in his 2003 memoir, *Lucky Man*—began seven years before his announcement, with a subtle trembling in the pinky of his left hand. He described the lack of control as if his digit were possessed by an evil demon. Using the language of classic dualist philosophy, Fox associated his physical tremor with his brain and his concern about his disease with his mind—as if his healthy mind were an independent entity totally distinguishable from his diseased brain. He described the experience. "My brain had issued a divorce from my mind." And then "my mind now had my brain's full attention."

Fearing the negative impact on his career, Fox attempted to hide his diagnosis by medicating himself with a variety of drugs prescribed by his neurologist. In his book, he describes the dilemma of being both an actor, whose entire job relies on exquisite bodily control, and a patient suffering from a chronic neurological illness that cannot be controlled: no matter how rich and famous you are, no matter how badly you might want your arm to move smoothly from here to there or for your disease to go away.

Over time, Fox's medications became less and less effective, at which point his neurologist, Dr. Allan Ropper, sent him to neurosurgeon Dr. Bruce Cook to perform an operation called a thalamotomy.

Coordinating the smooth movements of your arms and legs requires a delicate balance between several different groups of neurons that must work in perfect harmony. When any one of these malfunctions, it leads to shaky, uneven gestures. Imagine an orchestra playing a piece of music at 80 beats per minute. Now imagine a rogue French horn decides to play at 90 beats per minute. The result is cacophony. The solution is either to silence the renegade horn player or convince her to play at 80 beats per minute.

While it would be nice to just reset the timing of the neurons to abolish the tremor, the thalamotomy eliminates them. To this end, the neurosurgeon burns a small crater deep in the brain by passing a strong current through an electrode, which vaporizes the misfiring neurons. But how does the surgeon know where to find these unruly neurons? The trick is to first insert the electrode as close as possible using stereotaxis and then, while recording from that same electrode, move it around, searching for the signature aberrant firing patterns.

Each time a neuron discharges, it creates a small electrical field near its outer membrane. If an electrode is nearby, this tiny disruption in charge can be sensed, amplified, and then displayed on a computer screen. It kind of looks like a squiggly line dashing across the screen from left to right, like an EKG or the ball in the old-fashioned video game *Pong*. Since neurosurgeons in an operating room need to focus their visual attention on the surgery in front of them, they can't simultaneously stare at a screen. The solution is to send the signal through an audio speaker, which allows the surgeon to *hear* the neurons as they talk to one another. Each time a neuron fires, a popping sound echoes through the room. When neurons fire in bursts, it produces a crackling sound, like walking over a carpet of bubble wrap.

Back to Fox's surgery. As soon as Cook identified the rogue tremor neurons, he then passed a current through the electrode, thereby obliterating them—removing them from the orchestra, so to speak. Electrodes, you see, can work bidirectionally, either passively listening to electrical activity or actively stimulating. Stimulating at a low intensity activates or deactivates neurons, but if you crank up the power high enough, you can obliterate the small area of brain tissue surrounding the tip of the electrode. Fox's surgery was a success and the tremor in his left hand abated. However, tremor is only one of the many symptoms of Parkinson's disease. His other symptoms didn't follow in tow. In fact, they progressed.

Mostly retired from acting at this point, Fox has used his celebrity to help the Parkinson's community, becoming a patient advocate, increasing awareness, testifying before Congress in support of stem cell research, and raising hundreds of millions of dollars through the Michael J. Fox Foundation to find a cure. For this work, in 2010 he was awarded an honorary doctorate from the Karolinska Institute in Solna, Sweden, where Lars Leksell invented stereotactic radiosurgery as a treatment for this same disease.

———

Surgery for Parkinson's disease, and other forms of tremor, date back to the work of neurosurgeon Paul Clancy Bucy, who was born in 1904 in rural Iowa. Although he was accepted to Harvard, he couldn't afford the tuition. Instead, he attended the University of Iowa and then apprenticed at the University of Chicago under Percival Bailey, one of Cushing's disciples and another early pioneer of American neurosurgery. After traveling abroad to learn from the great neurosurgeons in Europe, Bucy spent time in the lab of John Fulton at Yale, whose experiments on monkeys, you may recall, inspired Moniz to develop the frontal lobotomy and Delgado to invent his brain stimulation electrodes. Bucy settled back in Chicago and went on to establish the department of neurosurgery at Northwestern University.

Bucy was best known for developing a surgical treatment for tremors, in which he simply removed the parts of the brain that initiate movements. However, while the surgery did indeed eliminate the tremors, it also rendered most patients paralyzed, and its complication rates were high. It was kind of like treating a cold by slicing off the nose.

It was inconceivable to surgeons of that era that the proper target for treating Parkinsonian tremor might be found in the circuitry of the basal ganglia. Walter Dandy, the famous neurosurgeon from Johns Hopkins, had erroneously concluded that in the basal ganglia lay the seat of consciousness. He had drawn this conclusion from witnessing patients who lapsed into a coma after the basal ganglia were damaged. What he failed to recognize was that other parts of the brain were damaged as well. So a coma was caused by the totality of the damage, rather than just by injury to the basal ganglia.

Bucy, the world expert in surgery for Parkinsonian tremor at the time, put it bluntly: "Nothing in my experience leads me to believe that it is possible to abolish tremor by any procedure which does not interrupt the pyramidal (motor) tract or destroy that portion of which it arises." The gauntlet had been thrown down and no other options were considered. None, that is, until Irving Cooper entered the scene.

CURING THE INCURABLE

Irving S. Cooper, born in Atlantic City on July 15, 1922, studied medicine at George Washington University. He was inspired to pursue a career in clinical neuroscience by Walter Freeman, the lobotomist whose charismatic and theatrical lectures enthralled many a medical student. Cooper studied neurosurgery at the Mayo Clinic in Minneapolis, where he also received a doctorate in neurophysiology. He settled in New York City and began his career at New York University, operating mostly at Bellevue, the city's overcrowded public hospital.

In October 1951, Cooper performed a surgery on a patient with Parkinson's disease to relieve a violent tremor in his left arm. Intending to follow Bucy's lead and cut the motor fibers on the right side of the brain, Cooper inadvertently damaged a small artery called the

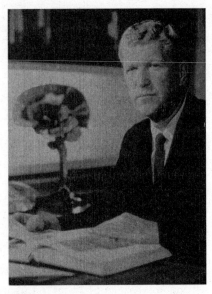

Irving Cooper.
National Library of Medicine

anterior choroidal. Unable to repair the injury, he sacrificed the vessel. He knew that this mishap would likely cause a debilitating stroke, so he decided to abort the operation and give his patient time to recover. Much to Cooper's surprise, when his patient awoke, not only was the man not paralyzed, but his tremor had miraculously disappeared!

Cooper immediately appreciated the significance of this serendipitous discovery and, like a man possessed, spent the remainder of his life trying to prove to the world that it was possible to abolish tremors without inducing paralysis. In his autobiography, *The Vital Probe: My Life as a Brain Surgeon*, Cooper described the Sisyphean effort it took trying to convince the medical establishment of the validity of his discovery.

Cooper's second case, a man named Raymond Walker, had suffered from viral encephalitis as a teenager: the kind made famous by Oliver Sacks in his book *Awakenings*. When Cooper met Raymond, he was lying rigidly contorted like a pretzel, unable to voluntarily control his arms or legs or even communicate. Even worse, his entire body would undulate with a violent and unrelenting five-beats-per-second tremor.

Raymond had been institutionalized in a psychiatric hospital, having attempted suicide on several occasions by thrusting his head through the glass pane of a window, thereby breaking it, and then moving his neck from side to side against the remaining shards in a desperate attempt to sever an artery in his neck.

In his book, Cooper writes that he battled with the morality of offering an experimental, high-risk, and unproven therapy to such a patient in such a state. However, he reasoned that it was his moral obligation as a physician to try to provide Raymond with some relief. So he obtained consent from Raymond's sister and scheduled the surgery.

Cooper wheeled Raymond into the operating room and placed a clip on the choroidal artery, disrupting its flow. When his patient awoke from the operation, the tremor was gone. "Jesus Christ, Aldo, it worked!" Cooper shouted to his assistant, Dr. Aldo Morello. But the euphoria was short-lived. A few hours later, Raymond slipped into a coma.

Nowadays, this patient would have been rushed for a CAT scan to determine the cause. But Cooper, unable to avail himself of this modern luxury, instead rushed Raymond back to the operating room, only to find an epidural hematoma—the same clot that overwhelmed Natasha Richardson, Ray Chapman, and my young horseback-riding patient. He promptly evacuated it.

Raymond continued to improve, eventually relearning how to walk, feed himself, and bathe. Amazed and reveling in his newfound abilities, Raymond loved to pull himself out of bed, bum some change from the nurses at the front desk, walk down the hall to the vending machine, buy a cold bottle of Coca-Cola, and down it in one long, rapturous swig—an activity he repeated over and over again. Madison Avenue could not have imagined a better advertising campaign.

Cooper performed the same operation on the other side of Raymond's head. (His first operation had only taken care of the tremors on half of Raymond's body.) To Cooper's shock and dismay, it had no effect. The tremors persisted, as if Raymond's brain had become resistant to Cooper's surgical trickery.

Cooper immediately performed an angiogram to see if the blood vessel was occluded, only to discover that the silver clips had slipped off. Without hesitation, he took Raymond back for his fourth operation and replaced the clips, which immediately resulted in complete cessation of all tremors on both sides of Raymond's body. On June 21, 1952, Raymond Walker, having undergone an Oliver Sacks–like awakening—this time in the hands of a neurosurgeon and not from a dose of L-dopa—walked out of the hospital, found a job, and returned to a normal life, freed from the shackles of his rigid, quivering incarceration. His once-divorced mind and body—to use Michael J. Fox's metaphor—had now resolved their irreconcilable differences.

Raymond's case was so miraculous that when Cooper tried to let his colleagues know of his success, he was immediately accused of being a self-promoting charlatan. Modern medicine had no place for such miracles. These events, contemporaneous with the alleged astonishing cures for psychiatric illness advertised by Walter Freeman, were met with similar skepticism by many members of the neurosurgical community. Cooper then performed the same operation on eleven more patients: six improved, five were unchanged, and one died. In 1953, when Cooper, then thirty years old, presented his results in Atlantic City to the American Academy of Neurology, he faced, not praise for his contribution, but bitterness, incredulity, and scorn.

Cooper's story, as it turns out, was a bit more complicated than his record of it might appear. In his memoir, he paints himself as an unappreciated genius trying to set the record straight. But his breakthrough contains several important asterisks.

The first is an ethical one. To prove his theory, Cooper continued tying off the anterior choroidal artery in dozens of patients without first performing any experiments in animals to ensure that he fully understood the associated risks of this new, potentially dangerous surgical procedure. He had no idea whether occluding the artery in his next patient would lead to the same miraculous result, paralyze them, put them into a coma, or just kill them outright.

As we now know, the anterior choroidal artery provides the blood supply to a part of the basal ganglia that coordinates movement, which explains its success. However, in 20 percent of the population, this same artery also supplies the pathways for movement that were cut in Bucy's procedure, meaning that in those 20 percent it would paralyze them. In other words, while Cooper's surgery might help 80 percent of his patients, the remaining 20 percent would be permanently harmed. From Cooper's perspective, a 20 percent risk of paralysis was certainly preferable to the 100 percent risk of paralysis resulting from Bucy's procedure.

Cooper eventually recognized that the risks of his operation were too high. His solution was to directly target the area in the basal ganglia fed by the artery. This is the area where the stroke was occurring that stopped the tremors. If he could only place a probe there and create a precisely contoured lesion, he thought, he might avoid the 20 percent risk of paralysis that accompanied his arterial ligation.

Although Cooper's logic was sound, his execution was ill-conceived and ultimately only garnered more criticism. He had deduced, based on limited anatomical studies, that the ideal target was a part of the basal ganglia called the globus pallidus. Rather than take advantage of the stereotactic systems already available at the time, Cooper decided to develop his own system based on X-rays and Dandy's ventriculography technique. Although he claimed his procedure was more elegant, it was, in fact, highly imprecise. Nevertheless, Cooper performed his procedure, which he called chemopallidectomy, on five more patients. To his utter delight, all were improved.

Cooper once again announced to the world that he had developed a new surgery that could eliminate tremor without causing paralysis. This time his arguments were more convincing. He quickly wrote up the results in a paper that he published in *Science*. In another strange twist, one of Cooper's patients passed away, for reasons not related to this surgery, providing Cooper with the rare opportunity to obtain an autopsy so he could examine the brain. The results revealed that the lesion caused by Cooper's surgery was not in the globus pallidus after all but rather in the nearby thalamus. In other words, his so-called *pallidotomy* (a lesion in the globus pallidus) was actually a *thalamotomy* (a lesion in the thalamus). Cooper once again benefited from remarkable luck, since this unintended target also happened to provide reliable tremor relief.

While he had discovered a novel surgical treatment for Parkinson's disease, his process relied more on serendipity than scientific rigor. Moreover, his enthusiasm for vindication served to further undermine his credibility. Cooper eventually applied to the National Institutes of Health to fund his research. As a part of the review process, the NIH appointed an expert in the field to evaluate his work. Whom did they choose? None other than Paul Bucy.

Bucy arrived in Cooper's office in New York, and Cooper did his best to convince the eminent neurosurgeon that the thalamotomy worked. He produced Raymond Walker and several other patients for Bucy to examine. Cooper had carefully documented each of his cases, including videos of their symptoms before and after surgery, and he presented Bucy with all the evidence. He lectured to Bucy for several hours, describing the rationale behind his procedure, illustrating the known pathways of the basal ganglia and thalamus and providing his reasoning for why his thalamotomies were so successful.

Bucy remained stone-faced throughout, never saying a word. When he returned to Washington, he submitted his recommendation. Cooper's application was denied. Moreover, Bucy remained skeptical of Cooper's results for the remainder of his life. Was it jealousy? Competition? Honest skepticism? Who knows, but the denial of Cooper's application to the NIH didn't stop patients from coming to Cooper for treatment. In fact, once word got out that his surgery was successful, come they did—in droves.

So what ultimately made Irving Cooper leave his private practice in New York City to set up shop in the Home for Incurables in the Bronx? At the time, St. Barnabas had a staff of only four doctors, and none of them were surgeons. It served a community that consisted entirely of chronically ill patients. Cooper candidly described St. Barnabas as "Dante's Inferno, surrounded by gutted apartment buildings and filthy streets." It seems that Cooper had become disillusioned with Manhattan. His private practice job was too demanding and required that he treat all types of neurological illnesses, which took him away from his true passion: the thalamotomy.

Cooper depicted his new situation as follows:

> *I was given a desk, a chair, a dictaphone, a telephone and a secretary. . . . No budget, no benefits, no tenure. Just opportunity. Virgin territory where I could pursue my dream. I was limited in facilities but unbounded by constraints other than my own judgement, my own morality, and my own ambition—which was inextricably tied to making the patient well. The only acceptable reason for my self-exile to the Home for Incurables, the only result that would justify my actions to others as well as myself, was to bring patients thought to be incurable into that unimaginable architectural relic, and to ease their suffering, relieve their incapacitation, unlock those frozen still by their own musculature, and, ultimately, to cure some of the incurable.*

The last phrase, "to cure some of the incurable," says it all: Cooper viewed himself as a savior of abandoned souls. And he was willing to sacrifice the prestige and safety net of private practice in an affluent zip code to affirm his faith in his surgery and achieve professional salvation. The Home for Incurables was the ideal place for Cooper's evangelistic goal of converting the nonbelievers in the neurosurgical community into embracing what he saw as his miraculous achievement.

When Cooper arrived, not a single functioning operating room could be found. He retooled an old barber's chair into an operating table and worked in a room that was originally designed for catheterizing old men with enlarged prostates. But that was all he needed. Over the next six years Cooper performed more than 1,000 thalamotomies for a variety of different movement disorders, most commonly for Parkinson's disease. Patients and visiting professors would fly in from around the world like pilgrims coming to Lourdes, not only to undergo the procedure but also to watch and learn how to perform it. Nevertheless, for many years Cooper remained a pariah within the medical community, labeled a fraud and accused of manipulating his results. Cooper eventually prevailed—not because his arguments were convincing but because his procedure actually worked.

He spent the rest of his career in the Bronx, if not exactly offering a complete cure for the incurable, then at least alleviating a great deal of suffering. The patients who sought him out were desperate for relief. They wanted to believe in Cooper's procedure, despite being told it was voodoo. Their faith was rewarded with astonishing and seemingly inexplicable improvements in their symptoms.

But as much as I wish that miracles were real, Cooper's success was grounded in science, even if it relied on dubious methodology. We now understand the precise circuitry underlying movement disorders and have identified the most effective neurosurgical targets for their relief, one of which remains the one discovered by Cooper. And it was this exact thalamic area of Michael J. Fox's brain that Cook vaporized with his electrode some thirty years later.*

PUNCH-DRUNK

THE CASE OF
MUHAMMAD ALI

Cassius Marcellus Clay Jr., better known as Muhammad Ali, started boxing at twelve. By eighteen, he had won a gold medal in the 1960 Olympics, and at twenty-two, he became the world heavyweight champion. Many

---

*For the sake of historical accuracy, it should be noted that Cooper was not the first neurosurgeon to consider surgery on the basal ganglia to treat tremors. Russell Meyers, while working at SUNY Downstate Medical Center in Brooklyn, showed that removing parts of the basal ganglia could ameliorate postencephalitic Parkinsonian tremor. By 1949, even before Cooper's first operation, Meyers had performed this operation no less than fifty-eight times and reported a 62 percent success rate. Spiegel and Wycis, the inventors of stereotaxis, were also investigating this surgery contemporaneous with Cooper, as were a few other neurosurgeons in France and Japan.

consider Ali to be the greatest heavyweight boxer of all time. *Sports Illustrated* called him the greatest sportsman of the twentieth century.

In 1984, when he was forty-two, Ali began experiencing tremors, slowness of movement, slurred speech, and fatigue. He consulted with neurologist Stanley Fahn at Columbia's Neurological Institute of New York, who diagnosed him with Parkinson's syndrome, which at the time was attributed to the repeated blows to the head he received during his career as a boxer. The term "syndrome" was used rather than the more familiar "disease," since at the time it was unclear if he had the traditional form of the disease or if it was a boxing-related phenomenon.

Despite his obvious symptoms, Ali lit the Olympic cauldron in Atlanta in 1996, openly revealing his disorder to the world. In 1997, he established the Muhammad Ali Parkinson Center at the Barrow Neurological Institute in Phoenix, which, at the time of this writing, has already raised over $100 million for research. In 2002, he testified alongside Michael J. Fox in front of Congress to request additional funding for stem cell research, a possible pathway to cure Parkinson's. Sadly, on June 3, 2016, Ali passed away from septic shock, most likely from pneumonia. He was seventy-four.

Ali, like Fox, began showing symptoms of Parkinson's disease at an unusually early age. This led many to suppose that it had been precipitated by his boxing. As we previously discussed, multiple concussions or even subconcussive head injuries over an athlete's career can cause a disease called chronic traumatic encephalopathy, or CTE. In professional football players, CTE leads to early onset dementia, aggression, and depression. But before it was recognized as a disease plaguing football players, CTE was first diagnosed in boxers.

The original term for this was "punch-drunk," a label first used in 1928 to describe the slurred speech, unsteady gait, and mental slowing in some aging boxers. In 1937, the more scientific moniker, "dementia pugilistica," replaced the term "punch-drunk," and many of the earliest recorded cases also had Parkinson's-like altered movements in addition to disorders of mental processing.

In 1967, the Royal College of Physicians in England commissioned a study on the long-term effects of boxing on the brain. The results were published in 1969 in the book *Brain Damage in Boxers: A Study of Prevalence of Traumatic Encephalopathy Among Ex-Professional Boxers*. In it, the author, Anthony Herber Roberts, found that as many as 40 percent of the boxers eventually developed some sort of movement disorder resembling Parkinson's disease. In another landmark paper, "The Aftermath of Boxing," published in *Psychological Medicine* in 1973, boxers' symptoms were catalogued, and their brains were examined postmortem. Not only were a majority of those studied found to have abnormal pathologic changes, but almost a third of the study's participants demonstrated tremors and slow movements.

When Ali was first diagnosed, his neurologists felt certain that boxing *must* have contributed in some way to his disease. I spoke recently with one of them, who reiterated this same idea, particularly since Ali's Parkinson's didn't really start, as most cases do, with a tremor. Instead, he showed a slowing in his reaction times, trouble with speech, and a gradual decline in his mental processing speed. These symptoms were indeed more reminiscent of CTE than Parkinson's.

So it's likely that boxing played some sort of role in Ali's Parkinsonian symptoms. But then, why was his form of CTE so different from a football player's? Well, it's possible that something about the injuries from boxing damage the deeper structures of the brain more than structures closer to the surface. CTE and dementia pugilistica might just be two different points along the spectrum of the same disease, in which repetitive head trauma interacts with an individual's unique biology to cause a set of symptoms that are distinct in each athlete. Although an autopsy would have settled the matter, Ali refused: perhaps his final act of loyalty to his beloved sport. Maybe he was afraid that the findings would confirm the link between boxing and his tremors, which might stain the sport's reputation.

Another unanswered question is this: Why was Ali never referred for neurosurgery? Michael J. Fox underwent a thalamotomy, so why didn't Ali? Certainly, he had the resources and guidance to do so.

When questioned about this decision, Ali's neurologist commented that when the boxer was first diagnosed, brain surgery was primarily used to treat refractory tremors. Ali was never all that bothered by his tremor. His minor shakes responded well to L-dopa. The more bothersome symptoms were his hesitant speech, his cognitive slowing, and his delayed reaction times, none of which could have been improved by a thalamotomy. In fact, they might have gotten worse. Simply put, Ali was never really a good candidate for surgery.

But there was another reason. According to his neurologist, Ali wasn't interested in brain surgery since he "didn't want to have wires sticking out of his head." In the last few decades, Irving Cooper's thalamotomy procedure has been replaced by deep brain stimulation, the same surgery done to treat the Eldritch twins' obsessive-compulsive disorder. However, when used to treat Parkinson's disease, the electrodes are targeted to a different part of the brain.

A thalamotomy causes permanent injury to the thalamus. Its effects are irreversible. Deep brain stimulation relies on electrodes that deposit a small current in the brain. They can be turned on and off, so the effect can be undone. But having electrodes implanted in your brain just *sounds* scarier and conjures images from a horror movie. It's no coincidence that Dr. Frankenstein's monster, at least in the films, had electrodes protruding from either side of his neck. They were symbols of surgical manipulation: of being a partially human experiment gone awry like a creature from *The Island of Dr. Moreau*. According to his neurologist, Fox was similarly concerned that he might appear disfigured after surgery, which is one of the reasons he decided to have a thalamotomy rather than deep brain stimulation, both of which were options at the time.

These fears remind us of the neurosurgeon-as-mad-scientist trope created by the memories of Freeman's ice pick lobotomy but with a new twist. Once electronics and computers are linked to the brain, a new fear emerges: that of increasingly sophisticated computers becoming Skynet sentient and taking over the world with Terminator-fueled aggression and Matrix-esque enslavement of the human population. Now, with ChatGPT on everyone's minds, and AI becoming more prevalent and sophisticated, and algorithms deciding what you see, buy, and think, depending upon what you clicked on yesterday, it's hardly surprising that we all worry that the computer part might become sentient and try to take over. Or, what if the electronics get hacked?

Allow me to reassure you that, at least for the moment, such fears vis-à-vis the DBS device are completely unfounded. Deep brain stimulators are subcutaneous, meaning they are placed *under* the skin. There are no wires sticking out. If someone with a brain stimulator were standing next to you, you'd never know it. As for the possibility of the device getting hijacked, either by a sentient AI or a human, while it *might* be possible to remotely activate the device, the effect would be only to impair the victim's movements, perhaps paralyzing or incapacitating them. While this might cause some harm if they were driving a car or swimming, it would be impossible to use a Parkinson's stimulator to control anyone's behavior, since the electrodes are not implanted in the parts of the brain that regulate thought or emotion. That said, I'm fairly certain this won't stop some Hollywood writer from creating a terrifying scenario involving a terrorist hacking the president's brain implant to launch our nuclear arsenal unless Jack Bauer can stop them within the next twenty-four hours.

What most people don't know is that Muhammad Ali *did* visit a neurosurgeon to discuss the possibility of having surgery for his Parkinson's disease, but it wasn't to get a brain stimulator and it wasn't undertaken at the recommendation of his neurologists. Ali flew down to Mexico to meet with Dr. Ignacio Madrazo Navarro. Madrazo, one of Mexico's most well-known neurosurgeons, was promoting an experimental surgery not FDA approved in the United States. Madrazo would remove the dopamine-producing cells from the adrenal glands and then transplant those same cells back into the basal ganglia—a sort of "self-to-self" brain transplant. Once in place, the cells could theoretically replenish the missing dopamine and reverse the disease. Doctors perform heart transplants, kidney transplants, liver transplants, and corneal transplants. Why not brain transplants?

It's not so crazy. Brain transplants are indeed possible, and the preliminary feasibility studies were done over fifty years ago by Dr. Robert J.

White, the chief of neurosurgery at Cleveland Metropolitan General Hospital. With support from the NIH, White showed that he could keep a monkey brain alive for several hours after removing it from the skull by giving it enough oxygen. He was even able to record electrical activity from his brain-in-a-vat. These preliminary experiments led to his tour de force simian head transplant surgery, which he successfully achieved on March 14, 1970, with the help of a large team of thirty other doctors, nurses, and technicians—a surgery he called a cephalic exchange. This was not exactly a brain transplant, since the entire head—skull, face, neck with all the blood vessels included—had to be reattached to maintain circulation. These poor monkeys were able to chew, swallow, and even track objects with their eyes. But they survived for only a few hours. Thank goodness, really.

Following these controversial experiments, White became the subject of protests and even death threats. His experiments were considered unholy, sacrilegious, cruel, and an affront to animal rights activists. Yet his motivations remained altruistic, and his methods were based on years of careful experimentation with the goal of finding a way to help patients suffering from spinal cord or brain injuries. Perhaps surprisingly, White was a devout Catholic. He became a close advisor to Pope John Paul II and was even awarded a papal knighthood. He was also nominated for a Nobel Prize, one of only a few neurosurgeons to be so nominated. On that list are other familiar names like Victor Horsley, Otfrid Foerster, Harvey Cushing, Walter Dandy, and Wilder Penfield. Emil Theodor Kocher, the Swiss neurosurgeon who performed the first successful pituitary adenoma surgery through the nose, did win a Nobel Prize, but it was for his work on thyroid surgery. So far, no Nobel prizes have been awarded in neurosurgery except the one for the frontal lobotomy, which, as we discussed, was given to a neurologist.

Since whole brain transplants were not only ineffective but unethical, physicians then tried transplanting small pieces of the cerebral cortex from one animal to another. This never worked because the complex neuronal connections between the host brain and the grafted brain generally failed to rewire. More recently, scientists have successfully transplanted small balls of human brain cells, called organoids, into the brains of very young mice whose immune systems are weakened to prevent cellular rejection. In this unique scenario, new circuits can indeed form, and the foreign neurons will integrate and begin to function. While this represents a step forward, it is still a far cry from performing a full brain transplant from one human to another.

Given that the root cause of Parkinson's motor symptoms is a loss of dopamine-producing cells in a specific part of the brain, the substantia nigra, replacing those cells with healthy dopamine-producing cells is a simpler strategy. The grafted cells don't need to reestablish complex connections; they merely have to survive long enough to start pumping out dopamine. After studies in animals showed that the idea held promise, efforts in humans soon followed. Dr. Madrazo's team had performed one of the first such trials, which is what drew Ali's attention, but the results were inconclusive. Ultimately, Ali chose not to proceed.

In their most recent attempts, scientists can now chemically cajole skin cells into making dopamine, and these transformed cells can then be transplanted back into the substantia nigra. Since the same patient is both donor and recipient, this strategy avoids immune rejection. Using skin cells and not fetal cells also avoids sticky ethical concerns for those who argue that a therapeutic use for fetal tissue might promote abortions. Another strategy has been to package the gene that codes for dopamine inside a virus, which can be injected into the substantia nigra in the hope that the virus will infect the neurons there and reprogram them to start producing dopamine. This so-called gene therapy for Parkinson's, while promising, has also met with mixed results and is still considered experimental.

While brain stimulation can control and mitigate the motor symptoms of Parkinson's disease, it's not the last word on ameliorating this degenerative disease. Unfortunately, Parkinson's doesn't just alter movement; it also impacts cognition. In advanced stages, issues arise with the chemicals that relay information between neurons, and abnormal proteins appear throughout the brain that gum up the machinery, like the plaques and tangles in Alzheimer's disease. Nevertheless, a surgical cure for the tremors and slow movements of Parkinson's is likely imminent once we can find a durable method to raise dopamine levels in the substantia nigra. We are getting awfully close, and given the importance of serendipity in advancing neurosurgical treatments for Parkinson's disease, the answer may emerge from where we least expect it.

FOCUSED ULTRASOUND

The latest technology to gain traction in the treatment of Parkinson's disease is called focused ultrasound. In the same way that stereotactic radiosurgery delivers concentrated energy to the brain in the form of radiation, focused ultrasound does the same with sound waves. In fact, focused ultrasound, in some sense, achieves the ultimate goal of neurosurgery: to alter the anatomy and physiology of the brain in a completely noninvasive manner.

The strategy behind focused ultrasound is reminiscent of that used by stereotactic radiosurgery: a machine that resembles an MRI scanner transmits hundreds of tiny ultrasonic waves through the skull, which all converge on a single point. While each individual wave by itself would be insufficient to damage biologic tissue, the sum of their energy, at the point where they meet, creates a small spherical crater in the brain.

To understand how focused ultrasound works, let's quickly review the science. Sound waves—what we hear with our ears—are produced when particles in the air collide. Picture microscopic billiard balls crashing into one another. Sound waves travel through the air like waves rolling across the ocean. A sound's volume depends on the height of the wave, and its pitch depends on the frequency, meaning how many waves pass by each second. Imagine a bobbing buoy floating in the ocean. If we stare at the buoy, it moves up and down. If we measure how many times the buoy bobs up in any given period, we arrive at a number equal to the frequency of the passing waves. For sound waves, if we measure the number of waves that roll by each second, then we are measuring a value called hertz.

The human ear can hear sounds ranging from 20 to 20,000 hertz—that is, sound waves that oscillate between 20 and 20,000 times per second. Sounds above 20,000 hertz are called ultrasonic. Dogs can hear sounds up to 40,000 hertz, cats up to 60,000 hertz. Bats and dolphins can appreciate ultrasound waves as high as 200,000 hertz. A dog whistle, for example, is in the 30,000-hertz range, which is above what humans can hear but well within a dog's range.

When we think about the medical uses of ultrasound, what probably pops into our heads is the profile of a baby in utero. That's fetal ultrasound. When the military uses the same technology to find hidden submarines, it's called sonar. However, ultrasound waves produced at high enough frequencies—around 700,000 hertz—can do much more than help expecting parents figure out what color to paint their baby's bedroom walls. It can actually heat up and vaporize living tissue.

Now let's say the device that shoots out these super-high-frequency sound waves is curved. Its destructive beams of sound can be concentrated and aimed at a target, such as a tumor deep in the brain. This concept, of blasting a small crater in the brain with focused sound waves, was developed in 1962 by an engineer at Columbia University, John G. Lynn, who teamed up with neurosurgeon Tracy J. Putnam. Putnam, who studied at Harvard College and Harvard Medical School, trained under—you guessed it—Harvey Cushing. He was considered a triple-threat physician, since he was also highly accomplished in neurology and psychiatry.

When Lynn began the collaboration, Putnam was the head of both the departments of neurosurgery *and* neurology at the Neurological Institute of New York at Columbia, the only physician ever to hold both posts. Putnam was such a renowned figure in neurosurgery at the time that he was consulted to operate on the sixteen-year-old son of acclaimed author John Gunther, who chronicled his son's heroic but losing battle with glioblastoma in *Death Be Not Proud*.

Putnam was also famous for having co-discovered the drug phenytoin, also known as Dilantin, which for years was the most effective treatment for epilepsy. Then, at the height of his career, which began with so much promise, Putnam was mysteriously fired from his job as director of the Neurological Institute. Too much infighting between the two departments was the hospital administration's explanation. It had been a mistake to have one person lead both neurology and neurosurgery.

After losing his position at Columbia, Putnam packed up and moved to California, publishing only a handful of articles for the remainder of his career. He continued to work in private practice, but he did so in relative anonymity. For years afterward, Putnam's precipitate collapse and disappearance from Columbia was shrouded in mystery. What had happened to one of the nation's most celebrated and influential neurosurgeons?

In 2008, Dr. Lewis P. Rowland, then chair of neurology at the Neurological Institute, finally shed light on the matter. Rowland first described the historical context. During the years leading up to World War II, Jewish immigrants had begun flooding into the U.S. to escape European anti-Semitism. Once here, they began filling the limited positions offered in medical training programs, particularly in the Northeast. A concomitant rise in anti-Semitic sentiments in America led to a flagrant backlash against the rise in Jewish applicants, who were derided for poaching so many of the medical training spots.

Just before Putnam took the helm of the Neurological Institute, Columbia imposed quotas on medical school admissions. They were not the only school to do so. Some schools even labeled applications from Jews with the letter H to denote their Hebraic origin, reminiscent of the J the Nazis forced Jews to sew onto their clothing before sending them off to concentration camps. Jewish trainees, once 47 percent of the class at Columbia in the 1920s, dwindled to a paltry 6 percent in the 1940s. Putnam, who was also the vice-chair of the National Committee for the Relocation of Foreign Physicians, ignored the edict set forth by the administration at Columbia and began hiring prominent German Jewish neurologists to work at the Neurological Institute.

Rowland uncovered a letter written by Putnam in which he claims to have been ordered by Charles P. Cooper, then president of Presbyterian Hospital, to fire all "non-Aryan" doctors from his service or else resign his post. The dictum was later corroborated by the chair of cardiothoracic surgery. Putnam refused to comply, and his disobedience likely played a role in his untimely dismissal and may even have contributed to his inability to find a subsequent post suitable to his stature.

Although Putnam's departure undoubtedly hindered the development of focused ultrasound at Columbia, the technique he helped pioneer flourished elsewhere. At the University of Illinois, two brothers, William and Francis Fry, founded a bioacoustics research laboratory. Together they built the first fully functional focused ultrasound machine, which they tested on hundreds of animals. Their device, as opposed to Putnam and Lynn's single probe, employed four transducers, making it more precise.

The Frys' first design had several significant limitations. The skull proved to be a huge hindrance, as it absorbed and distorted the sound waves. Moreover, the high-frequency sound waves intensely heated the scalp, leading to severe burns. As a solution, they figured that if they could cut open the skin and remove a piece of the skull, it might solve their problems, but for this they needed to collaborate with a neurosurgeon.

The Frys found the perfect collaborator in Russell Meyers, a Cornell graduate, who was the chief of neurosurgery at the University of Iowa.* Together, they performed the first focused ultrasound surgeries on a human patient with Parkinson's disease. The treatment required two separate surgeries, each lasting some six hours. Their work captured the public's imagination and was featured in the December 2, 1957, issue of *Time* magazine.

Over the ensuing fifty years—which brings us to the present day—advances in mathematics, engineering, physics, and computing power have led to the development of the modern focused ultrasound device, which is

---

*This is the same Russell Meyers who first operated on the basal ganglia for Parkinsonian tremor.

currently produced by the Israeli company Insightec. This modern machine relies on 1,024 individual transducers that emit sound at frequencies around 700,000 hertz. It has a built-in cooling system that continuously bathes the scalp in frigid water to prevent skin damage. Moreover, it no longer requires a craniotomy for the sound waves to pass into the brain. Instead, each transducer sends a pulsed wave with a slight delay, which allows them to be precisely shaped through the skull. Except for requiring a shaved head, the device is as minimally invasive as neurosurgery gets.

Focused ultrasound treatment is delivered inside an MRI magnet, which can measure temperature inside the brain, allowing the surgeon to see the exact size and shape of the damaged area—a process known as MR thermography. MR-guided focused ultrasound is now employed around the world to treat a host of illnesses, including essential tremor, Parkinson's disease, epilepsy, chronic pain, obsessive-compulsive disorder, and stroke.

Even more groundbreaking is focused ultrasound's ability to selectively open the blood-brain barrier. You will recall that this is the protective filtration system that prevents many of the drugs and therapies that we currently administer orally or intravenously from entering the brain. For instance, one of the reasons that GBM, the deadliest form of brain cancer, remains so resistant to treatment is that many of the most effective chemotherapies and immunotherapies can't reach the tumor due to the blood-brain barrier. If we could temporarily incapacitate it, which we are now able to do with low-intensity focused ultrasound, then thousands of chemotherapies that were previously found to be ineffective might become potential cures.

In fact, any drug that might work against any brain diseases—be it Alzheimer's disease, Parkinson's, Huntington's disease, multiple sclerosis, or epilepsy—but which in the past has been impossible to administer due to the impenetrability of the blood-brain barrier, might now be administered as a pill or through an IV and focally absorbed into the brain with focused ultrasound. Where this new technology will lead us is not yet fully understood, but in principle it could impact nearly every disease currently treated by neurologists and neurosurgeons.

FOURTEEN

WHAT IS IT LIKE TO BE A BRAIN?

Many of us have had to deal with an aging relative who develops severe memory loss or dementia. In some circumstances, such as advanced Alzheimer's disease, our loved ones may no longer recognize who we are. They may forget some of the most important moments in their lives. We say they are "no longer the same person" or have become "a shadow of their former selves." Yet, we still care for them and love them, despite these radical changes in the person they've become, because they not only look the same but our memory of who they used to be remains constant.

But at what point did they cease to be who they were and become someone else? How many neurons do we need to lose before our identities disintegrate? And if our identities can be so profoundly altered by changes in our brains—specifically, changes that are occurring daily as a natural part of the aging process (remember we lose about 50,000 neurons every day)— what does this tell us about the mind and our sense of self, which we tend to think of as continuous and invariable?

A classic philosophical thought experiment—the Ship of Theseus—may shed some light on this conundrum. First attributed to the ancient Greek philospher Heraclitus, who relied on it to provoke his students into thinking more deeply about the question of identity, the Ship of Theseus goes something like this: A shipbuilder is hired to maintain a wooden boat, whose planks decay with each passing year. Periodically, he replaces a few of the rotten boards with new ones. After several years, when every single plank of wood has been replaced, is the ship, which looks the same, still the same ship? If the answer is yes, then how is the identity of the ship determined if not by its physical components, which are now completely different from the original ones? If the answer is no, and it's now a new ship, then at what point in time did it cease being the former ship and start becoming the new one?

The point of this exercise is not to arrive at the correct answer but rather to contemplate the nature of identity. And one way to make sense of identity is to acknowledge the importance of time. At any moment in time, only one version of an object exists. As time passes, all things change. The ship from a few seconds ago is already different from the one that exists currently, which is slightly more decayed. Only the *idea* of the ship remains constant.

The same can be said of our identities as individuals. The number of neurons in our brains diminishes as we age. The structure of our brains is always in flux. As we learn and we forget, we form and eliminate connections. Therefore, we are physically never exactly the same person we were a moment earlier. You, having read that last sentence, are different from the person you were before you read it. Yet the *idea* of you—and of the self— remains constant. In this way, the invariability of our identities and the unity of the self can be seen as mental constructs rather than as immutable entities in the physical world.

But are mental constructs as real as physical objects? Do they exist in the same way? You can imagine a horse with five heads and twenty legs and even draw a picture of it, but does this new creature now exist in any meaningful way? Not really. Similarly, the notion that the "self"—our identity— remains the same over time is an illusion.

Even as I write these last few sentences, I realize that I am distinguishing between a mental world and a physical world, as if they were two separate things: the mind and the brain. Michael J. Fox did the same when he attributed his tremor to a problem in his brain but his *concern* about the tremor to his mind. Yet my firsthand evidence as a neurosurgeon has led me to the conclusion that the brain and the mind are one and the same. Psychosurgery and brain stimulation, as done by Sheth and Pouratian for depression and by VanSickle for OCD, show us that altering the brain can have a profound impact on our emotions, our behavior, and our personality. The mind and the brain only *seem* like two different things because we use two different words to refer to them, not because they are unique entities.

So if I know better, then why do I, too, dichotomize the mind and the brain in my descriptions?

Because the separation between mind and brain is built into our language. We have one word for mind and another word for brain, so we just assume that they exist apart from each other. The same can be said of words that describe mental states, like "love." The feeling of love corresponds to my brain being in a particular state, one in which I feel an attachment to another person or to a thing. You can love your spouse just like you can love a parent, a dog, or chocolate. But I assure you that your brain is not in the same state during each of these experiences. We have no clue what the *experience* of love is, which may explain why poets have spent the last two thousand years trying to describe it.

Until recently, our species—and our language—developed without any knowledge that brain states exist, so we have no words that describe them as physical entities. For thousands of years, we were aware only of our *experience* of those states, so we created words for the mental stuff, and in doing so, we constructed a world of psychic interactions, which may very well be an illusion. When I say it's an illusion, I don't mean it doesn't exist at all, but rather that it's a fairy tale—just a story we tell ourselves to make sense of it all, like the horse with five heads and twenty legs.

The separation between the mind and the brain reflects our commonsense view of the world, the one embedded in our language. This school of thought is called dualism, and it's attributed to the ideas of the French philosopher René Descartes. Dualists claim that the brain and the mind formed from two completely different substances. The brain is part of the physical world and as such observes its rules, better known as mathematics, physics, and chemistry. Dualists posit that while the mind can *interact* with the brain and may even *require* the brain to exist, the mind and the brain are two different real but separate entities. Unlike the rules that govern the physical world, the ones that govern the mental world are not so easily described. This is where our feelings, desires, and perceptions play out and create our subjective experience of the world—in other words, our consciousness.

From the dualist's perspective, my father the psychoanalyst operated on the mind and his tools were his words, just as I operate on the brain and my tools are my hands. Thoughts can impact the physical world, since we can intend to move our bodies and then cause them to move. The physical world can, in turn, impact our thoughts. For example, drugs that alter the brain's chemistry can relieve depression, help us relax, or make us hallucinate. Dualism is fundamental to the religious notion of the soul, and it's also arguably the basis for our belief that we possess free will and the capacity to control our decisions.

The philosophical viewpoint opposing dualism is determinism, also known as monism, reductionism, or scientific realism. Determinism presupposes that matter is all that exists in the universe. Our brains are physical substances, and the mind not only relies on the brain but is simply another word for the brain's experience of its different physical states. From this perspective, the mind is also subject to the physical laws that govern all matter—as opposed to being influenced by our will or by our choices. Our mental experiences are merely *what it is like to be our brains* at that moment in time, in that distinct physical state. According to this theory, the same laws of nature that describe what happens in the physical world can also explain the inner workings of the mind. If you endorse the tenets of determinism, then you accept that neurosurgeons can alter the mind—including thoughts, beliefs, feelings, and perceptions—merely by manipulating the brain. This perspective, which I believe is more consistent with what I have experienced as a neurosurgeon, eventually leads to some unnerving conclusions about free will.

From the die-hard determinist perspective, the laws of physics that dictate the movement of billiard balls on a table also dictate our thoughts. So every idea or choice that we make has already been determined by the prior state of all the atoms and electrons in our brains, each of which can be described and predicted. From this perspective, the future is inevitable and unalterable. As such, free will cannot exist, since each successive state of our physical brains has already been scripted based on the state of the brain in the prior moment and the immutable laws of physics.

But not all scientists are willing to jettison the possibility of free will. Not even determinists. Some, who call themselves compatibilists, believe that quantum mechanics—the laws that govern the subatomic world—introduces a degree of randomness and unpredictability, which provides them with the hope that free will may still exist. But the quirky laws of the quantum realm do not hold in our macroscopic world. For example, we cannot be in two places at the same time, nor can we be in two states simultaneously—both alive and dead like Schrödinger's cat—so there is no reason to think that some of these unorthodox laws apply in our Newtonian domain while others do not. Moreover, even if the future is uncertain and probabilistic, the unfolding of events along a particular path may be so highly likely as to be unalterable by force of will. Unless of course we imagine that the mind can alter events in the quantum realm and influence the location, movement, and energy of subatomic particles, which is improbable and without any known mechanism.

Other compatibilists, desperate to preserve the possibility of free will, have proposed that free will and determinism might coexist through a mechanism called downward causation, whereby complex systems like the weather or the flow of traffic can influence the behavior of its components in ways that cannot be predicted. Similarly, the brain's connections may be so complex that predicting the firing patterns of each of its neurons becomes impossible.

Anyone who gets caught in a surprise downpour after forecasts of a sunny day, or who finds themselves stuck in traffic when their Waze app promised clear roads, realizes that predicting the actions of complex systems is not a perfect science. But just because the weatherman is often wrong doesn't mean that raindrops have free will. And since the brain is infinitely more complex than traffic patterns in the busiest city, it's not surprising that human behavior would be even harder to predict. The inability to predict the future of complex chaotic systems does not erode determinism.

If we accept the fact that human experience is generated entirely by the firing patterns of the neurons in our brains, and if those neurons exist only in the physical world, then how can an immaterial entity, such as the self, influence them? Simply put, it can't. There is no little person inside your head pulling the strings, creating movements, or generating your ideas and or beliefs. You are nothing more than ion fluxes in a sea of chemicals. And what you imagine to be your identity—just like the Ship of Theseus, with its rotting planks—lacks permanence. It exists only for that specific moment in time.

The reductionist view of the brain also raises this question: If the exact wiring pattern of your brain could be reproduced faithfully in a computing machine made of either carbon or silicon, would that then *be you*? The determinist in me answers, first, yes, and then no. Within a millisecond of the creation of this new you, the two yous—merely by occupying two different physical spaces and interacting differently with the universe—would instantaneously diverge into two separate entities.

If I remove a part of your body—let's say an arm or a leg—you obviously remain the same person. But what if I remove the part of your brain that's responsible for recognizing your spouse or for regulating your sense of ethics and morality? If these aspects of your personality change drastically because you undergo brain surgery, are you still the same person? Remember, you look the same and you inhabit the same body.

The determinist in me responds that since you never had an immutable identity, the question makes no sense. If I remove part of your brain and you suddenly turn around and murder your spouse, you are no more or less the same person you were before your murderous rampage than if you caught them cheating with your neighbor and decided to settle the score.

Many of these fundamental questions about who we are and how our mental reality is constructed can be studied by neurosurgeon-scientists during brain operations. These inquisitive neurosurgeons can record from neurons, or make them fire, and see how these physical brain events correlate with human experience. And of all the diseases we treat, there is one, more than any other, that has provided us with the single greatest opportunity to unravel the mysteries of the mind-brain problem. This disease is epilepsy.

THE CASE OF FYODOR MIKHAILOVICH DOSTOEVSKY

Dostoevsky, one of the most widely read Russian authors, was best known for his depictions of the absurdity and tragedy of the human condition, which is not surprising, given his biography. Born in 1821, at sixteen he lost his mother to tuberculosis. Two years later, his father died of a stroke. He found a job as an engineer, a career that brought him little satisfaction. So he turned to writing, expressing his melancholy outlook through his now classic books: *Crime and Punishment, The Idiot,* and *The Brothers Karamazov.*

Dostoevsky had his first seizure when he was seven. In his teen years, his epilepsy progressed. He described his battle with his disease with exquisite revelatory detail in his letters, essays, and novels. Since his death, a great many writers have speculated about Dostoevsky's epilepsy and its impact on the psychological themes he explored in his books. Sigmund Freud's essay "Dostoevsky and Parricide" ascribed the writer's seizures to hysteria rather than to a brain disease. We now know that Dostoevsky suffered from a form of epilepsy called temporal lobe epilepsy, most likely coming from the right side of his brain.

Most striking about Dostoevsky's seizures was that they would begin with feelings of extreme ecstasy and religiosity, filling him with an unwavering conviction of the existence of God. These religious visions were as real to him as reading this book is to you now.

But what if Dostoevsky had lived a thousand years earlier and become a prophet rather than a writer? What if he had used his eloquence to convince us that he had witnessed the presence of God? Indeed, hyper-religiosity is a well-described symptom of a particular form of epilepsy. The phenomenon is so common that it has its own name, Gastaut-Geschwind syndrome, and we even know the location in the brain from which these seizures arise: the right temporal lobe.

Patients with Gastaut-Geschwind syndrome can have a variety of different experiences. These include intuitions of God's presence; the sense of being connected to the infinite; and hearing God's voice or seeing religious figures, such as saints, demons, apostles, and saviors. Other well-described phenomena that can accompany seizures are called autoscopic phenomena, described as the experience of leaving one's own body and viewing it from an external perspective (also called an out-of-body experience). Epileptic visions can also be demonic and include compulsions to commit crimes and even murder. (Did the devil make him do it, or was it a seizure?)

It's even possible to trigger religious convictions by directly stimulating the brain. Wilder Penfield described this very phenomenon in the 1930s. During many of his awake operations, Penfield noted that when he stimulated the temporal lobe, he could trigger what he called "experiential phenomena." The most common of these consisted of reliving a prior experience, as if the brain contained an archive of recordings from the past. Sometimes these memories included religious visions; other times they involved a sense of clairvoyance.

If religious instincts and fortune-telling abilities can be activated through brain stimulation, can they also be deactivated? Again the answer is yes. If seizures can be eliminated with medical treatment, so, too, can religious visions and religious convictions. Imagine, then, what would have happened to Dostoevsky had he lived not one thousand years earlier but a century and a half later, when a few doses of an anti-seizure medication might have alleviated his epilepsy—and extinguished his divine revelations. Would he still have become a writer? Would his books have had the same impact on the Western literary canon? Or would his writing have been even more profound if his mind had not been clouded by his disease?

THE SACRED DISEASE

Neurons in the brain communicate with one another through one of two mechanisms: excitation or inhibition. When a neuron fires a discharge, it sends signals to several other neighboring neurons. These signals, in turn, either excite or inhibit the surrounding neurons, causing them either to fire their own discharge (excitation) or to *not* fire a discharge (inhibition).

In patients with epilepsy, somewhere in their brains, there exists a group of interconnected neurons that has a lower discharge threshold, which means these neurons are more likely to fire. Once these hyperexcitable neurons are set off, the neighboring ones also become excited, creating a chain reaction that spreads through the brain like fire through dry brush, overwhelming the brain's inhibitory restraint mechanisms.

One can imagine a patient with epilepsy as having a desiccated patch of leaves in the forest of their brain, which, if the sun hits it just right, will ignite and spread, taking down even the healthy trees. Unlike the trees in a wildfire, however, neurons completely recover after a seizure with little to no permanent damage (except in the rare instance when the seizure doesn't stop, a condition called status epilepticus).

When a seizure arises in the motor area of the brain, it triggers uncontrolled movements in the body. If a seizure starts in the part of the brain dedicated to language, the patient will not be able to speak. Since seizures can occur in almost any location in the brain, the symptoms of epilepsy can be as varied as the range of human experience. Visual and auditory hallucinations, unusual smells, a sense of déjà vu, heightened anxiety, and even guilt are other well-described epileptic phenomena. These manifestations start independently of the free will of the patient. The patient does not *choose* to have a seizure at that moment, and the resulting behaviors are out of the patient's control.

In its most severe form, a seizure can engulf the entire brain, causing a grand mal seizure. During such an episode, the patient falls to the floor, all four limbs pulsing in uncontrolled rhythmic, paroxysmal movements. A patient having a grand mal seizure will grunt, scream, salivate, and lose control of their bladder. Witnessing such an event for the first time is terrifying, particularly if it happens to someone you know. The disease hijacks the brain's machinery.

Ancient cultures had little understanding of the causes of epilepsy, so they placed its trigger *outside* the body, in the spiritual realm. From their perspective, the same mystical forces that caused the sun to rise or the seasons to change or earthquakes to strike also triggered epileptic fits. Originally called the "falling sickness" or the "sacred disease," patients with epilepsy in ancient times were alternately viewed as being possessed by demons, touched by the divine, or punished for sinful transgressions.

Hippocrates, the ancient Greek father of medicine, was the first to propose—in a moment of early prescience—that seizures might come from the brain. But like so many revolutionary ideas that start out as heresy and then turn out to be true, Hippocrates's theory was promptly refuted and then forgotten, only to be replaced by more popular but misguided ones. Accordingly, early treatments for epilepsy were directed not at the brain but rather at the spiritual world and included the ingestion of a variety of witches' brews with mystically potent ingredients such as seal genitals, hippopotamus testicles, tortoise blood, and crocodile feces—giving new meaning to the saying "Sometimes the treatment is worse than the disease."

In the United States at the time of this writing, 3.5 million people live with epilepsy. Fortunately, the state of medicine has come a long way from those primitive remedies. Two-thirds of patients will respond to any one of over a dozen of our present-day medications. For the nonresponders, however, epilepsy remains a devastating disease. Attacks can occur at any moment, rendering some patients unable to attend school or work. After a seizure, patients remain stuporous for minutes to hours. They emerge disoriented, as if from a deep sleep, sometimes requiring days to recover. Their memories of events surrounding the seizure are erased, leaving gaps that undermine not only the temporal continuity of their experience of reality but the integrity of their sense of self. As the disease progresses, many notice a steady decline in their mental capacity.

The social stigma of epilepsy can be paralyzing. While we no longer believe that epileptics are possessed by demons, the seizures themselves can be so horrifying to witness that people with epilepsy often become increasingly withdrawn and isolated, afraid to leave their homes lest they have a seizure in public. They cannot drive lest they crash. They cannot swim lest they drown. They become so terrified of having a seizure that they generally shy away from taking on any responsibility that might require sustained alertness.

At the beginning of the twentieth century, in several American states, patients with epilepsy were forcibly sterilized. Some states even passed legislation prohibiting epileptics from getting married. Throughout much of the last century, epileptics were often institutionalized and not allowed to attend school. Many had difficulty holding down jobs and were even denied some of the basic human rights that define citizenship.

Outwardly, patients with epilepsy appear normal, but their life expectancy is reduced by roughly ten years. To make matters worse, there is a constant fear of a condition called SUDEP, which stands for "sudden unexplained death in epilepsy." One out of every 1,000 epileptics will suddenly die in their sleep, a result of a seizure impacting the center in the brain that regulates heartbeat and respiration.

But what many people don't know is that there is a cure for some forms of epilepsy. Perhaps not a surprise to anyone at this point, that cure is brain surgery.

THE ALMOND AND THE SEAHORSE

The first surgery for epilepsy was performed in 1886 by Sir Victor Horsley—the same British neurosurgeon who invented stereotactic surgery and attempted the first pituitary surgery. Horsley, born in 1857, was descended from artists on his father's side and physicians on his mother's. Wavering between the two careers, he settled on the latter. After spending a brief stint researching rabies in Paris with Louis Pasteur, Horsley began his career in 1886 at the National Hospital in Queens Square, where he served as its in-house surgeon.

In one of Horsley's first operations, he excised a piece of scar tissue that had built up in the brain of a young man in the wake of a traumatic depressed skull fracture. The injury triggered the onset of seizures, so the precise location in the cerebral cortex requiring removal—located just under the displaced skull bone—was already apparent. The surgery was a success, and the patient's fits were cured.

Horsley was only twenty-nine years old at the time. It's difficult to imagine the bravery it must have taken to attempt such a feat. In 1886 the field of brain surgery did not yet exist, and only a handful of such surgeries had ever been successfully performed. Cushing at that same time was not yet even in college. Horsley subsequently undertook two other epilepsy operations, both of which were successful—a remarkable statistic for that era. His cases inspired several other surgeons, including German neurologist-neurosurgeons Fedor Krause and Otfrid Foerster, to attempt similar operations.

The most difficult aspect of epilepsy surgery was (and remains) locating the initiation site of the seizures, since the epileptic brain often appears completely normal to the surgeon's eye. As a result, most successful surgeries in those early years required that there be traumatic scars in the brain, if only so the surgeon could see where to cut. If no scar were found, the surgeon could try stimulating the brain with electrodes—to trigger seizures—and then to remove those areas of the brain where the stimulation had been effective.

Into this field strode Wilder Penfield, who, as we stated earlier, studied with Krause and Foerster before bringing their techniques back to the United States and then Canada, where he further refined and improved upon them. As the director of the Montreal Neurological Institute, Penfield pioneered the field of epilepsy surgery before the invention of the MRI—meaning that the seizure-triggering area of the brain, unless caused by a tumor or a skull fracture, was unknown. Identifying the precise place in the brain from which the seizures arose was thus a critical first step in any surgery before it could even be offered. This involved a careful interview of the patient with the goal of relating their specific symptoms with the known distribution of those functions in the brain. If patients saw visual hallucinations at the start of their seizures, for example, the visual cortex was the presumed culprit. If abnormal movements or sensations preceded a seizure, then they were likely coming from the brain's motor or sensory areas.

Working with the electrophysiologist Herbert Jasper, Penfield began recording from the surface of the brain with electrodes to find the abnormal discharges, which he knew to be characteristic of diseased epileptic brain. To minimize the known suppressive effect of anesthesia on his patient's brain waves, Penfield would keep them awake during the procedure. Once these abnormal neurons were identified, he could then excise them in an attempt to cure his patients. One conclusion Penfield drew from this work was that not all brain regions were equally prone to cause epilepsy. He quickly noticed that the most common source of seizures was in the temporal lobe. Thus, many of his surgeries involved removal of that specific part of the brain.

But the results of his first temporal lobe surgeries were disappointing. While some patients improved, total relief from all seizure activity was uncommon. An observant scientist, Penfield soon realized that his outcomes were better when he removed two small structures, the amygdala and the hippocampus, which sit in the deepest part of the temporal lobe. At the time, no one had a clue what they did. It was their shape, under the microscope that gave rise to their names. In Greek, *amygdala* means "almond" and *hippocampus* means "seahorse."

Penfield's awake epilepsy operations were widely publicized throughout Canada. In the 1990s, to boost national pride, he was featured as the subject of a short video that highlighted the work of famous Canadians. These vignettes, called "Heritage Minutes," appeared on Canadian television and in movie theaters. In Penfield's segment, the narrator tells the story of a woman with epilepsy who always smelled burnt toast before the onset of her seizures. Such an experience is called an aura, and it generally precedes the onset of a full-blown seizure. Apparently, frequent moviegoers in Canada during that time were often heard joking about that woman who always smelled burnt toast.

The pianist George Gershwin, composer of *Rhapsody in Blue* and *Porgy and Bess,* had similar symptoms near the end of his life, only his were constant: an incessant odor of burnt rubber. Further testing revealed a tumor in his right temporal lobe: a glioblastoma irritating his brain and causing his seizures. By the time doctors discovered the tumor, in 1937, it had progressed to the point of requiring emergency surgery, which was performed at Cedars of Lebanon Hospital (now Cedars-Sinai) in Los Angeles by neurosurgeon Howard Naffziger, who was the chair of surgery at the University of California at the time.

Nafziger had trained with Cushing back when he was still at Johns Hopkins and even served alongside him during World War I. Given both Gershwin's prominence and the dire nature of his situation, Naffziger reached out to Cushing for advice, who, nearing the end of his career, recommended Nafziger contact his former student, Walter Dandy. Dandy was on vacation on a private yacht owned by the governor of Maryland at the time, somewhere in Chesapeake Bay. Eventually, the White House got involved and called in the U.S. Navy, which sent a small ship to retrieve Dandy, bring him ashore, and fly him on a private plane across the country. Alas, by the time Dandy reached Los Angeles and Gershwin, it was too late. Gershwin was too far gone and ultimately expired.

———

Penfield was initially quite conservative with his epilepsy operations. Upon opening the skull and inspecting its surface, if he found no visible evidence of where the seizures might be starting, he would halt the operation for fear of unnecessarily harming the patient. He literally shepherded patients through the ordeal of an awake brain operation and then did absolutely nothing, leaving them not only with a large scar and a monthlong recovery but also little hope for improvement. Moreover, these aborted operations were not uncommon, occurring almost 20 percent of the time.

As it became more evident that the amygdala and hippocampus were the primary offenders in many cases of temporal lobe epilepsy, removing them became routine. Soon Penfield's cure rate rose as his number of abandoned operations declined. But what was the function of these two odd-looking parts of the brain, and how did patients fare once they were removed? Most of his patients' cognitive abilities and personalities were seemingly unchanged after surgery. But how was this possible? Did the amygdala and hippocampus serve no purpose, or had the epilepsy damaged these structures to the point where they were now no longer functional?

This next piece of the puzzle fell into place—not from Penfield's conscientious inquiries, but rather from a surgery performed by a less judicious neurosurgeon named William Beecher Scoville.

JUST A SMALL MEMENTO

THE CASE OF
HENRY GUSTAV MOLAISON ("H.M.")

Henry Gustav Molaison, born in Connecticut in 1926, got into a bad bicycle accident when he was nine. He struck his head and was knocked unconscious. A year later he had his first seizure, which consisted of a forty-second attack during which he seemed to zone out and exhibit what doctors now call automatisms, or repetitive movements, such as the opening and closing of his mouth and the crossing and uncrossing of his legs. These seizures occurred intermittently until he turned sixteen, at which point they took a turn for the worse. He began having frequent generalized tonic-clonic (formerly known as grand mal) seizures, in which he would collapse to the ground in convulsions. In response, his doctors increased the dosages of his anti-seizure medications, but to no avail.

By age twenty-seven, Molaison was no longer able to work. It was at that point that he was sent to the chief of neurosurgery at Hartford Hospital in Connecticut, Dr. William Beecher Scoville. Scoville, a descendant of *Uncle Tom's Cabin* author Harriet Beecher Stowe, had studied at Yale and at the University of Pennsylvania. He obtained his neurosurgical training at Massachusetts General Hospital and then went on to study under James Poppen at the Lahey Clinic and then Walter Dandy at Johns Hopkins. Scoville invented a retractor still used in spine surgery today that bears his name. He's also credited with almost single-handedly founding the largest international neurosurgical society, now called the World Federation of Neurological Surgery.

One of Scoville's other interests, besides spine surgery, was psychosurgery: in other words, the frontal lobotomy. Scoville not only performed the operation, but he also tried to improve it—to enhance its anti-psychotic effects while minimizing its sedating and personality-altering sequalae. With these good intentions, he conceived of a new operation based on little to no experimental evidence. Instead of disconnecting the frontal lobes, as in the frontal lobotomy, Scoville first tried a procedure he called an orbital undercutting, but then he eventually began removing the hippocampus and the amygdala, the same deep parts of the temporal lobe targeted by Penfield during his epilepsy operations.

Scoville was aware of Penfield's pioneering work and the success he'd achieved removing the amygdala and hippocampus to treat epilepsy. So when Henry appeared in his clinic with an unrelenting seizure disorder,

Scoville decided to try on Henry's bike accident–induced seizures an operation he had originally designed to treat mental illness. Scoville mused that if Penfield had some success removing the hippocampus and amygdala on one side of the brain, perhaps removing them on both sides would be even more effective. In Scoville's own words, "This frankly experimental operation was considered justifiable because the patient was totally incapacitated by his seizures, and these had proven [resistant] to a medical approach."

Now, when Penfield performed his hippocampal surgeries, he would record electrical signals directly from the brain and remove only diseased tissue. If abnormal signals were not identified, Penfield would abort. During Scoville's operation on Henry, he, too, took the time to record electrical activity from both hippocampi. But although he failed to notice any abnormal electric discharges typically found in an abnormal epileptic brain, he forged ahead and removed both of Henry's hippocampi.

When Henry awoke from anesthesia, he seemed all right at first. On further examination, however, the effects of Scoville's double hippocampal removal became apparent. Henry was no longer able to form new memories. For example, if Henry met someone new, he could sustain a brief, pleasant conversation. But if his attention was distracted long enough, maybe fifteen to twenty seconds, he'd look back at the same person and see them as if for the first time, completely unaware of the earlier conversation. Henry, in other words, now lived in the eternal present—able to focus only on the current moment, with no sense of the past. He had been transformed into the character played by Guy Pearce in the Christopher Nolan movie *Memento*, who was coincidentally based on Henry.

In the movie, Pearce and his wife are attacked by a mysterious individual. His wife is killed, and Pierce is hit on the head and loses his short-term memory. His character tries to track down his wife's murderer, using clues he leaves for himself: a few short phrases tattooed on his body and a handful of fading photographs on which he has jotted down some helpful notes. Pearce's character—absent his memory—becomes like a leaf blown about by the wind, with no sense of self or free will when he's not following the clues that he'd previously left for himself or that were provided by those around him.

The only silver lining to Scoville's surgical debacle was that it did for memory what Broca and his patient Leborgne did for language. The hippocampus was henceforth proven to be the critical part of the brain responsible for laying down new memories. Since the brain has two hippocampi, one on each side, the loss of only one hippocampus doesn't cause amnesia. This explains why Penfield's unilateral operations were not problematic. Also, it's important to note that injury to both sides—as occurred in Henry's ill-conceived surgery—rarely occurs in nature, given the distance between the two hippocampi, so a *Memento*-like loss in our ability to record memories is quite rare. (That being said, herpes encephalitis, a viral infection of the brain, can be a rare cause of bilateral hippocampal injury.)

To his credit, Scoville asked Penfield's neuropsychologist, Brenda Milner, to examine Henry and try to unravel what exactly had happened to him. From her detailed study, Milner uncovered a fascinating fact about memory. Though Henry could not form any new memories about events or remember facts—which we now call episodic and semantic memory—he could learn new skills. This latter type of memory, called procedural memory, includes the ability to ride a bicycle or play the piano. Procedural memories, we now know, are stored in a separate part of the brain: the cerebellum.

Henry taught the world that there are different kinds of memories, and they are stored in different locations. Henry could practice a skill, like playing the piano or tossing a ring onto a peg, and he could improve over time with no conscious memory of how he had become so adept. He simply had no recollection of his rehearsals. One might conceive of Henry's experience of learning new skills as similar to those of Keanu Reeves's character Neo in the movie *The Matrix*, who downloads into his mind the ability to use kung fu but with no memory of the training.

Milner also discovered that Henry could still recall events from his childhood. But every memory from approximately three years before his surgery until the present moment was lost in an impenetrable fog. We now know the reason that Henry's older memories were preserved while the new ones were lost. The hippocampus, as it turns out, is not the final storage bin for our memories. Rather, it's the archiving mechanism that deposits our experiences into long-term storage, from where they can later be retrieved, another task also performed by the hippocampus.

Henry—or "H.M.," as he was known for the rest of his life to protect his identity—became a lifelong guinea pig. Not only was his injury highly unusual, but he was also the only one of Scoville's patients on whom the double hippocampal removal had been performed that didn't suffer from a severe psychiatric illness, so he was compliant and pleasant. He was institutionalized and scrutinized by generations of psychologists, some of whose careers were devoted entirely to studying him. As far as Henry's seizures were concerned, although they improved for a little while, the relief was short-lived. In retrospect, Henry probably didn't even have temporal lobe epilepsy but rather a form of generalized epilepsy. So the seizures weren't even coming from the parts of the brain that Scoville removed.

After more testing on Henry's brain, another curious fact emerged. Although his childhood memories were still accessible, they were clearly altered. While he could remember specific facts about his past—such as dates, events, and people—he had difficulty recalling them as stories, i.e., as facts and events distributed along a narrative timeline. When asked to describe his mother, for example, his response was "Just that she was my mother." Henry had lost his storytelling ability, which, as we shall explore in greater depth in the next chapter, like memory, is also critical to our sense of self.

Henry was also frozen in time. This, perhaps, was the most fascinating part of his new hippocampus-less world.

Our impression that we are the same person traveling through time is based on our ability to remember our past, which seems unchanged each time we mentally visit it. The feeling that time is passing while we remain constant is created by the continuous stream of events that we place in long-term storage. Our experience of time can even be understood as the sense that our memory banks are constantly filling with new experiences, which we draw upon to create the ever-expanding story of our past lives.

Researchers performed a study to examine Henry's sense of time. They would say, "Go," and then, a few moments later, "Stop," each time varying the interval between the two words. Sometimes it would be five seconds, sometimes a minute. They would then ask Henry to reproduce the same interval with the same words: "go" and "stop." Henry was quite good at it up to about twenty seconds, after which his sense of time completely broke down. The authors of the study concluded that "one hour to us is like 3 minutes to H.M.; one day is like 15 minutes; and one year is equivalent to 3 hours." Time, for Henry, had sped up. If we further extrapolate Henry's time contraction, his remaining fifty-five years of life would have seemed to him like only 165 hours—a mere seven days.

Which begs the question: When Henry looked in the mirror, was he surprised at how rapidly he had aged? This very question was asked of him, to which he responded, "I am not a boy." Like Rip Van Winkle waking up from a decades-long sleep, Henry was surprised to see the effects of time on his face, ravages of years he had no recollection of having lived. Scoville's experimental surgery, in other words, took much more from Henry than his hippocampus and his name.

History has not been kind to Scoville. His own grandson, Luke Dittrich, wrote a book highlighting his grandfather's central role in mutilating Henry's brain. In this remarkable family exposé, *Patient H.M.: A Story of Memory, Madness, and Family Secrets,* Dittrich uncovers evidence that Scoville may even have performed a lobotomy on his own wife (the author's grandmother), who was institutionalized at the time with mental illness. After her diagnosis and confinement, Scoville remarried. Once this first wife had recovered from his surgery, Scoville brought her home, where she passively lived out the rest of her days. Lobotomized, she was no longer bothered by living in the presence of her younger replacement.

Dittrich describes an interview with Henry in which a researcher asked him what he would have wanted to do with his life had he not been mutilated. Henry's response? "I would have liked to become a brain surgeon." When asked why he never pursued this dream, Henry said that he feared he would have made a mistake during surgery and hurt someone. In response to being asked what happened during his own surgery, Henry said that the surgeon must have made some sort of mistake.

But Scoville didn't make a mistake. He performed exactly the surgery he wanted to perform. Although he could have aborted, as Penfield no doubt would have done, he plowed ahead. As a colleague, I may be sympathetic, but I won't provide any excuses for his impulsive decision.

GUNTHER

After my residency was completed, I spent six months as a fellow at Yale New Haven Hospital, under the tutelage of Dr. Dennis Spencer, at the time the Harvey and Kate Cushing Professor of Neurosurgery and chief of Yale's department. Spencer, a tall, soft-spoken man, was known not only as one of the pioneers of epilepsy surgery but also for his unique well-kept appearance, more suited for the cover of a men's magazine than a hospital. Beneath his balding head, he wore small round glasses and maintained a thick white beard and moustache. His favorite accessory to his bespoke dark gray suits was a pocket watch, which he tucked into his front vest pocket. The final touch, a pair of black cowboy boots.

Hailing from a small farming town in Iowa, Spencer commuted daily as a child by horseback to a tiny country school serving only twelve students. Legend has it that he tried to build his own EEG machine at age thirteen. Suffice it to say, he'd come a long way.

Spencer had spent his entire career at Yale and been a resident there decades earlier when the program was still aligned with Hartford Hospital when Scoville was the chief. Spencer had even assisted Scoville in a few lobotomies, which were done on Saturdays, when the staffing was thin, so he could operate under the radar. Spencer remembered Scoville as a daredevil who would race to work in his Mercedes, well above the speed limit, arriving with a tail of police cars. Entering the parking lot at breakneck speed, he would bound up into the lobby and escape into the OR, asking the nurses to let the officers know he was stuck in surgery and indisposed. It was said that he had traveled to Italy to test-drive a Ferrari with Enzo Ferrari himself, who, after watching Scoville drive, refused to sell him the car, fearing that the surgeon "would be dead within a year." But Spencer was also emphatic that Scoville's motivations were always altruistic when it came to his surgeries. Scoville was always trying to do the best for his patients.

I asked Spencer if Scoville had ever spoken about Henry. He told me that Scoville had felt awful about how Henry's surgery turned out and never wanted to discuss it. To highlight Scoville's empathy, Spencer told me the story of a young man named Gunther, who suffered a horrible complication following one of Scoville's spine surgeries that had left Gunther a quadriplegic and unable to communicate.

The cause was neither Scoville's negligence nor his callousness but a rare event called an air embolus. This occurs when air enters the bloodstream, usually through a vein or a venous channel running through the skull that had not been adequately sealed with wax. All neurosurgeons train for such an event because it can occur at any time, during any operation. The most frequent scenario is when a surgery is performed with the patient sitting up, positioned with the head above the heart, which creates negative pressure within the veins.

Gunther was positioned this way, and air got sucked in through an open vein, which traveled up to a part of the brain called the brain stem, where it caused a stroke. The brain stem contains pathways for movement and sensation, all packed closely together. The density of important fibers makes damage to this area particularly devastating. It's called being "locked in," since the patient is essentially a prisoner in their own body—fully conscious but unable to move, feel, or speak.

After leaving Hartford Hospital, Gunther was placed in a nearby long-term care facility to live out the remainder of his life. His wife was so despondent with her husband's disability that she not only divorced him but even tried to kill him at one point.

How did Scoville deal with this tragic accident that had transpired under his watch? Rather than sweep the painful memory aside, Scoville faced his mistake. He would visit Gunther on the weekends for the next several years, just to bring him a few small gifts or to sit by his bedside to keep him company. Complications are not unusual for a busy neurosurgeon and are, unfortunately, a rare but unavoidable part of our business, albeit a part we don't like to discuss. What's unusual, however, was Scoville's ability to sustain his empathy and embrace his error rather than ignore it. Maybe visiting Gunther provided some sense of absolution for what had happened to Henry?

When a complication occurs during an operation, the hardest part of morning rounds is visiting that patient every day and seeing the result of your failure and the devastating consequences it has had on their life. Once their initial shock and disappointment pass, anger and resentment understandably creep into what was previously a sanguine and nurturing relationship. The focus of an injured patient's rage is, naturally, the surgeon, whose hands in some way must have faltered. While our first inclination might be to skip that room on rounds, if only to avoid a gut-wrenching confrontation with both the patient's disappointment and our own inadequacies, that urge must be overcome. This patient, above all others, is the one you must see every day—sometimes twice a day—to show them your concern and to keep the lines of communication open.

Once Gunther was discharged from Hartford Hospital and sent into long-term care, Scoville had no obligation to visit him again. He easily could have spent his weekends rounding on his satisfied patients or racing his cars through the Connecticut countryside rather than dutifully attending to Gunther as he did. Scoville clearly carried several scars with him throughout his life, gashes to his soul that never healed. Scoville is now primarily remembered more for his operation on Henry and his lobotomies, not as much for the retractor he invented. I asked Spencer what percent of Scoville's cases were lobotomies. His answer? "Less than five percent."

It may not be fair, but we are often judged more by our failures than by our successes.

When a neurosurgeon embarks on an operation, based on a hypothesis, and then convinces themselves, the patient, and their family that this is the proper course of action to solve the problem at hand, it can be difficult to suddenly change directions so late in the game. Mindset inertia can override cognitive nimbleness. When the unexpected occurs, if one remains humble and introspective, it is possible to pivot—right there on the spot—and pursue an alternative tactic that will lead to success, or at least mitigate the damage.

It is rare for a surgeon to completely abort an operation and close the head without doing anything. We even have a phrase for that: it's called a "peek and shriek," the implication being that the neurosurgeon was overly ambitious and tried to tackle a case for which they were not adequately prepared. When they saw what they were facing, they hightailed it out of there.

Think of it this way: if you are trying to summit Everest and the weather is nasty, sometimes the right decision is to cut your losses and return to base camp. But if you show up without the right equipment and training, you probably shouldn't have started the expedition in the first place.

When a neurosurgeon decides mid-operation that the best course of action is to abort, the resulting scar on the patient's head and the new divots in their skull serve as a constant reminder of the surgeon's misjudgment. At the same time, abandoning an operation because proceeding would likely do more harm than good not only shows self-awareness but puts the patient's interests first.

However, there are other reasons that a surgeon might abandon an operation in midstream.

I was once operating on a young woman, a mother of three, with epilepsy who had been suffering with seizures for most of her life. She wanted to be able to drive her children to school, to spend time with them and their friends without worrying that, at any moment, she might collapse to the ground and convulse, a situation that would not only embarrass her family but also frighten everyone present. She knew the risks of the operation she'd asked me to perform, but she also felt that she couldn't live this way anymore. The medications, which she was taking in ever-increasing doses, were making her sleepy and preventing her from working.

I planned a two-stage operation. In the first, I would incise a skin flap, open her skull, and then implant dozens of electrodes on and in her brain, encircling the presumed area that I thought was causing her seizures. The wires from the electrodes would then get tunneled through her scalp, and her removed skull bone would be replaced and the skin flap sutured shut. Once she was awake and in a hospital bed, these wires would then get hooked up to a computer to record her brain waves while we waited for her to have a seizure, which would, hopefully, provide me with a map of their site of origin. The plan was to do a second operation a few days later, in which I would remove the electrodes as well as any abnormal brain that might be triggering her seizures. In contrast to Penfield's surgery, where electrical recordings were briefly performed *in* the operating room, I had learned this alternative long-term recording strategy from Dr. Spencer at Yale.

We started the first of my patient's two operations and everything was going smoothly. The skin flap was opened and her craniotomy proceeded without a hitch. I was about to open the dura, the brain's thick, membranous covering, when I noticed that it seemed to be bulging out like an overfilled water balloon ready to burst.

I gently placed my forefinger on the timpani-tight dura. Normally, the dura would either be soft or maybe give a slight bit of resistance, but what I was feeling was *not* normal. It indicated that the pressure in her brain was unusually high. If I tried to take the next step and open the dura now, the brain would squeeze its way out like toothpaste, which would not only cause damage but also make it impossible for me to place the electrodes as planned.

I quickly ran through the list of possible causes for this sudden increase in pressure. Had a hemorrhage occurred? What else could possibly be going on? Was the patient waking up too soon? I ran through a mental checklist of possible causes. Her blood pressure was not that high. Her heart rate was normal. She was deep under anesthesia. Check, check, check. I called for the ultrasound—a pencil-like probe that allows us to see through the dura using sound waves, like a fetal ultrasound. I was looking for a blood clot, but the image I saw on the screen appeared unremarkable. Everything looked as expected—everything, that is, except the dura, which was extremely *not* normal.

So I decided to abort. I replaced the bone, closed the skin, wrapped the patient's head in a bandage, and woke her up.

She emerged from anesthesia perfectly—completely and utterly normal. I ordered a bunch of tests, which came back pristine. (To this day, I still don't know what happened or why the dura was so tense.)

Now I had to decide what to do next. Should I just give up on the surgery and her chance of a cure? Was it just not meant to be? Or should I give it another shot? Would she even trust me at this point?

In my mind, the decision was clear: I wanted another shot. Since I had no idea what had happened the first time, I had no reason to think it would happen again. Now all I had to do was to convince her and her family to let me give it a second try.

Not surprisingly, they had their reservations: "How do you know that what happened before won't happen again?" I didn't. But precisely *because* I hadn't found a cause, I had no reason to believe that this highly atypical event would repeat itself. I also knew that surgery was her best chance to stop her epilepsy, and I, for one, was not willing to give up so easily.

A few days later I took her back to the operating room and reopened the skin and the bone flap, using the same anesthesiologist, who gave her the same medications. To my relief, her dura was slack, and we proceeded with the operation. We implanted the electrodes, metaphorically erecting a fence around the presumed site of her seizures, as if corralling a wild stallion.

Sure enough, after a week the patient had three seizures, all originating in her hippocampus. This was a great sign, since hippocampal epilepsy is the most curable. We brought her back to the operating room, took out the electrodes, and working under the microscope for a few hours (just as Yaşargil taught us), carefully removed her hippocampus and her amygdala, the parts of the brain Penfield discovered to be the cause of most temporal lobe epilepsies. She woke up in perfect condition, went home a few days later, and has never had another seizure since.

FIFTEEN

WE TELL OURSELVES STORIES
IN ORDER TO LIVE

One of the basic organizing principles of the brain is that of crossed control. Simply put, the left side of the brain controls the right side of the body, and the right side controls the left. Yet such a description does not do full justice to the degree of separation between the brain's two hemispheres.

Although we may imagine we have a single brain, in truth our brain is divided into two completely independent hemi-brains, each a mirror image of the other, each capable of independent thought. Not only is one hemisphere of the brain able to control the other half of the body, but it can also think, feel, analyze, believe, and act on its own. In fact, sometimes the two hemispheres of the brain can, in a sense, be at war with each other, like the devil and the angel whispering contradictory suggestions into each ear (although this analogy is misleading, since it presumes that you and your brain are two different things).

Our consciousness, then, is fashioned out of a minimum of two separate but independent brains. More accurately, we are segmented into dozens if not hundreds of segregated mini brains. How do we know this? Because of an operation neurosurgeons perform called a corpus callosotomy, named for the corpus callosum, the thick fiber bundle that connects the two sides of the brain, which can be transected to prevent seizures from spreading from one hemisphere to the other.

The corpus callosum is like the fiber-optic cables that cross the Atlantic, connecting the United States with Europe: a superhighway for information. Its function is to ensure that any data processed on one side of the brain becomes immediately available to the other. Our natural assumption is that the callosum unifies our consciousness and therefore, without it, our minds would fracture into two separate conflicting identities, like a patient with a split personality disorder. So, what happens when a neurosurgeon disconnects the two hemispheres? Does the surgery cleave the individual's personality into two? Does all sense of self disintegrate? Or does a battle erupt for control?

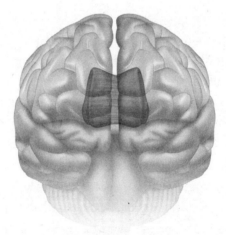

The human brain viewed from the front with the corpus callosum, connecting the two hemispheres, highlighted in dark gray.

William P. Van Wagenen—or Van, as he was better known—was born in 1897 in Nunda, a small rural town in upstate New York. The son of a farmer, he attended Cornell University and Harvard Medical School on scholarships before studying neurosurgery under Harvey Cushing at the

Peter Bent Brigham Hospital in Boston. Van Wagenen was the lucky recipient of both Cushing's advice and financial support, which allowed him to head to Europe to study pathology and physiology in Germany, after which he settled down near his hometown to establish the department of neurosurgery at the University of Rochester.

In the 1920s, when Van began his practice, the morbidity and mortality of his profession were disturbingly high. He therefore often struggled with the uncertainty of his surgeries. Van's niece, Marjorie Dessauer, recalled one evening, after her uncle returned home from a long day in the hospital, hearing him utter the infamous phrase so typical of that era: "Operation successful, patient died."

Van, the only neurosurgeon in town, was often overwhelmed with the work. A researcher at heart, he was also a keen observer of his patients' symptoms and kept a sharp lookout for unusual cases that might help him understand how diseases of the brain impact its functions. He noticed that a few of his patients—specifically, those with brain tumors causing epileptic seizures—experienced a reduction in the frequency of their seizures when their tumors grew into the corpus callosum. The bigger the tumors got and the more they obliterated the corpus callosum, the more infrequent the patients' seizures became. Inspired by this puzzling phenomenon, he figured he might as well try cutting the corpus callosum in one of his epileptic patients who didn't have a brain tumor to see if it might help. Walter Dandy had already shown that it was possible to divide the back part of the corpus collosum, a procedure he developed to reach tumors deep in the brain, near the pineal gland. So Van went ahead and tried it, and, sure enough, it seemed to work.

The first few patients to undergo Van's callosotomy all noticed some degree of improvement in their seizures. More remarkably, none of them were even remotely aware that their brains had been bifurcated. They remembered having the surgery but came through it cognitively unscathed. To the casual eye, their personalities were also unaffected.

A few years later, in 1936, Van published his results. The mechanism, he surmised, was that the operation prevented seizures from spreading from one half of the brain to the other. Despite its apparent success, the operation was still viewed with skepticism by mainstream neurosurgery. Cleaving the brain in two just sounded too radical. Like Irving Cooper's thalamotomy or the transnasal approach to brain tumors, the idea was so at odds with conventional wisdom as to appear heretical.

It wasn't until almost two decades later that the potential of the corpus callosotomy was fully appreciated when another neurosurgeon, Joseph Bogen, reintroduced the operation to the world. Bogen had worked as a graduate research assistant at Caltech, where he was exposed to the work of the psychologist Roger Wolcott Sperry. Sperry's lab was studying the effect of dividing the corpus callosum in cats, and he found, as with Van's patients, that the animals appeared to behave as if nothing had happened. After careful testing, however, Sperry was able to demonstrate that if one looked closely enough, something had, indeed, occurred. Once cut off from its counterpart, each identical twin hemisphere of a cat's brain was capable of processing information independently of the other.

Bogen wondered if the two hemispheres of the human brain could also act autonomously if split apart. He decided that the only way to find out would be to repeat Sperry's cat experiments on human subjects. He dredged up Van Wagenen's original papers from the library and learned that the corpus callosotomy had been a reasonably effective treatment for epilepsy. Bogen thought that if he could find the right patient, he could justify doing the procedure and put the question to the test. Once the surgery was done, he could then enlist Sperry to ascertain whether what held true for cats also held true for humans. After all, while the bisected brains of cats could teach us a lot about the role of the hemispheres in movement or visual processing, they couldn't really get to the more interesting questions about consciousness or personality. You can't exactly ask a cat how it feels or what it's thinking. For these types of experiments, you needed human subjects.

The only catch was that Bogen was still a resident in training at the time. Besides the fact that he didn't have any patients of his own, he was still only learning how to operate. So Bogen had to convince his chief, Phil Vogel, the head of neurosurgery at White Memorial Hospital in Los

Angeles, to try it. Bogen even found the first subject, William Jenkins, who had been admitted through the emergency room with uncontrolled epilepsy. Bogen just happened to be on call the night Jenkins arrived.

W.J., as he became known in the medical literature, was a former World War II paratrooper whose seizures began after a German soldier smacked him in the head with the butt of a rifle. Bogen and Vogel practiced the surgery on a few cadavers before attempting the first operation on Jenkins. The operation, which took place in 1962, proceeded without a hitch. After Jenkins recovered, Bogen was relieved to find that, just as with Van Wagenen's patients, Jenkin's personality and memory appeared unchanged. Even better, his seizures got dramatically better. Based on this first successful experiment, Bogen and White went on to perform callosotomies on dozens more patients, each of whom were studied by Sperry and his graduate student at the time, a young PhD candidate named Michael Gazzaniga.

Just as the neuropsychologist Brenda Milner had done with H.M., Sperry and Gazzaniga intensively scrutinized Bogen's patients with careful cognitive tests. Their work, unraveling the consequences of the split-brain operations, won Sperry a Nobel Prize in 1981. In fact, these experiments, perhaps more than any others, have provided neuroscientists with an understanding of how the mind forms from the brain. But had it not been for Joe Bogen, who originally brought the idea to Sperry, it's unclear if the corpus callosotomy operation would have ever been revived. Gazzaniga writes about Bogen's critical role in initiating this line of research, simply stating, "It was he who launched the project." Without Bogen (and Van Wagenen before him), the split-brain studies might never have occurred, and we might still have little grasp of the distinct characteristics of the left and right hemispheres of the human brain.

But, mind you, the popular conception that analytical people are left-brained and creative people are right-brained is *not* firmly grounded in Sperry and Gazzaniga's results. Nor is it true. This convenient framework, which has been fed to and then absorbed by the public, is an oversimplified and inaccurate interpretation of their findings. What Sperry, Bogen, and Gazzaniga really uncovered was far more mind-blowing.

Splitting the human brain does not divide the personality. People with cleaved brains still act the same. They have no idea that the two halves of their brains are no longer in communication. This result, by itself, is already remarkable. Imagine taking a sophisticated machine like the human brain, with its billions of components, and slashing its most dense cable bundle, which ferries enormous amounts of information between its most critical components, and the result is—wait for it—nothing. Sure, a certain amount of redundancy in the system to keep the brain working, even if a few parts break down, makes some sense. But this much?

The reality is that while split-brain patients do not notice, in their day-to-day lives postsurgery, that the architecture underlying their essence has been dramatically altered, they are not quite the same as they were before. And teasing out these differences earned Sperry the Nobel.

Each half of the human brain, Sperry noted, can independently process information, draw its own conclusions, and control the behavior of the opposite side of the body. This was also true of cats. But how is it possible that we have two independent brains working simultaneously and autonomously and yet we still perceive the world as a unified self? If the brain is the substrate of the mind, then two brains should equal two minds and two selves. It's simple math, right?

The answer is that the corpus callosum and the connections it provides between the two hemispheres of the brain are completely irrelevant to our sense of self.

Even with an intact corpus callosum, the brain comprises not only two but rather *multiple* independent modules, each of which processes information separately, maintains its own beliefs and desires, and influences behavior. The corpus callosum merely improves the integration of each module's decisions and then ferries all that information over to the dominant left hemisphere, which, according to Gazzaniga, interprets the information and generates a coherent story to make sense of it all.

Gazzaniga, who founded the field of cognitive neuroscience after relocating to the department of neurology at Cornell Medical School, is currently the director of the SAGE Center for the Study of the Mind in

Santa Barbara. He has written several books describing the split-brain experiments and elucidating his theory.

Using a device called a tachistoscope, Gazzaniga was able to show images to only one or the other half of his subject's brains after Bogen and White had divided them. In one experiment, he showed a picture of a snow scene to the patient's right brain but not the left. Since the right hemisphere has no language ability, the subject was unaware of what their right hemisphere had seen. If asked, they would have denied they were shown anything.

Simultaneous with the snow scene, a picture of a chicken's claw was presented to the left hemisphere. His subjects *could* describe the chicken claw, since language abilities are housed in the left hemisphere. When asked what they saw when the claw was shown to the left half of their brains, his subjects responded appropriately: a chicken claw. The subjects were then shown a few pictures of various objects and asked to choose the one most related to what they had just seen by pointing at it either with the right hand or the left, each of which, as we know, is controlled by the opposite hemisphere.

So what happened? The right hand, which is controlled by the left language-bearing hemisphere, correctly pointed to the picture of the claw, because it saw the claw image. The left hand, controlled by the non-lingual right hemisphere—the side which saw the snow scene but could not express what it had seen since it possesses no language abilities—correctly pointed to the picture of the shovel. Remember, in these studies, each hemisphere is also oblivious to what the other hemisphere has seen. When one of Gazzaniga's subjects was asked why they had pointed to two different images, one hand pointing to the chicken claw and the other hand to the shovel, they responded as if it were obvious, "The chicken claw goes with the chicken, and you need a shovel to clean out the chicken shed!"

Since the left language-bearing hemisphere was unaware that it had been shown a snow scene, it needed to fabricate a reason why the left hand was pointing to a shovel after being shown a chicken claw. In other words, the subject's left hemisphere was observing the right hemisphere's independent actions and, since they were under the illusion that they were a unified self, fabricated a logical explanation. They *made up a story* to explain their strange behavior, which had been motivated by the subconscious processing of the snow scene that was shown to the right hemisphere. Remember, the image of the wintry landscape never even entered the subject's conscious awareness, since the information could not cross the missing corpus callosum and reach the left side.

This idea—that the motivation for our behaviors might emerge from subconscious processing that occurs below the level of our awareness—is disquieting, to say the least. It implies that our behaviors are controlled not by us, not by a volitional self, but by autonomous sub-compartments within our brains. Which also implies that, in an eerily real and verifiable sense, we lack control over at least some of our behaviors, and perhaps all of them—not because we are robots or puppets but because we are aware of only a minute amount of the work our brains are doing at any given moment. Most of the brain's deliberations occur under the radar. Who we *think* we are is but a small fraction of who we *really* are.

That we then retroactively fabricate stories to justify our behaviors is also unnerving, since it means that we may be constantly fooling ourselves into believing that our behaviors are self-motivated and that we have free will. Yet this model of brain organization appears to be one of its most fundamental organizing principles. Having been raised in a psychoanalytic household, aware of the invisible powers of what Freud described as the unconscious mind, I am perhaps less shocked than most by all of this.

Here is another example: if Gazzaniga showed a scary image to the right brain, by flashing it quickly off to the patient's left, the subject would say they saw nothing, since the information never reached the left side of the brain, where language resides. Yet, when questioned about how they were feeling, the subject would say they felt afraid. When asked *why* they felt afraid, they might initially claim they had no idea, but soon enough they'd start making up reasons. They might claim they suddenly felt they couldn't trust Gazzaniga, or they'd claim they were worried their elderly father was going to die. In other words, once their left, language-producing hemisphere got involved, the subjects would create a false narrative to make sense of their emotion, as if the feeling of fear was internally generated—even though it had been planted in their right hemisphere by Gazzaniga.

This impulse—to find cause and effect and create a logical and coherent story out of our autonomous behaviors—was one of Gazzaniga's most startling discoveries. He demonstrated, in the lab with human subjects, that our narrating modules—our *false* narrators, if you will—are situated in the left hemisphere, and their sole function is to make sense out of chaos: to generate a fable of autonomy and the illusion of free will.

Gazzaniga called this brain process the "Interpreter," but it could just as easily be called the "Editor" or even the "Storyteller." Human consciousness may be nothing more than what it is like to have a brain composed of multiple subconscious modules that control our behaviors while another module, quill in hand, becomes our own personal Shakespeare, busily composing compelling but ultimately fabricated narratives to make sense of our behaviors.

Did I choose to become a neurosurgeon from an Oedipal urge to one-up my father the psychoanalyst? Perhaps. That story could make sense. Or did I imagine that a career in neurosurgery might provide me with a certain status in society so I could enjoy a sense of safety that my mother, the Holocaust survivor, never felt? Sure. That's a good story, too. Or did I really have no choice in the matter, as a puppet of a myriad of programmed and constantly updating algorithms running in my brain's CPU? Clearly, I am arguing for the latter, but this is most certainly *not how I feel*. On the other hand, did my upbringing impact the organization and the circuitry of my brain? Certainly, but my autobiographical descriptions do not truly describe what's really going on and may, in the end, be completely inaccurate. In a very real sense, we all have our own built-in personal biographer on retainer whose job it is to keep the timeline of our life stories tight, the plot plausible, and the action moving forward—only the writing style is fiction, not journalism.

THE WIZARD OF I

The feeling that we go through life as the captain of our own ship, capable of making our own decisions and directing our behaviors, seems as obvious to us as any belief we hold dear. Yet the illusion of a single unified commanding self may just be an adaptive byproduct of evolution. We feel like there is an "I" in charge because it's useful for us to feel this way. What better way to ensure that the physical package carrying and protecting our DNA—namely, our bodies—survives long enough to pass on that code to the next generation, other than to make us feel unique and that our purpose in life has some sort of higher meaning?

As we already discussed, most of the brain's processing unfolds subconsciously, performed by a multitude of smaller modules. They each make their own calculations, spit out an independent solution—suggestions for what to do or how to think—each of which is compared to all other options, and then the winning idea leads to a specific choice or behavior. You can think of it as a Darwinian survival-of-the-fittest idea. Once the choice is made or the behavior occurs—the person you marry, the career to pursue, or merely what you are going to eat for breakfast that day—the brain creates an after-the-fact illusion that the winning idea was intended all along.

This concept may seem contrary to common sense, but let's think about it for a minute. We don't really know how or why ideas pop into our heads when we think a thought. Most ideas just appear. We *experience* our thoughts, and then we imagine that we created them. If I ask you to think of five books you have read, you could probably generate a list. But why did you choose those specific books and not five others? And why did you choose them in that specific order? The truth is that you don't really know. Maybe you visualized their covers or you remembered a plot point, but each title just emerged into your consciousness from out of nowhere.

Further neurosurgical evidence supporting this model of brain organization can also be found in a set of experiments performed decades ago by the Spanish neurophysiologist José Manuel Rodríguez Delgado, the scientist working at Yale who stopped the charging bull with his stimoceiver. In the 1950s, Delgado enlisted the help of two MGH neurosurgeons, William H. Sweet and Paul Chapman, to implant his stimoceivers into a few human patients to treat schizophrenia and epilepsy. In one of these patients, the stimoceiver triggered an involuntary head turn. Unbeknownst to the patient, each time Delgado pushed the button and the electrode stimulated their brain, their head would turn slightly to the side.

When asked why he was turning his head, the patient would create a story to justify his action, as if Delgado were not the puppeteer pulling the strings. "I'm looking for my slippers," he would say, or "I heard a noise," or "I'm restless." The patient unconsciously tried to convert his involuntary actions into intentional ones. This is just another example of Gazzaniga's Interpreter module in action. After we experience our body doing something, whether triggered spontaneously from a module within our brain or externally by an electrode, we fashion a story that ascribes free will to the behavior.

Brain modules can communicate with each other in two different ways: either internally, using the brain's circuitry, or externally, by providing cues to other modules via the body. The internal messaging system, of which the corpus callosum is just one of many fiber bundles, connects modules into larger networks, which are distributed throughout the four lobes on both sides of the brain. These networks process information in two distinct ways: serially—meaning they extract simple features first and then pass the information on to the next level, where more complex integration occurs—and in parallel, meaning that several networks are working simultaneously on the same bits of information.

Modules also communicate with each other externally through our behaviors, such as subtly turning the head or moving the hand or making a quick glance to the side. These movements, which go unnoticed to all but the most careful of observers, can be picked up by other internal brain modules, which sense them and then process the information. Gazzaniga called this process "cuing," since one module in the brain gives a physical cue to another.

External cuing is going on constantly; we're just clueless about it. Modules in our brain communicate with each other using the body to telegraph ideas. If you are a gambler who can read another person's tells or a wife who sensed her husband was cheating simply by the way his eye twitched that one time, you've experienced the power of unconscious cuing to advertise hidden thoughts or feelings to anyone, or to any brain module, sensitive enough to pick them up.

Here's an example of how our brain's modules might interact with one another: if you were having a conversation with a friend, your interpretation of their facial expressions and their emotional state draws on networks housed in your right hemisphere. Making sense of the actual words and sentences they are speaking, however, engages networks lateralized more heavily on the left side of your brain. To put it all together, you need to integrate both networks. In a normal person, the corpus callosum unifies these geographically separate networks. For the split-brain patient, however, external cuing plays a bigger role, since their callosum is absent.

Depending on the task at hand, certain of the brain's networks may be more or less important than others in processing and unifying a complex behavior, but most activities will simultaneously engage multiple networks that must work together. There does not appear to be a "master" hemisphere, nor a master module surrounded by subservient ones, or emissaries, as has been hypothesized. Instead, the brain's organization runs more like a democratic assembly of differentially specialized modules and networks, each constantly speaking with and debating against its partners to advance the overall interests of the republic. As the demands of the task shift, the dominance of the network specialized for that task also shifts. Like any complex organization, it houses many specialized departments: one dedicated to manufacturing, others to production, marketing, sales, and research. The only difference is that the brain lacks a CEO. However, we create the Oz-like illusion of a capable CEO—the "I" of us—at the head of Me, Inc., to lull everyone, including ourselves, into the false sense that a strong figure stands at the helm of our organization, making smart decisions.

Modules themselves are made up of dozens of smaller units, called cortical columns, a discovery first made in 1978 by neurobiologist Vernon Mountcastle, while working at Johns Hopkins. Each of these columns, in turn, consists of several thousand neurons. The idea that the brain contains some 150,000 identically wired microchips, like a bowl full of jelly beans, was nicely summarized by Jeff Hawkins in *A Thousand Brains: A New Theory of Intelligence*. Hawkins describes how each of these small, identical processing units absorbs sensory information, analyzes the data, and then produces an output. At any given moment, these columns are busy at work, independently calculating, generating maps of the outside world, making predictions about what to expect, reacting to experiences, and then adjusting their maps and generating more data. The information produced by each column is fed into the larger modules, which in turn interact with other connected modules in its network.

If we reverse engineer the brain's organization, the implication is that when we are born, the neocortex, containing the brain's neurons, is composed of a relatively homogeneous sea of identical microchips ready to start processing. The final organization—modules connected into widely distributed networks that perform both serial and parallel processing of information—is created from the inputs that flow into the brain during the first years of life, when the brain is still capable of a remarkable amount of reorganization.

This rewiring ability, called plasticity, not only allows the brain to develop during childhood but also forms the basis of learning throughout life. Information flows into specific areas of the brain through our hardwired sensory nerves—visual information into the occipital lobe, auditory information into the temporal lobe, and sensory information into the parietal lobe. Internally generated data from the body also creates sensations such as hunger, fear, pain, and anxiety, which bombard the brain with more inputs.

Together, these data streams modify the connections in the neocortex, which transforms the previously homogenous bowl of identical microchips into a structured organ whose wiring diagram becomes increasingly complex, eventually looking like a map of the New York City subway system on steroids. All of this occurs mostly before age six, although some reorganizing can still take place for a few more years. After a while, to continue the computer analogy, the motherboard is at capacity, so it can't fit in any more expansion units. You can still load new software and store new documents, but the hardware is fixed.

But the slate of the neocortex is not completely blank at birth. Some connections are pre-wired, both by our genetics and by hundreds of thousands of years of evolution. Take our fear of snakes and other predators, along with—according to Noam Chomsky, for one—our ability to learn language. But, for the most part, the infant brain is incredibly flexible and programmable. This malleability is perhaps most evident through another surgery done for epilepsy called the hemispherectomy, in which a neurosurgeon removes an entire half of the epileptic's brain.

If we go back to our dry-leaves-in-the-forest metaphor as the trigger for an epileptic seizure, in some such situations, mostly in young children, the tinderbox of dehydrated undergrowth lies not just in one small area of the brain, like the hippocampus, but threatens an entire hemisphere. In other words, half of the forest is desiccated and ready to explode into a giant conflagration, and one small spark can set the whole thing off.

The hemispherectomy operation differs from the corpus callosotomy in that, in the former, the neurosurgeon removes half the brain, while in the latter, the two hemispheres are divided but remain in place. We perform a hemispherectomy on our epileptic patients only if all their seizures are coming from one—and only one—hemisphere. The result is usually a total relief of seizures: in other words, a cure. Meanwhile, the corpus callosotomy is *not* intended as a cure but rather to prevent the spread of seizures from one side of the brain to the other, thus preventing localized seizures from becoming generalized.

Children in whom an entire hemisphere is diseased are often impaired: weak on the side of their bodies contralateral to the damaged brain. If the problem strikes the left side of the brain, their language development may be delayed. The treatment for this devastating situation is as radical as the affliction, which is to surgically remove half the brain. While a hemispherectomy may sound like a barbaric operation, without this treatment the child would be sentenced to a life of uncontrolled seizures. The healthy hemisphere would be constantly bombarded by a barrage of electrical surges from its diseased twin, and it would therefore never have a chance to develop normally.

The hemispherectomy was originally conceived of as a treatment for malignant brain tumors by Walter Dandy in 1928, which, as we discussed, proved ineffective. The first hemispherectomy performed specifically for epilepsy was completed in 1938 at the hands of Canadian neurosurgeon Kenneth G. McKenzie. After spending a year training with Harvey Cushing, McKenzie became Canada's first surgeon to specialize in neurosurgery. His first patient, a young girl of sixteen at the time of her operation, had been born prematurely. During her delivery, the right half of her brain was injured, leaving her both paralyzed on the left side of her body and suffering from frequent, uncontrolled seizures, all of which originated in the damaged right hemisphere. When the seizures became so severe that she had to leave school, McKenzie offered to perform a hemispherectomy. The operation was so successful that she was soon able to stop taking her medications and eventually returned to a relatively normal existence. Since then, this life-altering operation has undergone some technical modifications, but the end result remains the same: a person with only one rather than two halves of their brain.

So what happens to a child who loses half their brain? Remarkably, cognitive, emotional, and behavioral development is almost completely unchanged by this radical surgery. Occasionally, motor abilities regress slightly on the side of the body opposite the hemispherectomy, particularly if the hemispherectomy is performed after age ten, when the brain is less plastic, but the rest of the brain's higher-level processing abilities—the patient's mind, if you will—remains mostly intact. The fact that a hemispherectomy patient feels the same *after* their operation is even more mind-bending than the fact of the callosotomy patient being unaware that their brain was cleaved in two. Would the space shuttle still fly if you removed half its components? No way. Not a chance.

Studies have shown that once the hemispherectomy is complete, the remaining hemisphere *develops much faster* than if the surgery hadn't been performed. But if the mind and the brain are the same, why don't these patients have half a mind? Because, as we have discussed, a mind is not a physical object. It's a concept, just like justice or peace or honesty, none of which can be cleaved with a scalpel.

Hemispherectomy patients reorganize their brains. They use what modules they still possess to create new networks. In fact, their remaining hemisphere becomes more interconnected than would a normal brain. Their plasticity goes into overdrive. So long as there are enough modules in the one remaining hemisphere, and the storyteller module can develop, the hemispherectomy patient can create an illusory self using whatever remaining brain machinery is still in place.

You and I will never know what it's like to live with one hemisphere, just as we will never know what it's like to have our brains split or what it's like to experience the world through any other person's eyes. We will only ever know what it is like to be ourselves, using however many neurons we happen to have at our disposal at the time.

DEUS EX MACHINA

If you are still not entirely convinced that free will may be an illusion, here are some other examples of experiments done during a neurosurgical operation that may prove more convincing. Around 1983, a neuroscientist named Benjamin Libet, working at the University of California, San Francisco, formed a partnership with neurosurgeons Bertram Feinstein* and Grant Levin. Together they performed a series of experiments at Mount Zion Hospital in San Francisco. The results and their interpretation are still being debated to this day.

Here is the crux of their first experiment: Feinstein was doing a surgery for Parkinson's disease, in which the patient was awake and able to communicate. Meanwhile, Libet would touch the patient's hand—tickling it with a feather or poking it with a pin. At the same moment as the tickle, Feinstein would stimulate the part of the brain that processes sensation. Libet would then ask the patients which sensation they felt first, the feather tickle or the brain stimulation.

Libet knew how long it took for each of these stimulations to reach conscious awareness when done independently. The stimulation of the brain should have been felt very quickly, while the pinprick or tickling of the hand should have been delayed, needing to travel up the arm, across a synapse or two, and into the brain before being recognized. He discovered that, contrary to what he expected, patients always felt the object touching their hand first, well before the sensation triggered by the brain stimulation. In fact, it wasn't even close.

Many different interpretations of these experiments have been suggested, but Libet's explanation for this mental time warp was that the patient's brain fooled the patient into thinking the tickling occurred before its neuronal signals reached the brain, essentially rewinding the brain's internal clock backward by a few hundred milliseconds. In Libet's words, the brain "refer[red] the sensation back in time," which misled the patient into believing that the event happened prior to the moment when the brain processed the incoming signals.

---

*Bert Feinstein, who trained in Canada with Wilder Penfield, was at the time married to Dianne Feinstein, the future mayor of San Francisco and Democratic senator from California.

Libet's experiments, like Gazzaniga's, show the brain plays tricks on the mind, reordering the timing of our perceptions to create a story that ultimately makes sense. Try this. Put your arms straight out in front of you. Now tickle your left index finger with your right one. Pay attention to when you *see* the fingers touch and compare that moment to when you *feel* them touch. Both the sight and the feeling seem to occur simultaneously. But if you think about it, there must be a delay between when the fingers touch and when the sensation reaches your brain.

After the touch receptors in your finger fire, the signals travel up your arm, across a synapse, into your spinal cord, and then into your brain, where more synapses are crossed until a large enough group of neurons in your sensory cortex are activated to achieve conscious perception. For you to see the fingers touching, in contrast, the photons from the event travel at the speed of light and hit your eye, where they activate neurons in your retina, which then send the signals back through a synapse in your thalamus into your visual cortex, where the image is processed. Is it possible that the timing of these two very different yet quite complex events is identical? Probably not. Yet they seem both instantaneous and simultaneous.

One of the most fundamental rules of the physical world is the temporal sequence of cause and effect. Our brains are wired to presume that all effects have causes. If no cause is obvious, we make one up. We perceive the march of time as linear and methodical, but our brains may be artifactually speeding up or slowing down time to create the illusion of a stable temporal metronome. As you recall, H.M. had lost his internal metronome, after having both his hippocampi removed, and so time for him marched at a different pace than it does for the rest of us.

Libet performed another experiment in which he examined the question of free will. Back in the 1960s, Hans Helmut Kornhuber and Lüder Deecke at the University of Freiberg described a phenomenon called the *Bereitschaftspotential*, or "readiness potential." Basically, if you record brain waves from a part of the brain called the supplementary motor area, or SMA, while asking a subject to move their finger—or perform any motor task—those recordings will show that the neurons begin to fire a few hundred milliseconds before the movement occurs. This finding is not that surprising, since the decision to move your finger should happen before its actual movement, as a matter of common sense. The early brain activity reflects the moment you make the decision and prepare to move, but before you actually move.

Libet recorded the readiness potential with scalp electrodes while his subjects looked at the second hand of a clock, to make a note of the moment when they consciously decided to move their finger—to set a time stamp of the onset of their conscious decision to move. When Libet compared the moment that they decided to move with the readiness potential, he found that the readiness potential preceded not only the physical movement *but even the conscious decision to initiate the movement.* Again, it wasn't even close: the brain's electrical activity occurred a few hundred milliseconds before the subjects decided to move.

The implication is that some part of your brain—a module or network if you will—determines that your finger should move before you are even aware that you have made that decision. The results of these experiments indicate that even when we think we control the choice to act—a behavior as simple as moving a finger—the brain is deciding for us when to make the move. After making the decision, without our being aware of the internal impetus, the brain then convinces us that we were in control of that decision.

Philosophers have debated the significance of this experiment and its relevance to the question of free will. Some have proposed that the delay described by Libet allows for the conscious mind to decide *against* a behavior that might be recommended by the brain—to choose *not* to do something. Such an interpretation empowers us with the ability to veto any module whose suggested behavior we don't like. Instead of free will, it allows for "free won't." There is no widespread agreement on how to interpret Libet's findings, but taken at face value, these results confirm a model of brain organization whereby subconscious computing modules are making

decisions and controlling our behavior without our knowledge or awareness.

A few decades later, neurosurgeon Itzhak Fried picked up Libet's work
and advanced it one step further. Fried is an Israeli who was raised in Tel
Aviv. He came to the United States to earn his PhD at UCLA and then got
his medical degree at Stanford. Fried studied with both George Ojemann
and Dennis Spencer and now divides his time between UCLA and Tel Aviv
University, where he performs epilepsy surgery and brain research. Fried
essentially repeated Libet's experiments, but this time he inserted electrodes directly into the supplementary motor area (SMA). This area, if you
recall, is the source of the readiness potential: those brain waves that pre-
cede volitional movement, from which Fried could now record the activity
of individual neurons. (Libet, in contrast, had placed electrodes on the
scalp, so he was recording the activity of thousands of neurons in a slightly
delayed fashion compared with Fried's setup.)

Fried inserted his electrodes, like Feinstein, to treat a disease, not to
experiment, but he used the opportunity to learn more about the brain. For
Feinstein, the disease being treated was Parkinson's disease. In Fried's
case, it was epilepsy. Fried wanted to see if Libet's findings held up to closer
scrutiny when recording individual neurons in an unanesthetized human
brain.

Fried's experiment was simple. With electrodes recording from neurons in the SMA, he asked his patient to push a button at the precise moment when they made the decision to move their fingers. As Libet had
previously discovered, the neurons in Fried's patients were firing well before they made the decision. In fact, in some cases this activity preceded
the desire to move by more than a full second—a far greater interval than
had been reported by Libet and Feinstein. Fried then identified another
area of the brain, called the anterior cingulate gyrus, which, like the SMA,
contains neurons that fire in anticipation of the desire to move. It appeared
there was a whole circuit within the brain, not just one area, that was involved in volition.

Fried went yet a step further. As we already discussed, if the motor cortex of the brain is stimulated, the finger will move involuntarily. In this situation, the patient feels their finger twitch, but they know that they didn't make it happen. The trigger was provided by the neurosurgeon, who touched an electrode to the brain and activated the neurons that moved the finger. This time, however, instead of stimulating the part of the brain that causes movements, Fried stimulated the SMA, the part of *the brain that makes the decision to move.*

He wasn't sure exactly what would happen. Would the stimulation not only trigger the movement but also convince the patient that they had made the decision to move? Or would it still seem like some external force had caused their finger to move? In other words, was it possible to trigger the movement earlier in the timeline so that the patient might think they had decided to move their finger, when, really, it was the neurosurgeon who was in control?

Fried performed the experiment and found that SMA stimulation could indeed trigger the *desire* to move, as if he could control the patient's will. In another set of related experiments performed in France, researchers stimulated a different region of the brain, within the parietal lobe, which has strong connections to the SMA. The French researchers also placed electrodes in their subject's muscles, so they had an objective measurement of when the muscles twitched. They found that low-level stimulation made their subjects feel an overwhelming desire to move, even if no movement occurred. A stronger stimulation made them feel that they had *already* moved, even though no movement occurred.

These findings, together with Fried's, demonstrate the existence of a network of modules consisting of the anterior cingulate, the SMA, and part of the parietal lobe that somehow act in unison to create not only the decision to act but also the sense that the action was intended in the first place. Just as brain stimulation in one location can create an overwhelming certainty that God exists, in another location it can create a false sense of free will.

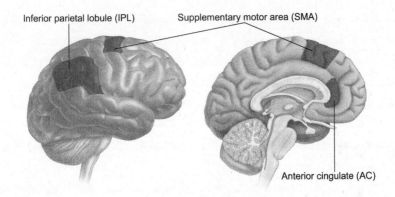

Inferior parietal lobule (IPL)   Supplementary motor area (SMA)

Anterior cingulate (AC)

The inferior parietal lobule, supplementary motor area, and anterior cingulate gyrus are important components of the freewill network of the brain.

So, what happens when a neurosurgeon removes these areas of the brain? Such a surgery in a normal person would be unethical and has never been performed. However, if a patient has a tumor or a scar in the brain causing uncontrolled seizures arising from these freewill areas, surgery to remove those parts of the brain becomes a necessity. When the SMA is damaged, patients develop a syndrome in which they are not paralyzed but lack the ability to *willingly* move their limbs. If you ask them if they want to move, they will answer yes, but then they'll be unable to initiate the movement *even though the pathways for movement are all still intact.* If the SMA on their left side is removed, the same thing happens to their ability to speak: they want to communicate, but they are unable to utter a word, even though all the language areas controlling speech are still intact. After a brief period of inertia, the brains of those with SMA damage, thankfully, rewire themselves and their ability to speak and move—or, rather, their ability to decide to do so—returns.

I've removed the SMA a few times, to treat either tumors or epilepsy. When my patient emerges from the operating room with a new paralysis or an inability to communicate, the sudden shock of the new deficit is still disconcerting. Even though I may understand on an intellectual level what has happened and that recovery is likely, I still have to manage the fear, anxiety, and stress on these patients and their families until they return to normal.

Since SMA removal doesn't cause a permanent loss of volition, most researchers have concluded that free will does not reside within the SMA. Rather, they believe that the SMA acts as a final gateway in an extended network that underlies our sense of autonomy.

But what would it be like if you lost the freewill center of the brain anyway? Does this question even make sense if free will doesn't exist?

Damage to the parietal lobe part of the freewill network, in the location where stimulation triggers a desire to move, results in a syndrome called apraxia. Patients with apraxia retain the ability to move but lose the ability to willingly carry out complex tasks. For example, if you ask a patient with apraxia to pick up the phone, they may stare at it, unable to figure out what to do. Yet, if the phone rings, they will reflexively pick it up to answer it. The ringing is an external source that motivates an overly learned and reflexive behavior. You don't need free will to answer a ringing phone. A robot can be programmed to perform this task every time it senses a ring. The motivation to pick up the phone without its ringing—let's say to check on an aging parent—is internally motivated, not externally, a product of a volitional force that has been eliminated. As another example, a patient with apraxia may be unable to blink on command; yet, if an object comes near their eye, they will still reflexively blink.

Alien hand syndrome, yet another affliction of the brain, provides additional clues to what it might be like to lose a part of the brain's volitional system. These patients lose control of one of their hands, which behaves as if it were controlled by an external force. Patients with alien hand syndrome have been known to button their shirts with one hand while unbuttoning it with the other. They feel as if a part of their body is under the influence of another's will.

So, what do we find when we do an MRI scan on a patient with alien hand syndrome? No surprise: we often see damage in the freewill network of the brain—either the SMA, the anterior cingulate, or the parietal lobe. In some cases of alien hand syndrome, the corpus callosum is also injured, since it connects the freewill network on one side of the brain with its mirror image network on the other side.

How can we explain alien hand syndrome in the context of the Gazzaniga paradigm of the brain, in which multiple modules subconsciously determine behavior? In this scenario, alien hand syndrome lends itself to an alternative explanation: a failure of the brain's storytelling instinct to include the actions of a subgroup of modules. In plain terms, there might be a disconnection between the freewill network and the storytelling network. While the behaviors triggered by most of brain's modules are interpreted as being volitional because we tell ourselves we have moved our hand or our leg, the apparently random and unwanted actions caused by a disconnected subgroup of modules don't fit nicely into the story. This would create the perception that someone else, or thing, is in control of your body. Which, by the way, it is, since there is no you in the first place to be in control.

HOW MEMORIES ARE STORED IN THE BRAIN

The prevailing theory of how memories are stored in the brain was for many years based on the work of psychologist Karl Lashley, one of Roger Sperry's mentors. As far back as the 1920s, Lashley performed experiments on rats and tried to find the location where a memory, which he called an "engram," was kept by destroying different parts of the rats' brains. He was never successful at finding such a place, so he concluded that the brain was equipotential. Any one part, he surmised, could take over the function of any other, and memories could be stored everywhere and anywhere.

This theory was later abandoned, in part because of Brenda Milner's groundbreaking studies on Scoville's patient H.M. and Penfield's epilepsy patients. Some thirty years after Lashley, a new model slowly emerged in which the hippocampus was understood as the gateway that inputs memories into specific areas of the neocortex for long-term storage, from which they can be accessed by the hippocampus when needed. The neocortex, you may remember, is just another name for the surface gray matter of the four lobes of the brain, where the neurons are located.

Let's take our ability to recognize faces, a unique function of the right temporal lobe. Damage to this area causes prosopagnosia, a syndrome that was delightfully detailed in Oliver Sacks's book *The Man Who Mistook His Wife for a Hat*. Meanwhile, the tip of the left temporal lobe stores the names of certain categories, like animals or tools. These types of memories are called declarative, which refers to memories of facts (also called semantic memory) and events (also called episodic memory). But *how* exactly does the hippocampus input memories of people's faces and their identities into long-term storage in the neocortex?

One possibility is that the memory of a face could reside in a widely distributed network of neurons, each of which responds to a unique visual characteristic of the seen image. For example, one neuron might be unique to that person's eyes, another to their mouth, another to their smile, and another to their hair color. If this "network theory" were correct, each face would trigger a distinct but widely distributed population of neurons to fire, each neuron reflecting some singular feature of the face. Another face with similar eyes but a differently shaped mouth would trigger the same eye neurons but different mouth neurons.

An alternative theory posits that the memory of a face could reside within a single cell that stores the entirety of that one person's face. In this case, recognition of any one face would require activity in only that one neuron. This hypothesis came to be called the grandmother cell theory, since it implied that there was a neuron somewhere in your brain that would fire every time you looked at, or thought about, your grandmother. By extension, if this neuron were removed, you would no longer recognize her.

Another possibility is that both theories are correct. While the visual components of a face might be processed by a widely distributed network of facial feature neurons, the individual's facial *identity* might not enter consciousness until a single neuron dedicated to that one individual's face begins to fire.

Into this debate strolled Itzhak Fried, the Israeli neurosurgeon working at UCLA. In collaboration with an engineer, he designed his own set of electrodes that could record individual neurons in the human brain, and which he implanted in and around the hippocampus of his epilepsy patients. Not only could these electrodes localize the source of his patients' seizures, but—working alongside a group of psychologists and physiologists—Fried could record the activity of individual neurons while his patients viewed and remembered pictures of famous faces to see what exactly the neurons were doing.

In one experiment, he showed a patient a picture of Jennifer Aniston while recording data from dozens of different neurons near the hippocampus. To his amazement, only one neuron started firing every time the patient looked at Aniston's face. No matter what she was doing, which direction she was looking, or what clothes she happened to be wearing, that one single cell would fire. If he showed a picture of Bill Clinton or Halle Berry, the Jennifer Aniston cell would not fire. A different cell would fire for Bill and yet another one for Halle. If Fried showed the patient the words "Jennifer Aniston," the Jennifer Aniston cell fired. If he played a recording of someone saying the words "Jennifer Aniston," it fired.

Fried's discovery showed that the grandmother cell theory, although not entirely accurate, appeared to be a closer description of what was going on in the brain when we scan a crowd or our social media feed for known faces, compared with the distributed memory network theory, at least in the location of the brain in which he was recording. Given that Fried could record from only a limited number of neurons, it would be unlikely that he just *happened* to find the *exact cell* that responded to the picture he chose to show. Out of the billions of neurons and millions of possible faces, the odds were incredibly slim. For this reason, he concluded that each neuron in that area responds to between 50 and 150 different distinct individuals—not just to their faces but to the *idea* of that individual, presented either as their picture, their name, or their description.

As for the timing of the neuron's activity, Fried's findings resembled those of Libet. When Fried asked the subject to think about Jennifer Aniston, the cell would fire almost a full second before the person was aware of whom they were thinking about. The brain was active first, creating the *idea* of Jennifer Aniston before the patient was conscious that they were thinking about her. Perhaps a more accurate description of our thoughts might be afterthoughts, since ideas exist in the physical substrate of our brains—the neuronal networks—well before we are consciously aware of them.

Fried's findings are far from conclusive, since he couldn't record every neuron in the brain while his patients remembered every possible face and object. But his results do point to a mechanism, at least in the hippocampus and its neighboring regions, whereby neurons are tuned to fully formed ideas, not just features or attributes. Not playing favorites with grandmothers, he renamed these cells "concept cells," since they fired in response to certain concepts, and they did so selectively and invariably.

But the hippocampus is not where ideas are stored; it's only the gateway to long-term storage. It's like the librarian who knows where all the books are located and can access them or replace them based on a filing system. Another way to think of the hippocampus is like a keyboard on your computer. When you tap the letter *c*, it appears on your computer screen—not because the letter *c* exists inside the keyboard's button but because when you strike the c button, this triggers an electrical signal that then passes into the hardware of your computer, where multiple circuits are activated that produce a *c* on your screen. The letter *c* is not stored in the keyboard, nor is it stored on the screen. Rather the keyboard and the screen are gateways for the input and output of the letter *c*, which is brought into existence on the hard drive of your computer. The cells identified by Fried in the hippocampus may be similar.

But how exactly are memories put into long-term storage in the neocortex and then retrieved?

———

One possible answer came from experiments performed by another neurosurgeon, second-generation Egyptian Kareem Zaghloul, who graduated from MIT and then the MD-PhD program at the University of Pennsylvania. Currently working at the National Institutes of Health, Zaghloul, like Fried, performed his experiments on epilepsy patients during their surgeries. Unlike Fried, however, Zaghloul was able to record neurons in both the hippocampus (the gateway) *and* the neocortex (the storage bin) simultaneously. He discovered that new memories were formed *only when neurons in both structures were reverberating at precisely the same frequency.* Likewise, the act of remembering also required simultaneous oscillations of the same neurons in the hippocampus and the neocortex as when that memory was first created and stored. Moreover, each memory, or engram, was encoded by a population of neurons firing in a specific sequence, so memories were stored not just in one neuron but more like a dozen of them.

One way to think of this is to compare neurons to the keys on a piano. While a piano has only eighty-eight keys, it can produce an infinite number of melodies and harmonies, depending on the order in which the keys are struck. Likewise, a small set of neurons can fire in many different patterns. If neurons are like keys on a piano, then playing one melody—let's say "Twinkle, Twinkle, Little Star"—would encode one memory, and another melody played with the same notes—maybe "Ring Around the Rosie"—would encode a different memory. In this way, the same small group of neurons could store several different memories when activated in a different sequence.

While one memory—let's say learning how to ride a bike for the first time—might activate a group of neurons in one sequence, falling off the bike and skinning your knee might activate those same neurons in a different order. With such a storage technique, the same group of neurons could, in theory, store multiple different memories by firing in different patterns, just like a piano, with its fixed keyboard and notes, can produce an infinite number of songs.

If we could learn to "play" the brain like we play an instrument, it might be possible to replay any memory whenever we want. Or whenever anyone else wants, for that matter. Say your therapist wanted you to relive a repressed memory. No problem! Likewise, if a jury needed to determine whether a suspect had committed a crime, the suspect's memory could be forced back, relived, and (hopefully) result in a confession.

Inserting a new memory of an event that never occurred, on the other hand, would be much more difficult, since the neurons and their firing sequences would have already been linked to specific memories. However, it might be possible to mix and match prior memories into a new sequence of events, like taking a jigsaw puzzle of the Eiffel Tower and rearranging the pieces to form a new picture of, say, Big Ben. The new memory would not be nearly as clear. It might be blurry and vague, but, in theory, new fuzzy memories could be created out of a composite of older ones.

Erasing a memory, on the other hand, would be much easier. Once the location of the group of cells that form the nexus of a specific memory is known, elimination of these cells should, in principle, wipe out the memory as well. One could imagine the selective erasure of a memory as a useful treatment for post-traumatic stress disorder. Or if you don't want to remember your ex-girlfriend anymore—let's say after a bad breakup—all you'd have to do would be to find those cells where that memory was stored and have each one removed.

If you remember the Jim Carrey movie *Eternal Sunshine of the Spotless Mind,* this is exactly what happened. Carrey has the memory of his girlfriend erased to ease the pain of their split. However, if the same group of neurons store several different memories, as Zaghloul's research hints, it's likely that other memories would be lost as well. The issue is moot for the moment, since we are not yet able to expunge individual neurons from the human brain while leaving adjacent ones intact, but in principle it shouldn't be that difficult.

Indeed, altering our ability to recognize loved ones by changing the brain's anatomy has already been documented. A deficit like prosopagnosia, the inability to recognize faces, provides some clues. If you remember the story from Oliver Sacks's book, his patient, Dr. P., grabs his wife's head on the way out of the office and tries to put it on his own head, mistaking her for a hat. If the brain can be altered so drastically that you not only forget the appearance of your spouse's face but also mistake it for an inanimate object, what's keeping any object, person, or event from being rendered unrecognizable or erased?

If we define ourselves by our memories, our personalities, and our decisions, all of which can be easily adjusted by tinkering a bit with the brain, what does that say about our concept of the self as stable and unchanging? And if free will is an illusion created by modules in the brain that can be altered by a stroke so that our bodies begin to act out with seemingly uncontrolled behaviors—as in alien hand syndrome—or triggered with brain stimulation, then what exactly is the nature of the human consciousness?

Perhaps the clearest way to put it all together is to accept that we are, in some sense, in the predicament faced by Neo in the *The Matrix*. If you recall, Neo is given a choice by Morpheus to either take the red pill and see the world as it really is—an illusion created by a computer—or take the blue pill and continue to live with a veil of oblivion over his eyes. We are very much living in a Matrix-like simulation created by the modules in our brains, only our situation is even more dire than the one faced by Neo. At least he still had a self with agency and free will, should he choose to empower it by taking the blue pill. We do not have this option. Both our identity and our agency are also parts of the simulation. There is no escape, except perhaps to accept our fate and live accordingly. It makes you wonder if perhaps the Buddhists are onto something?

Subjectivity remains an impenetrable safe whose contents may, in the end, turn out to be empty. And the breadth and wonder of human consciousness may be no more than a bedtime story that we tell ourselves in those brief few moments before we drift off to sleep.

SIXTEEN

THE TERMINAL MAN

n *Transcendence*, Johnny Depp uploads the contents of his brain to a so-phisticated computer after he learns he has months to live. In *The Matrix*, Neo and his crew plug their brains directly into a terminal and control an avatar body in a virtual world. These science fiction scenarios depict an actual technology being developed today called a brain-computer inter-face, or BCI. In its most general sense, a BCI is a linkage between the hu-man brain and a computer.

Although the term "brain-computer interface" was first coined by UCLA professor Jacques Vidal in 1973, the first mention of the potential compatibility between brains and computers appeared decades prior in the stories of Edmond Hamilton, a pulp science fiction writer who wrote for the magazine *Weird Tales*. In 1926, his fanciful story "The Metal Giants" described a mechanical brain, comprising tubes and wires, that could rep-licate the electrical activity of the human brain until, magically, a lightbulb flashes and it becomes conscious. But the desire to connect a brain to a computer—and the limitless possibilities that might emerge from such a union—has not merely been fodder for countless science fiction books and movies. Even as I write this, several start-up companies are actively racing to bring such devices to market.

BCIs can be separated into two broad categories. In the first, the brain's electrical signals are routed from the brain and directed into a computer. We'll call this an *output* BCI, since information flows *out* of the brain. What would this look like in practice? Well, instead of using a keyboard or a mouse to input information, the user, whose brain is plugged in, need only think about what they might want to accomplish, and it would happen instantaneously.

One obvious application for an output BCI is the restoration of movement to a paralyzed limb. If your brain was linked to a mechanical arm, for example, it could think, *Move arm!*, and the mechanical arm would move. Such a device is called a neuroprosthetic. (Think Peter Weller in *RoboCop* or Matt Damon in *Elysium*.) When the function of the artificial limb is enhanced, it has a different name: neuroaugmentation.

For example, why limit the design of a neuroprosthetic to what nature gave us? Why not design one to be even more flexible and superhuman, like the appendages attached to Doctor Octopus in the *Spider-Man* comics and movies. An output BCI could also drive a car or fly a plane. Taken even further, a more complex output BCI might one day extract fully formed ideas or even sensations directly from the brain, as in *Strange Days*, where Ralph Fiennes's character wears a skullcap called a SQUID to record his experiences so he or someone else might relive them.

In the other direction, an *input* BCI takes information out of a computer and inserts it directly into the brain. Such a device could also be a neuroprosthetic, such as the visor that restored vision to a blind Geordi La Forge in *Star Trek*. Once again, the SQUID in *Strange Days* also counts as an input BCI, since the device functioned bidirectionally. Or take the 2018 movie *Upgrade*, in which a paralyzed man has a chip implanted in his nervous system that gives him superhuman abilities. Since information is flowing *into* his nervous system, this, too, would be considered an input BCI.

One crucial defining attribute of an input BCI is that it must interface directly with the brain. For this reason, the cochlear implant and the retinal implant, which restore lost hearing and vision, respectively, don't count as true BCIs because they input information into peripheral sensory nerves and organs rather than directly into the brain.

Science fiction movies aside, the most common BCIs, which already exist and have been described herein, are the deep-brain-stimulating devices that treat Parkinson's disease and OCD. These therapeutic input BCIs are what we call neuromodulatory, since they alter the brain's existing circuitry. As for neuroprosthetic BCIs, as of 2023, there are very few on the market, although several are currently in development. More critically, since BCIs require an interface between the brain and a computer—and since that interface often involves opening the skull and inserting electrodes—neurosurgeons have become their gatekeepers.

In fact, neurosurgeons have been involved not only in implanting BCIs in their patients' brains but also in designing and testing them. Unlike in science fiction movies, where BCIs provide superhuman abilities, current BCI research is primarily focused on their medical applications, such as helping a blind or paralyzed accident victim reconnect with the outside world by providing the means to hug their children, browse the internet, watch a movie, or simply maneuver their way around the house. (No need to worry about sentient AI computers taking over our planet or supervillains with octopus arms destroying our cities . . . at least, not for now.)

HACKING THE BRAIN

The language of the brain and that of a computer are quite different. The former involves neurons, which sum the excitatory and inhibitory activity of 100,000s of its neighbors. Once a certain threshold is reached, the neuron fires an action potential and becomes one of the 100,000 inputs into another adjacent neuron. Groups of these connected neurons, each firing at a specific rate and in a unique sequence, create the brain's code. Computers, on the other hand, rely on electronic circuits that can be in one of two binary states, reflected in 1s and 0s, that indicate whether current is either flowing or not flowing. For brains to communicate with computers requires a sort of Google Translate function between the two that does not yet exist. Although we are making progress, it's not as if we possess a brain-to-machine Rosetta stone to guide us. In fact, we still don't fully understand exactly how neuronal firing patterns code for information.

So how do BCI devices untangle this coding mystery? The trick is to provide the computer with simultaneous access to both the brain's code— the firing activity of a group of neurons—and the body's actions that those neurons are controlling. Then all the computer needs to do is find a way to link the brain's neuronal signals with the behavior. In this way, computers create their own Rosetta stone, so long as the physical behavior they are controlling can be broken down into discrete units. These units are then simultaneously fed back into the computer so it can solve the translation problem on its own.

For example, imagine you are sitting at a table with a cup on it. Let's put some tea in that cup. Your brain says, *I'd like to take a sip of that!* When you reach your hand out to grasp the cup, the neurons in the part of your brain that control your arm and hand will fire in a precise pattern to make that happen. If the cup—once you sip the tea and place it down again—is now sitting in a slightly different location, but you are still thirsty and want to reach for it again, the pattern of neuronal activity will be slightly different, since your arm must move to a new location. If someone brings you a large mug of tea instead of a cup, your fingers may need to open a little wider, so the firing pattern will again be slightly altered.

Now say we implant recording electrodes in the area of your brain that moves your arm and hand, and we then record the activity of the neurons there. We can also place sensors on your arm and hand that measure both the movements of the joints and the positions of your arm, hand, and fingers in space. This way, all we have to do is feed both streams of information back into the computer simultaneously, and it will learn how an arm works. How? Simple: we program the computer to connect the different variations in movement with the different firing patterns of the neurons. The experiment is then repeated many times, using cups of different sizes, locations, directions, heights, etc. This allows the computer to eventually machine learn, by observing and comparing the two data streams, how the brain codes for different arm and hand movements.

What is machine learning? Machine learning means that, in time, the computer will be able to predict exactly where the limb is going, as well as the precise size of the object it must grasp, simply by listening to the brain's electrical signals. The computer literally teaches itself how to make the translation from firing pattern to arm movement, and it is programmed to learn these skills on its own. Not even the programmer fully understands how the computer is doing the translation. That's why it's so easy to do. The computer does all the hard work by self-teaching.

Now imagine this BCI is attached to a robotic arm. Using the signals recorded from your brain, the computer could command the mechanical arm to grasp the cup, and the movements of the motorized limb would then mirror the movements of your actual arm, precisely and instantaneously, no matter how fast you moved it or in which direction. From your perspective, you would be controlling both your real arm and the robotic one as if the latter were attached to your body. If your arm was paralyzed, the BCI-powered robotic arm could be worn on a harness and become a prosthetic. If your legs were paralyzed, a similar device would allow you to walk again.

Though these devices might sound like science fiction, they are not. They already exist.

Eyes, on the other hand, are a different story. Think of it this way: BCI-powered arms and legs require pulling information *out* of the brain to power a mechanical limb. Eyes are the opposite. To power a BCI eye, the information must go *into* the brain. As you might expect, it's much more difficult to put stuff *into* the brain than to pull stuff *out*.

When your eyes see an object, tens of millions of neurons in the brain fire in a unique spatial and temporal pattern to produce that experience. Alas, for a computer to even attempt to master the activation sequence of every neuron involved in the visual perception of an object would require the ability to record from all those neurons simultaneously, which is far beyond our current capabilities. If we then wanted to make you see that object by stimulating your brain, we would need to trigger each of those neurons to fire in exactly the same pattern. Although the engineering complexity of these tasks seems almost impossible to imagine, let alone to conquer, the first attempts to create a neuroprosthetic BCI tried to do precisely this: restore vision to the blind.

LET THERE BE LIGHT!

The idea behind a visual BCI is fairly straightforward. A video camera is mounted on a pair of glasses. The moving images it captures are transformed into electrical impulses that are then fed directly into the visual cortex, the area of the occipital lobe that processes vision. But wait! Didn't we just explain that we don't have the technical capacity to tackle such a complicated problem of engineering? So, why even try? It turns out that the visual cortex—as German neurosurgeons Fedor Krause and Otfrid Foerster discovered back in the early 1920s—exhibits a particularly unusual phenomenon when stimulated with an electrode.

Krause and Foerster—the same neurosurgeons whom Penfield visited early in his career—discovered that if they stimulated the visual cortex with an electrode, their patients would see small pinpoint flashes of light. Move the electrode a bit to the side, and a flash of light appeared in a slightly different location. If the electrode were then returned to its original position and re-stimulated, the flash would once again appear in the original location.

Krause and Foerster coined a name for this phenomenon, calling these artificially induced visual perceptions "phosphenes." Just to be clear, the sparks of light seen by their subjects were not real. Subjects *experienced* them as if they existed in the outside world, but the flashes existed only within the circuitry of the brain. No one else in the room could see them.

Wilder Penfield expanded on these studies through careful investigations of his epilepsy patients at the Montreal Neurological Institute. Remember, these patients had to be kept awake during their surgeries, which offered Penfield a unique opportunity to explore this phenomenon, and what he discovered was this: depending upon where he placed his electrode in the occipital lobe, he could produce phosphenes in specific zones in his patient's field of view. If he wanted them to see a flash in the upper outer quadrant on the right, he would stimulate the bottom half of the left visual cortex. (Everything in the brain is reversed. In the visual cortex, it's also upside down.)

It didn't take long for others to realize that if you could stimulate the visual cortex with several electrodes in a specific pattern, you could, in theory, create an image made up of multiple phosphenes *even if the patient were blind*. What would this type of "vision" look like? Think of the designs that emerge just after fireworks explode, when the bursts of light pause, briefly suspended in the air. Or think of the stars that outline the constellations against the blackness of the night sky. As long as a subject's blindness was caused by damage to the eyes and not to the brain, the visual cortex could still produce this type of vision.

Why? Because the *experience* of vision does not come from the eyes. It comes from the brain. In fact, you don't really need your eyes to see because *seeing doesn't happen in the eyes or in the optic nerves*. It occurs in the visual cortex of the brain.

It took a few more decades for researchers to realize that they could use the signals coming out of a video camera to control the distribution of phosphenes, which, in turn, could enable a blind person to see the outside world in the form of patterned flashes of light. Precisely what this would look like and how it would appear to the user was, at that time, unclear. In its natural state, our visual cortex does not process vision via phosphenes. Rather, our neuronal circuitry is designed to detect the edges and lines of our world, no matter their orientations, as well as lines moving in different directions. This is how our brains enable us to see visual scenery with exquisite resolution, luminosity, color, and depth. Phosphene-induced vision, by contrast, is the equivalent of trying to produce a Haydn sonata by banging two violins, a viola, and cello together. Sure, this may create some noise, but it's not going to sound like a well-rehearsed string quartet.

The first neurosurgeon brave enough to implant electrodes in the visual cortices of blind patients was Tracy Putnam, the fallen former head of the Neurological Institute of New York, who was cast out for being sympathetic to Jewish persecution. In 1962, Putnam was the chief of neurosurgery at Cedars of Lebanon Hospital in Los Angeles, soon to become Cedars-Sinai Hospital. At the time, Putnam had formed a relationship with a scientist named John C. Button, who was the real mastermind behind these experiments.

Together, Putnam and Button were somehow able to convince three blind patients to volunteer for their experiment. Under local anesthesia, Putnam placed them facedown on the operating room table and inserted four wires directly into their visual cortices through separate burr holes. These were the days before institutional review boards and ethical committees determined which human experiments were permissible. Putnam and Button could basically do whatever they wanted.

They later addressed the issue of consent in the paper they went on to publish, but not in a way that we, from our modern perspective, would find acceptable. They wrote: "[One patient] was extremely likeable and cooperative, and understood thoroughly the nature of the experiment." This compliant chap had volunteered, "to help the doctors invent a way for all blind people to see." While it's tempting to judge these men from a contemporary moral high ground, it's also unfair. These kinds of experiments were standard operating procedure at the time.

The four implanted electrodes were then connected to a handheld photoreceptor device using a few electrical components purchased at a secondhand electronics dealer for $9.45. And that's how the first visual prosthetic was born. With this off-the-shelf device, Button and Putnam were able to show that their blind subjects could identify the location of a light in a darkened room and even navigate through a simple obstacle course while essentially holding their primitive eye in their hands, just like you might prowl through your home with a flashlight after a blackout.

Although Putnam and Button's gadget was primitive, it was the proof of principle needed to stimulate more sophisticated attempts. A few years later, physiologist Giles S. Brindley and Walpole S. Lewin, the head of neurosurgery at the United Cambridge Hospitals in East Anglia, England, implanted a grid of eighty electrodes over the visual cortex of a fifty-two-year-old woman who had lost her vision due to a combination of progressive glaucoma and a retinal detachment. Using a radio frequency transmitter, Brindley and Lewin remotely activated each electrode and created discrete flashes of light in different regions of her visual field. Each spot, according to the patient, looked "like a star in the sky."

If enough electrodes could be implanted and stimulated with adequate control, their theory went, perhaps her vision could be restored if not crisply—say, like a high-definition LCD screen—then more like a 1980s jumbotron. Brindley and Lewin summarized their work thus: "Our findings strongly suggest that it will be possible, by improving our prototype, to make a prosthesis that will permit blind patients not only to avoid obstacles when walking, but to read print or handwriting, perhaps at speeds comparable with those habitual among sighted people."

The visual neuroprosthetics baton was then picked up by a scientist named William H. Dobelle. Working primarily with neurosurgeon John P. Girvin, the chair of neurosurgery at the University of Western Ontario, Dobelle created a device that relied on a sixty-four-contact grid of electrodes, which he began implanting in humans in 1973. One of his patients, a thirty-three-year-old man who had been sightless for over ten years, claimed he could now process "detailed visual information." Other implantees claimed they could now read braille five times faster than they could with their fingers. At long last, the idea of a visual prosthetic seemed to be more than mere fantasy.

---

n 1978, neurosurgeons Donald O. Quest and João Antunes implanted electrodes in the brains of two more patients at the Neurological Institute in
New York. Their devices remained in place for over twenty years. When
coupled with a video camera mounted on a pair of sunglasses, these devices
supposedly produced 20/1200 vision, which means their patients were able
to "see" six-inch characters from five feet away.

While the wires Putnam implanted could be inserted under local anesthesia, Dobelle's devices were so big that his patients had to be put under
general anesthesia. To give the surgeons access to the occipital lobes,
located in the back of the head, Quest and Antunes would position the subjects facedown on the operating table. Then they'd cut a large horseshoe-
shaped incision into the skin at the bottom of the back of the head and
remove a piece of bone the size of a bread plate. Earlier devices were only
implanted on one half of the brain, but later versions were implanted on
both sides so that the phosphenes could be produced throughout the patient's field of vision. After opening the dura and exposing the cortex, the
doctors gently slipped a small grid of electrodes between the two occipital
lobes. These electrodes had to be placed facing outward, toward the brain's
inner surfaces, since the visual cortex lies hidden in a cleft between the
hemispheres.

Each electrode was at-
tached to a wire—one for
each of the sixty-four
electrodes—and the resulting long fiber bundle was
tunneled through the dura
and bone. Each layer—dura,
bone, and skin—was care-
fully sewn shut. This cable
was then snaked under the
skin around the back of the

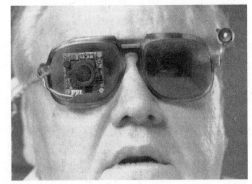

One of the first patients implanted with Dobelle's
visual prosthesis from his original publication.
Wolters Kluwer Health, Inc.

head toward a small round pedestal, or connector, which was screwed into the skull, where it protruded through the scalp. Into this plug was inserted another cable, which would link the electrodes on the brain directly with a computer worn on the patient's belt. This computer, in turn, was connected to a video camera mounted on a pair of glasses.

The visual information coming into the camera was sent to the computer, which transformed each pixel into an electrical impulse, which was then sent through the skull-mounted connecting pedestal to activate the individual electrodes resting on the brain. Since the location of the electrodes was slightly different in each patient, an individualized map had to be constructed by stimulating each electrode one at a time to determine where exactly the patient saw the flashes of light. Once this visual field-to-electrode-to-brain translation was systematized, the device became fully functional, and the patient could be trained to use their new synthetic eye.

The role of the neurosurgeon in these implants cannot be understated. The sterility of the procedure was critical and the risk of infection was high. One of the greatest hazards was that cerebrospinal fluid might track along the electrodes and seep through the skin, allowing bacteria to follow the same pathway back into the brain. The sockets needed constant cleaning to prevent them from getting infected. Nevertheless, these early visual BCIs remained functional for decades. At the time, no one knew if the brain would reject them or encase them in a dense scar, or if the patients would have continuous seizures from the irritation. Yet, none of these complications came to pass—at least, not often. Occasionally a patient would undergo a seizure, when stimulation amplitudes were cranked up too high, but on the whole the devices were well tolerated.

Although some patients developed infections, most did not, which indicated that once the surgical technique was optimized, it would be possible to have a human being live indefinitely with an electrical outlet sticking out of their head. This boded well for the future of BCIs.

Although Dobelle's visual prosthetic was crude and imperfect, it was nevertheless technically sound. More important, it was built from reasonably priced components, so it could be mass-produced and marketed, which is exactly what he tried to do. Dobelle was so inspired by his early success that he formed a company to sell a visual prosthetic to the blind community, which he thought would accomplish for the sightless what the cochlear implant had done for the deaf.

Unfortunately, Dobelle was less Steve Jobs and Bill Gates and more P. T. Barnum and Bernie Madoff. He also grossly underestimated the importance of neurosurgeons in his entrepeneurial endeavor.

WIRED FOR SIGHT

THE CASE OF
JENS NAUMANN

In 1967, when he was three, Jens Naumann emigrated with his family from Germany to Canada. He got his first job working for the British Columbia Railway at seventeen. One day, while hammering a pickax through some ice that had frozen around the tracks, he missed the rail by a few inches and dislodged a shard of metal that ricocheted into his left eye. He felt a searing pain as the vision in that eye went black. A few years later, in a cruel twist of fate, a piece of debris caught in the chain of a snowmobile broke off and flew into his other eye. In spite of multiple surgeries, Jens was left completely blind. Undaunted and compelled to overcome his disability, he became obsessed with the idea of regaining vision by any means necessary. After learning about Dobelle's work, Naumann volunteered to be the first person implanted with this now commercially available visual prosthetic.

William Dobelle was not a neurosurgeon. In fact, he wasn't even a physician. He was a laboratory scientist, more comfortable working with rodents in a research institute than with human beings in a clinic. Rather than remain under the auspices of a university and gradually develop his device, Dobelle formed his own self-funded company, which lacked any internal regulatory oversight or ethics committees. Instead of recruiting a large group of sophisticated collaborators to work full-time, he contracted with the specialists he needed—computer programmers, engineers, psychologists, and neurosurgeons—on an ad hoc basis to tackle each aspect of this incredibly complex and experimental undertaking.

Like the Music Man marching into town to great fanfare, Dobelle promised to restore sight to the blind. The only catch: each customer had to pay $100,000 cash. Dobelle claimed that the surgery would take only a few hours and could be performed under local anesthesia. He told them there would be no overnight stay. He trumpeted his ability to restore enough vision for the implantee to distinguish faces, drive a car, and lead fully independent lives. Such promises were irresistible to many members of the blind community—particularly those who had once had sight and then lost it later in life.

When Naumann stumbled across Dobelle's advertisement, he had been supporting his wife and eight children by selling firewood and tuning pianos. He saved what he could of his limited income, begged and borrowed from neighbors to make up the rest, and signed on the dotted line. He fully expected to be skiing, motorbiking, and even flying an airplane with his new robovision.

The first glitch in his plans appeared when he learned that the surgery wouldn't be performed in the United States, since the device was not yet FDA approved. Naumann found himself on a plane to Portugal, where he met up with two neurosurgeons hired by Dobelle, Drs. John P. Girvin and João Antunes. Antunes had left the Neurological Institute in New York by that time and become the chair of the department of neurosurgery of Hospital de Santa Maria in Lisbon.

Once Naumann arrived, he learned that, rather than the quick outpatient procedure he had been sold, his surgery would be a four-hour operation under general anesthesia with a five-day hospital stay. At this point, he was too far committed both psychologically and monetarily to back out. A few days later, Naumann was brought into the operating room and implanted with two seventy-two-contact grids of electrodes, one on each side of the brain.

It rapidly became evident that Dobelle had both underestimated the complexity of the neurosurgical aspect of his enterprise and overestimated the visual restoration it could provide. Naumann suffered for weeks with headaches. He had two seizures when the device was being programmed. Other implantees had frequent infections. Brain fluid leaked around the sockets, placing them at high risk for meningitis. Well before the Theranos debacle, Dobelle found that he, in Elizabeth Holmes fashion, had prematurely released a medical technology to the world that was far from ready for the marketplace.

And yet, when the device was first activated, and only one of the ninety possible phosphenes appeared in Naumann's visual field, the impact was overwhelming. Like a newly liberated prisoner after years held captive in a cave, Naumann was finally able to see light again. "I gasped," he writes. "There was a bright, white flickering light almost at my center of vision, surrounded by the most beautiful rings of color, as one would see on a perfect rainbow." Once all the electrodes were turned on and mapped, he could appreciate around fifty phosphenes in the bottom left part of his field of vision and thirty on the top right. So how good was his vision? He writes: "I saw the jagged outlines of the table's edges and was able to follow them around the entire span of the table, noting the lumps of dots angled, marking the backs of the office chairs surrounding the table [. . .]. A square-shaped blob of phosphenes marked the conference room telephone just a couple of feet from my right hand."

Walking into his home, he could count the windows in his kitchen, see the outlines of the doorframes, and even partially make out the faces of his children, each delineated by a few dots of light. In need of money, Dobelle requested that Naumann drive a car around an empty parking lot as a publicity stunt in front of a group of reporters. Naumann complied, reluctantly, admitting that at the time he didn't fully trust the system to keep him from crashing.

As rudimentary as Naumann's new eyesight was, the eighty points of light he could now see were a dramatic improvement over the perpetual midnight he had endured before his implant. He soon became both physically and emotionally dependent on his new vision, craving it like an addict. One morning he woke up and noticed that a few of the more prominent phosphenes were suddenly missing. It was subtle at first, but slowly, it became obvious that he was once again losing his sight. Each day, fewer and fewer stars appeared in his sky; eventually, only one or two remained.

The poor design and inadequate pre-implant testing of the device resulted in its eventual failure. To make matters worse, two years after Naumann's implant, Dobelle, now mired in debt, abruptly died of diabetes-related complications. When he learned of Dobelle's death, Naumann was both bitterly resentful at the man's incompetence and, ironically, also deeply grateful for his dedication to trying to help the blind community. For many years Naumann refused to have his implants removed. He continued to hold out hope that someday another brave visionary might pick up Dobelle's research and provide Jens with a few more years of artificial vision.

So where are we now? Several companies are currently working on visual prosthetics that have roughly the same basic design as Dobelle's, but the newer ones are fully implanted, meaning that communication between the electrodes and the computer is done wirelessly, without the need for a socket protruding through the skin.

The most advanced of these prosthetics is made by a company called Second Sight Medical Products. At the time of this writing, six of these devices have been implanted by two neurosurgeons, Daniel Yoshor and Nader Pouratian, currently the chairs of neurosurgery at the University of Pennsylvania and UT Southwestern. Scant published data on the outcomes of these trials exist, since the company is keeping its cards close to the chest. For now, they've released only a press report indicating that most of the subjects can distinguish a white square on a black computer screen and the direction of a moving bar of light. Whether these modest results are sufficient to provide enough vision to justify the risk of a brain implant remains to be seen.

It's unclear, in fact, whether phosphenes will ever provide enough res-olution to create useful vision. Missing from the field of visual prosthetics—and critical to its long-term success—is the ability to activate the intrinsic processing machinery of the visual cortex. We already know a remarkable amount about how the brain creates vision. If only we could rapidly acti-vate thousands of individual neurons in complex patterns, we might be able to create detailed visual perceptions. But how long until this is possible?

Currently, the only technology up to such a task would be optogenetics. Optogenetics uses light to turn individual neurons on and off. Such a sys-tem would require gene therapy to insert the optogenetic receptors into the neurons of the visual cortex, and then a surgeon would have to implant an array of millions of fiber-optic light threads tiny enough to illuminate one neuron at a time. Although such a device can be imagined, sadly, it cannot yet be built. We are still decades away. But the good news is that another implant device, originally created to compete with Dobelle's surface elec-trode BCI, called the Utah array, has facilitated giant leaps forward in the development of output BCIs—ones that can restore movement to the para-lyzed and even permit verbal communication in patients who have lost the ability to speak.

A BED OF NAILS THE SIZE OF A PEA

While Dobelle was working on his visual prosthetic, which relied on elec-trodes placed on the *surface* of the brain, another researcher in Utah, Rich-ard A. Norman, was pursuing an alternative strategy. He invented a small rectangular chip containing ninety-six tiny electrodes, each only a milli-meter long, which could be placed *in* the brain like a thumbtack. This de-vice, the Utah array, is roughly the size of a pea. Each of the pin-sized needle electrodes on its 4-millimeter surface can either stimulate or record from nearby neurons. When magnified, the array resembles a miniaturized bed of nails, like something a teeny-tiny yogi might lie upon while medi-tating.

After years of animal testing, the Utah array was first implanted in humans as an investigational device in 2004 and was FDA approved in 2021. Although originally designed to compete with Dobelle's visual prosthetic, the array was soon inserted into the motor cortex to help paralyzed

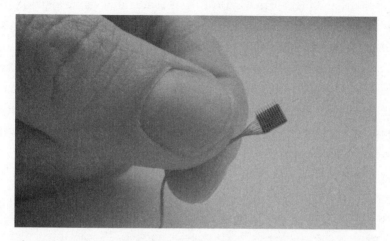

The Utah array, shown in this zoomed-in image, contains one hundred small electrodes designed to penetrate the human brain, each of which can record the signals from hundreds of nearby individual neurons.

Utah Array—©2023 Blackrock Neurotech, LLC

patients move robotic arms. It's currently being implanted in the brains of quadriplegics at several different academic institutions throughout the world. Dozens of patients have already had between one and four Utah arrays embedded in the motor and sensory parts of their brains. These patients have been able to control robotic arms to move objects and feed themselves, and one lucky implantee even got to fist-bump President Obama with his mechanical appendage.

Neurosurgeon Ali Rezai, currently the director of the Rockefeller Neuroscience Institute at West Virginia University School of Medicine, along with a team from Batelle, a nonprofit applied science and technology organization, are using the signals from the Utah array to reanimate atrophic muscles in paralyzed patients' motionless arm rather than bothering with a robotic one. A more recent breakthrough occurred at the University of

Pittsburgh, where neurosurgeon Elizabeth Tyler-Kabara* and her team were able to create a combined input/output BCI that not only could move a mechanized extremity but was also able to incorporate tactile feedback using another Utah array to stimulate the hand sensation area of the brain.

With the addition of touch, Dr. Tyler-Kabara's innovation improved the speed and accuracy of the arm by about 50 percent. Tyler-Kabara, an MD-PhD from Vanderbilt with degrees in biomedical engineering and neurophysiology, also showed that the same BCI used to control a robotic arm could be leveraged to fly a plane. After being hooked up to a flight simulator, using only the power of thought, her subject was able to control the ailerons and elevator of a virtual F-35 fighter jet to snake it through the walls of the Grand Canyon.

A commercially available movement-restoring BCI will likely be on the market within a decade. Such a device will be fully implanted, without a socket protruding through the skin, and it will send the brain's signals wirelessly to a phone-sized computer. This computer will, in turn, either electrically reanimate the flesh-and-blood atrophied muscles in the patient's own body or control a robotic limb.

Mechanical appendages may even offer certain advantages over the biological limbs provided to us by evolution. The limits of a robotic arm are constrained only by the imagination of the engineer. Not only could such an arm be stronger than a human arm; it could rotate a full 360 degrees in all its joints, or even function like an octopus arm. Such technology will eventually form the foundation of devices that will permit both the paralyzed and the able-bodied to control machines with their minds—not just cars or airplanes but also robots, spaceships, asteroid mining platforms, and even rovers on distant planets.

As enticing as it may be to enhance our abilities with a BCI, it's still

*Dr. Tyler-Kabara currently works at the University of Texas at Austin.

important to differentiate between a neuroprosthetic, which *restores* a lost function, and neuroaugmentation, which *enhances* already existing abilities. The latter device remains ethically questionable. The surgical implantation of a BCI is still a risky procedure. It would be a shame to damage an otherwise healthy brain and watch a previously normal patient leave the operating room weak and debilitated from the complications of an aspirational enhancement surgery. For the moment, BCI implants for neuroaugmentation remain decades away. Risking injury to the motor cortex of a paralyzed patient is one thing as long as there is a reasonable chance that the procedure will restore lost movement. Taking a similar gamble in an otherwise healthy brain is another matter altogether.

The Utah array, which penetrates the brain, has a small but real risk of either damaging the underlying neurons or causing a hemorrhage, even in highly skilled hands. My lab at Cornell employs the Utah array to record seizure activity in mice. We've had to abort a few of our experiments because the implant caused too much damage. For this reason, such arrays are now being placed using a robotic pneumatic tamping tool that rapidly plunges the array into the brain, which is surprisingly safer than a manual slow push.

It's a strange irony, the fact that we surgeons must rely on surgical robots to help us overcome the limitations of our own imperfect biology so that we can help our patients rely on a different set of limb-replacing robots to overcome the frailties of their imperfect biology. The human mind and its computing power may be the pinnacle of human evolution, but the dependence of the brain and our bodies on biology, miraculous though it may be, is a weakness that limits our abilities, both cognitive and physical.

CAN YOU READ MY MIND?

The holy grail of BCIs is to extract thoughts and ideas directly from the brain and then send them directly into a computer. That way, if you were injured and unable to move your lips, hands, or fingers, you could still communicate. Once your thoughts were digitized, they could be displayed on a screen, emailed to a friend, or maybe even inserted directly into another person's brain. My favorite science fiction novel that explores this idea is the Old Man's War series by John Scalzi, where future soldiers are implanted with a BrainPal, which allows them to access not only their weapons and ships' computers but also each other's BrainPals so they can engage in high-speed mind-to-mind communication. Before we discuss the current state of such technology, which is much further along than you might think, it's important to understand the difference between *thinking* and *articulating*.

As discussed, we have no clue how thoughts pop into our heads. Ideas arise from some unknown manner of subconscious algorithmic processing performed by hundreds if not thousands of interconnected brain modules. Once formed, these thoughts are then crunched through the brain's language modules and turned into words and sentences as I'm doing right now. But before I type out my ideas, they exist only in my head as a string of words. They haven't yet been communicated. To send my ideas out into the world, I must engage a few more modules—namely, those that move my lips, hands, or fingers. Only through these movements of the muscles of articulation can I finally release my ideas into the world. In other words, *movement* is the key to expressing thoughts.

Ideas can and often do exist only inside our heads, never to be unleashed. Or they can be shared with others in the form of spoken or written words. We can read quietly to ourselves or we can read out loud. I might *think* that my friend's new midlife crisis sports car is a complete waste of money, but I *don't* have to say it to him. This distinction between thinking and articulating is critical. It lies at the root of every current communication BCI, which records only the neuronal activity from the *motor* output parts of the brain—mouth, tongue, hands, fingers—not the thought fragments themselves before they are expressed. It's the outward *expression* of those thoughts, in other words, that language BCIs transmit.

If a BCI could extract your thoughts directly and deposit them into a computer without your consent, it might then be possible for a hacker or a powerful government to penetrate the computer's firewalls and gain access to them. This raises serious and justifiable ethical concerns. Our constitution guarantees inalienable rights, but the right to privacy of thought was never on the agenda. Our founding fathers never even remotely considered our inner lives alienable. But rest assured—and I can't stress this enough— BCIs in their current form cannot access our inner lives, so they cannot violate privacy.

UNLOCKING THE BRAIN

In 1997, French journalist Jean-Dominique Bauby was working as the editor in chief of French *Elle* when he suffered a stroke in his brain stem, the part of the brain that connects the cerebral cortex with the rest of the body. Unable to move his arms or his legs, unable to feel anything, and incapable of moving most of the muscles of his face, Bauby was in a state neurologists refer to as "locked in." It's estimated that there are some 80,000 locked-in Americans.

Despite his limitations, Bauby found a way to write a book, *The Diving Bell and the Butterfly*, which documented both his impaired physical condition as well as his vibrant inner mental life. How did he do this? Bauby used his only remaining function, his left eyelid. As an assistant scrolled through the alphabet one letter at a time, Bauby would wink when the correct letter appeared. The book took him only ten months to write, even with each word requiring almost two full minutes to compose.

Stephen Hawking, plagued by ALS, used a different technique. A computer would automatically move through a series of words and Hawking would twitch his thumb to access the right one. Once his thumb stopped working, he used a muscle in his cheek. His top speed was about 15 words per minute—a monumental effort, just like Bauby's. As tedious as it was, this system provided a way for Hawking's thoughts and theories to move out of his brain and into the world. Freeing the minds of the locked-in and the physically impaired is one of the primary goals of a communication BCI.

The first such device employed the same machine learning strategy we outlined earlier, but instead of moving a robotic arm, it moved a cursor on a computer screen. The goal was to create a mind-controlled point-and-click system. Electrodes implanted in the part of the brain that moves your arm and hand would record your brain waves as you think about moving a cursor across a computer screen. In front of you the letters of the alphabet are laid out in a grid on the screen. When the cursor hovers over the correct letter, you mentally select it by thinking about clicking a mouse button. Eventually, letter by letter, words and sentences appear on the screen as if you texted them out with one finger.

These devices reached a top speed of about 2 letters per minute.

The next generation relied on electrodes placed *in* the brain rather than simply on its surface. In fact, it used the Utah array just described to record the activity of individual neurons. How much faster could this one go? About twenty times faster, reaching a top speed of about 40 letters per minute—still shy of Hawking's pace but much faster than Bauby's. Yet the problem with these point-and-click methods was that they were still too slow. A new strategy was needed.

In *The Martian*, the 2011 novel by Andy Weir and the 2015 film directed by Ridley Scott, astronaut Mark Watney is trapped on Mars and needs to communicate with NASA to let them know he's still alive. Watney is isolated from humanity—locked-out if you will—on another planet. His first solution is a point-and-click strategy, rotating a camera head to select characters one by one. This painfully slow process is transformational, providing him with contact with the rest of humanity. Eventually he locates the buried Pathfinder Probe and, after hijacking its computer and downloading a program from NASA, he figures out how to message them more efficiently by typing on a keyboard.

A similar transition is occurring in communication BCIs.

The new generation still records from the same hand or mouth movement areas of the brain, but it uses a completely different strategy. Rather than moving a cursor on a screen to hunt and peck out individual letters one by one, these devices figure out which letters or words you're trying to say or write by associating your brain waves directly with spoken and written letters and words.

How? Well, it turns out that if you give a computer access both to the sounds that come out of your mouth as well as to the signals recorded from the part of the brain that moves your mouth, it can eventually figure out which sounds are associated with which signals using machine learning algorithms. The same can be true of the part of the brain that controls your hand movements. Every time you write a letter of the alphabet with a pen, your hand moves in roughly the same way and the neurons that move your hand fire in the same pattern. Therefore, the computer need only distinguish twenty-six different brain wave patterns to translate them into handwriting—one for each letter. The computer creates this transformation function using a machine learning algorithm, and then teaches itself through trial and error.

So how much faster are these newer methods compared with the point-and-click ones of the recent past? Neurosurgeon Jaimie Henderson, who co-directs the Neural Prosthetics Translational Lab at Stanford, implanted two Utah arrays in a quadriplegic's brain, specifically in the part that controls the hand and fingers, the use of which they lost after a spinal cord injury. After eleven training sessions—each one lasting three hours, during which the subject was asked to imagine writing letters in cursive using their paralyzed hand—they attained a rate of 90 characters per minute! That's six times faster than Hawking's point-and-click system. If you figure that you and I can text with our thumbs at roughly 115 characters per minute, these results are not too shabby. Astounding, really, if you think about it. It's as if Mark Watney had picked up his cell phone at the beginning of *The Martian* and texted NASA to say, "Hey, you guys left me here. Please come back. I'm getting hungry."

MR. WATSON, COME HERE

THE CASE OF
PANCHO

Pancho was a healthy twenty-year-old day laborer who worked at a vineyard in California. In 2003, while driving home, he was in a car accident. His injured stomach required surgery—a simple enough procedure, with few risks—but something went wrong. Pancho woke up almost completely paralyzed from his head to his toes. Eventually, Pancho learned to communicate through the tedious and drawn-out process of pecking out letters and words one at a time using his few remaining neck muscles. Picture a pencil-shaped pointer attached to his baseball cap. This jerry-rigged contraption produced a mere 5 words per minute.

Frustrated by his slow communication speed, Pancho volunteered for a clinical trial of a new BCI device developed by University of California, San Francisco, neurosurgeon Edward Chang. Chang is one of the rare neurosurgeons who is as skilled as a scientist as he is as a surgeon. In 2015, he won a Blavatnik Award, which celebrates the achievement of a handful of the nation's most exceptional young scientists in fields ranging from chemistry and astrophysics to molecular biology and nanotechnology. Chang remains the sole neurosurgeon on the list. In 2020 he was elected to the National Academy of Medicine. At forty-six he was named the chair of neurosurgery at UCSF and the co-director of the Center for Neural Engineering and Protheses.

Once inside Chang's operating room, Pancho lay with his brain exposed where Chang had opened his skull. Chang then implanted a 128-contact electrode grid the size of a postcard over the part of Pancho's cortex that controlled the movement of his lips and tongue. The wires from these electrodes were then tunneled under the skin to a socket implanted in his skull that protruded through his scalp. The researchers were thus able to plug a computer into Pancho's brain to record his brain waves as he mentally articulated a list of fifty different words.

Chang's BCI doesn't rely on electrodes that penetrate the brain like the Utah array; rather they sit on the brain's surface, like the ones used by Dobelle but with much finer resolution. These electrodes, in lieu of recording the activity within individual neurons, sample the collective activity of thousands of neurons and translate their electrical output into electrical signals. To program the device, Chang's team would show Pancho a word on a screen and ask him to say it. Although Pancho's stroke made speech impossible, the computer could nevertheless record the signals from his brain and—over the course of twenty-two hours spread out over a year and half—learn to link each of the fifty unique brain waves with each of those fifty different words. Once this digital Rosetta stone had been created, Pancho had only to think of one of the words, and it would appear on the screen as written text.

Chang and his team recorded their results in the July 15, 2021, issue of the *New England Journal of Medicine.* Their quasi-telepathic BCI could translate Pancho's thoughts into words at a rate of 15 words per minute. Just as Alexander Graham Bell's "Mr. Watson, come here—I want to see you" heralded the dawn of the telecommunications industry, so, too, did Pancho's first sentence—"My family is outside"—mark a giant leap in the annals of BCI communication. In each case, it's interesting to note, the first instinct of each speaker—Bell, whose wife and mother were deaf; Pancho, who was rendered mute—was to bring people together through the spoken word. (Or, as in Pancho's case, the imagined word.)

A few details of Chang's accomplishments are worth unpacking. First, Chang's BCI didn't actually read Pancho's thoughts because the recorded brain waves didn't originate in the part of the brain that processes thinking or language. Instead, Pancho had to imagine himself saying the words, which in turn activated the parts of his brain that would otherwise move his lips and tongue. The speech motor areas of the brain are much easier to decipher than those involved in intention, desire, feelings, and thinking.

We are still a long way from being able to access these inner recesses of human consciousness.

Second, after a year and half, Pancho's vocabulary was still limited to only fifty words; and his rate of speech—roughly 15 words per minute—while three times faster than prior attempts, was still markedly slower than the 150-words-per-minute rate of normal speech. However, with additional training and better computer algorithms, faster rates are inevitable. Also, keep in mind that the postcard-sized 128-contact-grid Chang used on Pancho's brain was far from state-of-the-art. Higher-density grids with thousands of electrodes that can record from smaller and smaller groups of neurons have already been developed. In fact, less than two years after Chang's breakthrough, neurosurgeon Jaimie Henderson implanted two Utah arrays in the brain of a paralyzed ALS patient. This was the same area of the brain as Pancho's, but recordings were made from individual neurons. His BCI decoded speech almost three times faster than Chang's— roughly 62 words per minute—which is not that far off from the normal rate of speech.

A few months later Chang upped the ante in the BCI "pace" race. Using a larger grid of 250 electrodes, his BCI translated a paralyzed patient's imagined words into synthesized speech at a rate of almost 100 words per minute, incorporating a vocabulary of over 1,000 words. Since the speech articulation areas are situated right next to the areas of the brain that control the facial musculature, Chang was able to harvest this information as well to control a cartoon face that could move its lips along with the synthesized speech and even generate facial expressions to convey the nonverbal, emotional components of speech. Rather than just projecting lines of text on a computer screen, this digitized reproduction of the patient's face appeared on a screen speaking in an audible voice, and its mouth and eyes moved with its own idiosyncratic expressions.

It's not hard to imagine that, as robotic technology advances, this digital doppelgänger could become a fully formed three-dimensional head and body that could move through the environment like the avatars in a James Cameron movie. With enough samples of their lost voice, the synthesized new voice could even sound just like them. If the patient's sensory cortex were implanted with a grid that stimulated the brain whenever their new synthetic body touched something, they could also interact with and feel the world as if they were physically present within their new body. If they wore virtual reality goggles that projected their robot's eye-cameras onto a heads-up display and used earphones to listen to the sounds collected in the robot's microphone ears, it would feel, to the paralyzed patient locked in their wheelchair, as if they once again inhabited the physical world. Their brain would be in one location, perched atop a wheelchair, trapped in the fractured remains of their former body, while their "mind" and "self" would be elsewhere, reborn and journeying the world in a new, artificial chassis.

Although the surface grid used by Chang cannot record individual neurons, its success implies that the fine spatial resolution of the Utah array may not be necessary. The neocortex, as you recall from Jeff Hawkins's description, comprises approximately 150,000 similar computational columns, each the size of a grain of rice. Therefore, we may need to record only the output of each of these neuronal assemblies rather than the

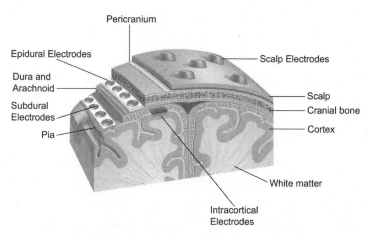

Individual electrodes can be placed on the scalp, as is done to record an EEG. Grids of electrodes can be inserted above the dura (epidural), below the dura and on the brain (subdural, as done by Chang), and intracortically (Utah array, as done by Henderson).

activity of every single neuron. The Utah array paradigm, while attractive from a conceptual standpoint to understand *how* the brain works, may be too granular for practical interpretation of *what* the brain is trying to say, metaphorically missing the forest for the trees.

For now, it remains to be seen whether smaller surface grids with finer resolution or larger arrays of intracortical electrodes will ultimately prove to be a more effective BCI design. What's certain is that future versions will only improve. Existing communication BCIs are primitive, like a telegraph machine transmitting Morse code. Imagine what we will be able accomplish when we develop the BCI equivalent of the telephone, much less video chatting.

But why stop there? Might it be possible, for example, to one day program a speech BCI that will allow communication to be *faster* than the normal rate of speech? Think about it: listening to a podcast at one-and-a-half or double speed is often a more efficient use of time and just as easy to comprehend. But if you tried listening at three or four times the normal speed, you might miss a lot. Is there an upper limit to what the brain can process? Is that limit fixed and hardwired, or is it merely what we are accustomed to interpreting? The reason we are comfortable hearing words spoken at 150 per minute is because that pace has been evolutionarily set by the limits of speech production. That's just how fast our mouths and tongues prefer to move. Speaking any faster is uncomfortable and hard to sustain, just as we can run only so fast based on the design of our legs and the strength and speed of our muscles.

But what if we were raised in an environment where speech was spoken at ten or twenty times the current rate? Would our brains adjust? This experiment has never been tried, but—given the known plasticity of the infant brain—my money says it would. It's a well-known fact that blind people can process speech much faster than the sighted. How? Their brains simply reallocate the part of the visual cortex that would otherwise process vision and use it to accelerate speech decoding. Some blind individuals have even trained themselves to echolocate like a bat by repurposing the circuitry of their unused visual cortex to perform a new function. The brain is not a hardwired computer, capable of only this and not that. It is instead a highly adaptable, multipurpose computing machine that gets programmed during our development for the specific world around us. Change the world and the brain will adapt.

One could even imagine creating a BCI that would allow a human brain to understand and program in raw computer code. Let's say a child is born congenitally deaf. Soon after birth, a two-way BCI could be implanted in their auditory cortex, the part of the brain that would otherwise be relegated to interpreting sound but now lies fallow. Instead of auditory information bombarding their primitive neuronal circuits—because it can't—raw code from the computer would instead be fed directly into the brain *as its connections form.* These tot bots would, I believe, be able to create the required circuitry in the brain to decipher digital language as rapidly and efficiently as you and I speak English. If the connection were bidirectional, they might even be able to write computer code as easily as we jot down reminders on a Post-it Note.

We're still a long way off from high-speed communication BCIs and super cyber-babies, but at the rate the technology is progressing, it's only a matter of time. If human progress has taught us anything, it's that science fiction can become science fact faster than you can say "driverless cars."

O BRAVE NEW WORLD

BCI implantation is still considered experimental, and it can be performed only at a handful of large academic medical centers. However, in a few years it may become as routine a part of a neurosurgeon's practice as operating on brain tumors. While I have not personally placed a BCI in any of my patients' brains, I have implanted dozens of responsive neurostimulators, devices that control epileptic seizures.

In responsive neurostimulation (RNS), a small computer is implanted in the skull and attached to two electrodes that are slipped onto the surface of the brain. The entire system is hidden beneath the skin, without protruding wires. Once the incision—made behind the hairline—is healed, the whole thing is completely invisible. The device records brain waves, analyzes the signals, and then runs them through a sophisticated algorithm that can anticipate when a seizure is about to occur. When it senses a seizure is imminent, it delivers a small shock to the brain, just as a pacemaker does for the heart, to abort the seizure before it begins. The RNS device is a modern version of Delgado's stimoceiver with one key difference: instead of relying on a human to trigger the stimulation, the device self-activates in response to its own built-in intelligence.

Since the entire system is subcutaneous, the infection rate is very low, and the RNS device can safely remain in place for decades. It is not hard to imagine a future BCI for movement, speech, or vision that is like the RNS device, with its self-contained computer and power source implanted in the skull, attached to high-density electrodes inserted in the brain. Such a device could communicate wirelessly with an external computer, a video camera, or a robotic arm and even be recharged through the skin.

Neurosurgeons Jaimie Henderson and Emad Eskandar,[*] while working at Stanford and MGH, respectively, have already created a fully implantable BCI that can transmit information recorded from a Utah array using radio frequency and Bluetooth, so no wires protrude. Patients are fully mobile, untethered from bulky computers. If Moore's law holds true, and the speed of computer circuitry doubles every two years, then BCI technology should also become progressively smaller and faster.

As devices become more delicate, neurosurgeons' hands may no longer be sufficiently precise to place them, as we saw was the case with the Utah array. Elon Musk's company Neuralink, for example, has developed a BCI

---

[*]Dr. Eskandar is currently the chair at Albert Einstein College of Medicine and Montefiore Medical Center.

consisting of over a thousand microelectrodes, which are inserted into the brain using an automated robotic surgeon, the R1, that pokes each tiny flexible electrode into the cortex like a sewing machine. In fact, as I write this, early human trials in quadriplegic patients have begun. Will this make my job obsolete? I really don't think so. Although Musk's goal may be to take humans out of the equation to increase precision, if the history of brain devices has taught us anything, it's that attempts to bypass neurosurgeons have not always ended well, for either the patients, the company, or the project. Luckily, Musk has a neurosurgeon advisor on his board: Dr. Matthew MacDougall.

One of the founding members of Neuralink was the Harvard- and MIT-educated neurosurgeon Benjamin I. Rapoport, who trained at Cornell. He has since cofounded his own BCI company: Precision Neuroscience. Rapoport's device, which he calls the Layer 7 Cortical Interface, is placed through a novel, minimally invasive surgery—performed by a flesh-and-blood neurosurgeon, I might add—and consists of one thousand tiny electrodes that rest on the brain's surface, like Chang's surface grid. This device appears to carry less surgical risk than Musk's. If it can be placed safely in unimpaired individuals, it might someday provide all of us with computer-assisted telepathic and telekinetic abilities. Further evidence of neurosurgical innovation: an Australian neurosurgeon named Thomas J. Oxley has designed a new type of BCI, the Stentrode, which can be implanted inside a blood vessel as an outpatient procedure under local anesthesia. The Stentrode uses the same interventional neuroradiology techniques that treat aneurysms and strokes. The surgeon inserts it like an IV into the patient's arm and then threads it up into the blood vessels overlying the brain. Once in place, the Stentrode records brain waves from inside the blood vessel, which are transmitted to a computer. After a few months, the Stentrode becomes fully incorporated into the wall of the blood vessel, providing stable information for years. It has already been used in association with eye-tracking software to create a point-and-click device that helps paralyzed patients with ALS surf the internet.

The future of visual prosthetics is less certain. It's unclear whether phosphenes will provide enough points of light to create a useful image. An alternative strategy for a visual prosthetic would be to use phosphenes as alerts that signal the proximity of a specific person or thing. For example, facial recognition software could identify an individual and activate a phosphene in a unique position in the subject's visual field when that person approaches, like an early-warning system such as the sensors in the deep ocean that foretell an impending tsunami by flashing a red light on the control panel in a monitoring station. You could imagine, for example, enjoying a moment of quiet on the couch at home when suddenly a phosphene flashes to let you know that your mother-in-law just entered the room. Alternatively, a brief sparkle in a different spot could also alert you to lean over, since your youngest child is moving in for a hug.

To create vision with as much detail as what we currently have, novel strategies for activating the visual cortex will be required. Possibilities include white matter stimulation, multifocal optogenetic activation, or leveraging the inherent plasticity of the developing brain. For example, let's say soon after the birth of a congenitally blind baby, we insert the digital data stream from an external camera into the white matter—that is, the input stream—of the infant's visual cortex. The baby's brain circuitry could learn to interpret the incoming visual data and provide its wearer with a representation of the external world just as our eyes do for us. This visual prosthetic could provide our implantee with vision in the normal spectrum or even enhanced vision into the ultraviolet and infrared range. But visual input can also be plugged into virtually any part of the baby's brain, not just the visual cortex. The visual cortex *becomes* the visual cortex only because it's processing input from the eyes. Any random part of an infant's proto-cortex could do the same job.

Although it's hard to imagine what this form of vision would be like, it's equally difficult to imagine how blind people hear the world with enhanced auditory capabilities or echolocation. We could also imagine a BCI that senses electric and magnetic fields—as birds and fish do—and inputs this information directly into the brain to create enhanced humans with perceptual abilities beyond our five senses. And their experience of these new extrasensory perceptions would be as normal to them as our experience of our five senses is to us.

Creative solutions in the adult brain might involve techniques to reintroduce plasticity with drugs that restore lost malleability. Virtually any sort of incoming information could be inserted into the chemically altered unused visual cortex, which would reprogram its circuitry to interpret these new signals. Or let's say the adult brain is more plastic than we think. If so, we could try placing such a device for several years in the brain of a blind adult to see if, over time, the signals become interpretable.

Plasticity in adults varies according to which part of the brain we're talking about. Regions such as the visual cortex, for example, are strongly hardwired by adulthood to interpret the visual signals that correspond to our existing world. Such rigidly fixed areas may not be the best targets for a BCI. On the other hand, other downstream areas—we call these association areas—integrate information from the primary sensory areas for vision, touch, and hearing and create our experiences and our long-term memories. These brain regions are malleable, so they can respond to new information and develop novel connections between the various sensory streams. Perhaps targeting our BCIs to these higher-order brain processing regions makes more sense in an adult, even for a visual prosthetic.

We may even have to rethink what vision is and learn to avoid our own biases. Re-creating in the blind what we know as vision so they can perceive the world the way *we* perceive it may not be the best strategy. For one thing, it may be impossible. But more important, there is no inherent reason visual information must be experienced as we do. The same visual information with the same level of detail, if processed in a different brain area, might elicit a completely different phenomenology, such as complex patterns of sounds, touch, or even smells, similar to the way a dog experiences the world in fine detail with its nose. In fact, if we were to insert visual data in an area of the brain whose function we don't fully understand, like the right frontal lobe, we might create a new sensorium unlike anything we can imagine. Such out-of-the-box thinking may be required for BCIs to fully realize their potential.

BCI technology is advancing so rapidly, in fact, that it's difficult to say where the field will be between the time I write these words and the time you read them. However, it's more than likely that, within five years or so, a fully implantable, commercially available device will help both paralyzed and locked-in patients move about, search the internet, or communicate using only their minds integrated with computers. As for telepathic BCIs that transmit thoughts, ideas, and emotions from one brain to another, these remain, for now, science fiction. They will require enormous breakthroughs in our understanding of how neurons in the brain create the abstract components of our mental world. At the same time, we are already living in an age when the BCIs of today were considered science fiction a few decades ago, so mark my words: in the blink of a mechanical eye, humans and computers will soon be integrated in ways we can barely imagine today.

We are standing on the precipice of the next great leap in human evolution, and if my hunch is correct, neurosurgeons will play a pivotal role in the forthcoming transformation of our species.

EPILOGUE

Modern neurosurgery owes an enormous debt of gratitude to the early brave pioneers who explored the hostile topography of the human brain to make the landscape more hospitable for us future settlers. We've come a long way since the days when most neurosurgeries ended in either failure or death. Like all human progress, our field has relied on each subsequent generation surpassing the accomplishments of its predecessors.

But revolutions in thought are rarely greeted warmly. The prevailing experts of the time will generally condemn new ideas as either too fanciful, too dangerous, or too much of a threat to existing authority. Neurosurgery is no exception. Walter Dandy's aggressive but curative surgeries were offensive to Harvey Cushing's meticulously safe ones. Irving Cooper's elimination of tremor without paralysis was disparaged by Paul Bucy as fraudulent and inconceivable, primarily because Bucy hadn't succeeded in doing so himself. Yaşargil's boss, Krayenbühl, refused to let Yaşargil operate on aneurysms for years following the latter's return from Vermont, in a futile attempt to perpetuate the power structure of the department. Stereotactic radiosurgery has supplanted surgery as the treatment of choice for most brain metastases, and coiling has replaced clipping to secure most aneurysms. Minimally invasive skull base surgery, which uses the nasal passages or the orbit as the gateway to the most-difficult-to-reach tumors, was rejected as a gimmick when first suggested. Now I, and many others, perform these surgeries routinely.

Each of these once-novel technologies and ideas eventually moved the field forward, regardless of whether they were initially appreciated or repudiated. Progress always marches on. The apprentice always becomes the master.

One of the goals of this book has been to unpack the myth of the neurosurgeon, to trace its origins and separate the authentic from the apocryphal. Since the days of Harvey Cushing, two competing stereotypes have emerged. The first, engendered by Cushing himself, was that of the brilliant, hardworking, unemotional, but daring surgeon-scientist with a Renaissance expertise in a variety of topics. Certainly, many of the larger-than-life forebears of the profession fit this mold. However, if we hold ourselves up to this archetype, we inevitably fall short. Neurosurgeons, no matter how talented and smart, will inevitably make mistakes. That is how we learn. But it is our obligation to critically scrutinize our decisions and continually improve, which is why we don't really hit our stride until mid-career.

In addition, the profession has traditionally been populated mostly by White men. We need to do better by welcoming more women and minorities into the specialty of neurosurgery. Trailblazers like Ben Carson, Alfredo Quiñones, and Karin Muraszko are far too uncommon. While women are now entering the field in greater numbers, diversity remains an issue.

The other, more bothersome stereotype is that of the mad scientist, which implies the possibility that a neurosurgeon may be driven by ego or malevolence to use their patients as guinea pigs. Hollywood has perpetuated this myth. It sells. I've tried to expose the truth that, historically, the perpetrators in this case—Burkhardt, Freeman, Moniz—were, for the most part, not neurosurgeons. The exceptions were Drs. Scoville and Poppen. The former performed experimental surgery on a desperate patient and robbed him of his most precious possessions: his memories and his life story. The latter lobotomized incarcerated criminals. Both of these surgeons were hardworking, respected members of the neurosurgical community. Both made valuable contributions to our field despite their indiscretions. Both show us that human fallibility is ever present, even among neurosurgeons.

The modern neurosurgeon-scientist could not be more different from the odd characters who inspired the mad scientist myth. In addition to my mentors, George Ojemann and Dennis Spencer, I profiled the work of Drs. Sameer Sheth, Nader Pouratian, Itzhak Fried, Kareem Zaghloul, Elizabeth Tyler-Kabara, Ali Rezai, Jaimie Henderson, and Edward Chang, who are only a handful of the many academic neurosurgeons currently making groundbreaking strides in neuroscience. As a result of their work, neurosurgeons will soon be implanting electrodes and injecting chemicals into the brain to rewire its circuitry, alleviating the symptoms of all manner of mental illnesses, not to mention restoring sight, movement, hearing, and speech to the disabled. These investigators are under intense scrutiny by the ethics committees at their institutions and take the issue of informed consent and the principle of beneficence very seriously, the latter being the mandate that all human experimentation be for the good of society. They are, most important, doctors first and researchers second.

I asked Chang if he thought that Pancho, the patient whose speech he restored with his BCI, was more a patient or an experiment. He thought about it for a while and then replied, "A patient." He likened implanting a BCI to any other neurosurgical operation done for the first time, like taking out a tumor through the nose when no one thinks you can or should. "We saw he had a big problem, inability to communicate, and we had a solution." Chang gets weekly emails from desperate patients eager to gain access to his restorative device. I asked him how that makes him feel. His answer: "It reminds me. We have to move faster."

Perhaps one of the greatest ironies in the history of neurosurgery emerged after Harvey Cushing's death. His autopsy revealed that, deep within the third ventricle of his brain, he harbored a small colloid cyst: a benign growth that, if large enough, might obstruct the flow of cerebrospinal fluid and become life-threatening. Luckily, Cushing's cyst never needed treatment. Had the cyst grown a bit larger during his lifetime, it could have been identified only by using Dandy's ventriculogram. Were surgery indicated, the most qualified person to perform such a surgery would have been Dandy himself, Cushing's protégé and nemesis. Which begs the question: Had Cushing not been so hard on Dandy, would Dandy have been as motivated to prove his worth to his disdainful teacher?

Neurosurgery training is rigorous, demanding, and emotionally draining. While it might be nice for the experience to be more nurturing, it's far from clear that such a soft and cushy environment would breed great neurosurgeons. Maybe the training needs to be this way? If the drummer Jo Jones hadn't thrown the cymbal at the teenage Charlie Parker's head during his botched solo, would the humiliated Parker have worked so hard to become Bird, the greatest alto saxophone player of all time? Don't get me wrong, I'm not arguing in favor of abusive training. We examined how this can foster insensitivity, isolation, and depression. Remember, Bird ended up addicted to drugs and died at a young age from an overdose. But if neurosurgery training is to become more nurturing, which it must and already is, it cannot become less rigorous. We need neurosurgeons who demand excellence from themselves, give their very best every time they show up for work, and are willing to sacrifice their personal liberties for the greater good.

Which brings us back to the cliché "It's not brain surgery." If neurosurgery is so difficult, does it follow that neurosurgeons are, on average, smarter than people in other professions? In 2021, the *British Medical Journal* addressed this precise question—namely: Who is more intelligent, neurosurgeons or rocket scientists, and are they smarter than the rest of the professional world? The authors examined 148 neurosurgeons and 600 rocket scientists and compared their answers in a panel of intelligence tests to those of the general population. The authors found that, contrary to public opinion, neither the neurosurgeons nor the rocket scientists scored any better than anyone else. The conclusion was that brain surgeons as well as rocket scientists are "unnecessarily placed on a pedestal."

However, I would argue—and I hope you would agree by now—that the authors of this study missed the point entirely. They asked the wrong question. It's not about intelligence. Neurosurgeons are not inherently smarter than anyone else any more than Navy SEALs are more physically elite. However, SEALs undergo intense mental and physical training that enables them to perform at a high level under extremely stressful circumstances. What makes brain surgery so difficult is that the training and the job are so challenging on so many different levels—physically, mentally, and certainly with respect to work-life balance—that few want to make the necessary sacrifices of time and personal interests to do the job.

Neurosurgery, like all fields of medicine, is, at its heart, a service industry. Like a priest or a nun, we swear an oath to dedicate ourselves to a higher purpose far greater than ourselves: the health of our patients. The soldier's creed holds true for neurosurgery as well: "I will always place the mission first. I will never accept defeat. I will never quit."

So the next time you use the phrase "It's not brain surgery" to compare the difficulty of a particular activity to what we do, maybe pause to consider your words. If you are describing a task—any task—that doesn't just require raw intellect but rather a combination of intense focus, dedication, discipline, humility, sensitivity, dexterity, physical stamina, confidence, and sacrifice . . . then maybe it is?

BIBLIOGRAPHY

Chapter 1. The Myth

Barnett, Randaline R., Kristin G. Weiss, Hengameh B. Pajer, Jo L. Goh, Dawn N. Kernagis, and Carolyn S. Quinsey. "Revolutionizing Neurosurgery without Wielding the Knife: The Legacy of Dr. Louise Eisenhardt." *Journal of Neuropathology and Experimental Neurology* 80, no. 9 (September 2021): 875–80.

Beil, Laura. "Dr. Death." Wondery. 3 seasons, 36 episodes. https://wondery.com/shows/dr-death.

Bliss, Michael. *Harvey Cushing: A Life in Surgery.* New York: Oxford University Press, 2005.

Carson, Benjamin, and Cecil Murphey. *Gifted Hands: The Ben Carson Story.* Grand Rapids, MI: Zondervan, 1992.

Casillo, Stephanie M., Anisha Venkatesh, Mallammai Muthiah, Michael McDowell, and Nitin Agarwal. "First Female Neurosurgeon in the United States: Dorothy Klenke Nash, MD." *Neurosurgery* 89, no. 4 (September 2021): E223–28.

Corley, Jacquelyn, Eliana Kim, Chris Ann Philips, Martina Stippler, Ann M. Parr, Jennifer Sweet, and Gail Rousseau. "One Hundred Years of Neurosurgery: Contributions of American Women." *Journal of Neurosurgery* 134, no. 2 (February 2021): 337–42.

Cushing, Harvey. "The Special Field of Neurological Surgery." *Bulletin of the Johns Hopkins Hospital* 16 (1905): 77–87.

Detchou, Donald K., Alvin Onyewuenyi, Vamsi Reddy, Andre Boyke, Nnenna Mbabuike, William W. Ashley Jr., and Edjah K. Nduom. "Letter: A Call to Action: Increasing Black Representation in Neurological Surgery." *Neurosurgery* 88, no. 5 (May 2021): E469–73.

Fulton, John. *Harvey Cushing: A Biography.* New York: Oxford University Press, 1947.

Hansson, Nils, and Thomas Schlich. "'High Qualified Loser'? Harvey Cushing and the Nobel Prize." *Journal of Neurosurgery* 122, no. 4 (2015): 976–79.

Johnson, Sharon. "Disabled in Professions Grow." *New York Times,* July 18, 1983. https://www.nytimes.com/1983/07/18/us/disabled-in-professions-grow.html.

Light, Richard U. "Remembering Harvey Cushing: The Closing Years." *Surgical Neurology* 37 (1992):147–57.

McClelland, Shearwood, III. "Alexa Irene Canady: The First African-American Woman Neurosurgeon." *Journal of the National Medical Association* 100, no. 4 (April 2008): 439–43.

——, and Kimbra S. Harris. "Clarence Sumner Greene, Sr: The First African-American Neurosurgeon." *Neurosurgery* 59, no. 6 (December 2006): 1325–27.

Muraszko, Karin. "Doctor with Spinal Bifida Defies Expectations." CNN, April 27, 2016. https://edition.cnn.com/2016/04/27/health/turning-points-dr-karin-muraszko/index.html.

Quiñones-Hinojosa, Alfredo, with Mim Eichler Rivas. *Becoming Dr. Q: My Journey from Migrant Farm Worker to Brain Surgeon*. Berkeley: University of California Press, 2011.

White, Robert J., Lee R. Wolin, Leo C. Massopust, Normal Taslitz, and Javier Verdura. "Cephalic Exchange Transplantation in the Monkey." *Surgery* 70, no. 1 (July 1971): 135–39.

Chapter 2. The Training

Csikszentmihalyi, Mihaly. *Flow: The Psychology of Optimal Experience*. New York: Harper and Row, 1990.

Fishman, Steve. "Skull's Angels." *Rolling Stone*, March 9, 1989.

Greenwood, James Jr., "Two Point Coagulation. A New Principle and Instrument for Applying Coagulation in Neurosurgery." *American Journal of Surgery* 1 (1940): 267–70.

Quest, Donald O., and J. Lawrence Pool. "A History of the Neurological Institute of New York and Its Department of Neurological Surgery." *Neurosurgery* 38, no. 6 (June 1996): 1232–36.

Results and Data: 2020 Main Residency Match. National Resident Matching Program, Washington, DC, 2020. https://www.nrmp.org/wp-content/uploads/2021/12/MM_Results_and_Data_2020-rev.pdf.

Schernhammer, Eva. "Taking Their Own Lives—The High Rate of Physician Suicide." *New England Journal of Medicine* 352 (June 2005): 2473–76.

Solomon, Robert A. "New York City at the Dawn of Neurological Surgery." *Journal of Neurosurgery* 125, no. 5 (2016): 1291–1300.

"Storage and Handling of Potassium Chloride Concentrate and Other Strong Potassium Solutions." National Health System Alert/PSA 01, October 31, 2002. www.npsa.nhs.uk.

Chapter 3. Penetrating Head Trauma

Centers for Disease Control and Prevention. National Center for Health Statistics: Mortality Data on CDC WONDER. Accessed April 2023, https://wonder.cdc.gov/mcd.html.

Cytowic, Richard E. "The Long Ordeal of James Brady." *New York Times*, September 27, 1981. www.nytimes.com/1981/09/27/magazine/the-long-ordeal-of-james-brady.html.

Gautschi, Oliver P., and Gerhard Hildebrandt. "Emil Theodor Kocher (25/8/1841–27/7/1917)—A Swiss (neuro-)surgeon and Nobel Prize Winner." *British Journal of Neurosurgery* 23, no. 3 (2009): 234–36.

Komisarow, Jordon M., Theodore Pappas, Megan Llewellyn, and Shivanand P. Lad. "The Assassination of Robert F. Kennedy: An Analysis of the Senator's Injuries and Neurosurgical Care." *Journal of Neurosurgery* 130, no. 5 (June 2018): 1649–54.

Levy, Michael L., Daniel Sullivan, Rodrick Faccio, and Robert G. Grossman. "A Neuroforensic Analysis of the Wounds of President John F. Kennedy: Part 2—A Study of the Available Evidence, Eyewitness Correlations, Analysis and Conclusions." *Neurosurgery* 54, no. 6 (June 2004): 1298–1312.

Menger, Richard, Piyush Kalakoti, Rimal Hanif, Osama Ahmed, Anil Nanda, and Bharat Guthikonda. "A Political Case of Penetrating Trauma: The Injury of James Scott Brady." *Neurosurgery* 81, no. 3 (September 2017): 545–51.

Rossini, Zefferino, Federico Nicolosi, Angelos G. Kolias, Peter J. Hutchinson, Paolo De Sanctis, and Franco Servadei. "The History of Decompressive Craniectomy in Traumatic Brain Injury." *Frontiers in Neurology* 10 (May 2019): 1–9.

Silverman, Willa Z. "Life and Death of a 'Non-Conformist': Thierry de Martel (1875–1940)." *Modern & Contemporary France* 5, no. 1 (1997): 5–19.

Sullivan, Daniel, Rodrick Faccio, Michael L. Levy, and Robert G. Grossman. "The Assassination of President John F. Kennedy: A Forensic Analysis—Part 1: A Neurosurgeon's Previously Undocumented Eyewitness Account of the Events of Nov 22, 1963." *Neurosurgery* 53, no. 5 (November 2003): 1019–27.

Warren Commission Report. National Archives. www.archives.gov/research/jfk/warren-commission-report.

Yan, Sandra C., Timothy R. Smith, Wenya Linda Bi, Ryan Brewster, William B. Gormley, Ian F. Dunn, and Edward R. Laws Jr. "The Assassination of Abraham Lincoln and the Evolution of Neuro-Trauma Care: Would the 16th President Have Survived in the Modern Era?" *World Neurosurgery* 84, no. 5 (November 2015): 1453–57.

Zwirner, Johann, Sarah Safavi, Mario Scholze, Kai Chun Li, John Neil Waddell, Björn Busse, Benjamin Ondruschka, and Niels Hammer. "Topographical

Mapping of the Mechanical Characteristics of the Human Neurocranium Considering the Role of Individual Layers." *Scientific Reports* 11 (February 2021): 1–11.

Chapter 4. Head-on Collisions

Ahmed, N., A. Soroush, Y.-H. Kuo, and J. M. Davis. "Risk Associated with Traumatic Intracranial Bleed and Outcome in Patients Following a Fall from a Standing Position." *European Journal of Trauma and Emergency Surgery* 41 (2015): 307–11.

Athiviraham, Aravind, Adam Bartsch, Prasath Mageswaran, Edward C. Benzel, Brian Perse, Morgan H. Jones, and Mark Schickendantz. "Analysis of Baseball-to-Helmet Impacts in Major League Baseball." *American Journal of Sports Medicine* 40, no. 12 (2012): 2808–14.

Attwood, Jonathan Edward, Gabriele C. De Luca, Terence Hope, and Deva Sanjeeva Jeyaretna. "Sir Hugh Cairns: A Pioneering Collaborator." *Acta Neurochirurgica* 161, no. 8 (2019): 1491–95.

Bandak, Faris A. "Shaken Baby Syndrome: A Biomechanics Analysis of Injury Mechanisms." *Forensic Science International* 151, no. 1 (June 2005): 71–79.

Bhattacharya, Bishwajit, Adrian Maung, Kevin Schuster, and Kimberly A. Davis. "The Older They Are the Harder They Fall: Injury Patterns and Outcomes by Age After Ground Level Falls." *Injury: International Journal of the Care of the Injured* 47, no. 9 (September 2016): 1955–59.

Brewster, Ryan, Wenya Linda Bi, Timothy R. Smith, William B. Gormley, Ian F. Dunn, and Edward R. Laws Jr. "The Neurosurgeon as Baseball Fan and Inventor: Walter Dandy and the Batter's Helmet." *Neurosurgical Focus* 39, no. 1 (July 2015): 1–6.

Brown, Joshua B., Christine M. Leeper, Jason L. Sperry, Andrew B. Peitzman, Timothy R. Billiar, Barbara A. Gaines, and Mark L. Gestring. "Helicopters and Injured Kids: Improved Survival with Scene Air Medical Transport in the Pediatric Trauma Population." *Journal of Trauma and Acute Care Surgery* 80, no. 5 (May 2016): 702–10.

Camp, Christopher L., Dean Wang, Alec S. Sinatro, John D'Angelo, Struan H. Coleman, Joshua S. Dines, Stephen Fealy, and Stan Conte. "Getting Hit by Pitch in Professional Baseball: Analysis of Injury Patterns, Risk Factors, Concussions, and Days Missed for Batters." *American Journal of Sports Medicine* 46, no. 8 (2018): 1997–2003.

Carniol, Eric T., Kevin Shaigany, Peter F. Svider, Adam J. Folbe, Giancarlo F. Zuliani, Soly Baredes, and Jean Angerson Eloy. "'Beaned': A 5-Year Analysis of Baseball Related Injuries of the Face." *Otolaryngology—Head and Neck Surgery* 153, no. 6 (December 2015): 957–61.

Casson, Ira R., Ozzie Siegel, Raj Sham, Edwin A. Campbell, Milton Tarlau, and Anthony DiDomenico. "Brain Damage in Modern Boxers." *Journal of the American Medical Association* 251, no. 20 (May 1984): 2663–67.

Chadwick, David L., Robert H. Kirschner, Robert M. Reece, Lawrence R. Ricci, Randall Alexander, Mia Amaya, Judith Ann Bays et al. "Shaken Baby Syndrome—A Forensic Pediatric Response." *Pediatrics* 101, no. 2 (February 1998): 321–23.

Chen, Xilin, Mark L. Gestring, Matthew R. Rosengart, Timothy R. Billiar, Andrew B. Peitzman, Jason L. Sperry, and Joshua B. Brown. "Speed Is Not Everything: Identifying Patients Who May Benefit from Helicopter Transport Despite Faster Ground Transport." *Journal of Trauma and Acute Care Surgery* 84, no. 4 (April 2018): 549–57.

Delgado, M. Kit, Kristan L. Staudenmayer, N. Ewen Wang, David A. Spain, Sharada Weir, Douglas K. Owens, and Jeremy D. Goldhaber-Fiebert. "Cost-Effectiveness of Helicopter Versus Ground Emergency Medical Services for Trauma Scene Transport in the United States." *Annals of Emergency Medicine* 62, no. 4 (October 2013): 351–64.

Duhaime, Ann-Christine, Thomas A. Gennarelli, Lawrence E. Thibault, Derek A. Bruce, Susan S. Margulies, and Randall Wiser. "The Shaken Baby Syndrome: A Clinical, Pathological, and Biomechanical Study." *Journal of Neurosurgery* 66, no. 3 (April 1987): 409–15.

Engelhardt, J., D. Brauge, and H. Loiseau. "Second Impact Syndrome: Myth or Reality?" *Neurochirurgie* 67, no. 3 (May 2021): 1–11.

Fox, William Lloyd. *Dandy of Johns Hopkins*. Baltimore: Williams & Wilkins, 1984.

Ganz, Jeremy C. "The Lucid Interval Associated with Epidural Bleeding: Evolving Understanding." *Journal of Neurosurgery* 118, no. 4 (April 2013): 739–45.

Garner, Alan A., Anna Lee, and Andrew Weatherall. "Physician Staffed Helicopter Emergency Medical Service Dispatch Via Centralised Control or Directly by Crew—Case Identification Rates and Effect on the Sydney Paediatric Trauma System." *Scandinavian Journal of Trauma Resuscitation and Emergency Medicine* 20, no. 1 (December 2012): 1–6.

Gladwell, Malcolm. "Conquering the Coma." *New Yorker*, July 8, 1996.

Guthkelch, A. N. "Infantile Subdural Haematoma and Its Relationship to Whiplash Injuries." *British Medical Journal* 2, no. 5759 (May 1971): 430–31.

Hadley, Mark N., Volker K. H. Sonntag, Harold L. Rekate, and Alan Murphy. "The Infant Whiplash-Shake Injury Syndrome: A Clinical and Pathological Study." *Neurosurgery* 24, no. 4 (April 1989): 536–40.

Hamel, Anissa, Maxime Llari, Marie-Dominique Piercecchi-Marti, Pascal Adalian, Georges Leonetti, and Lionel Thollon. "Effects of Fall Conditions and Biological

Variability on the Mechanism of Skull Fractures Caused by Falls." *International Journal of Legal Medicine* 1277, no. 1 (January 2013): 111–18.

Hawryluk, Gregory W. J., and Jamshid Ghajar. "Evolution and Impact of the Brain Trauma Foundation Guidelines." *Neurosurgery* 89, no. 6 (November 2021): 1148–56.

Jenecke, Cassandra Ann. "Shaken Baby Syndrome, Wrongful Convictions, and the Dangers of Aversion to Changing Science in Criminal Law." *University of San Francisco Law Review* 48, no. 1 (2014): 147–88.

Lynøe, Niels, Göran Elinder, Boubou Hallberg, Måns Rosén, Pia Sundgren, and Anders Eriksson. "Insufficient Evidence for 'Shaken Baby Syndrome': A Systematic Review." *Acta Pædiatrica* 106, no. 7 (July 2017): 1021–27.

Matur, Abhijith V., Laura B. Ngwenya, and Charles J. Prestigiacomo. "The Surgical History of Head Injury in Motor Vehicle Collision." *Journal of Neurosurgery* 135, no. 2 (November 2020): 594–600.

Park, Kee B., Walter D. Johnson, and Robert K. Dempsey. "Global Neurosurgery: The Unmet Need." *World Neurosurgery* 88 (April 2016): 32–35.

Punchak, Maria, Swagoto Mukhopadhyay, Sonal Sachdev, Ya-Ching Hung, Sophie Peeters, Abbas Rattani, Michael Dewan et al. "Neurosurgical Care: Availability and Access in Low-Income and Middle-Income Countries." *World Neurosurgery* 112 (April 2018): 240–54.

Sarani, Babak, Brandy Temple-Lykens, Patrick Kim, Seema Sonnad, Meredith Bergey, Jose L. Pascual, Carrie Sims et al. "Factors Associated with Mortality and Brain Injury After Falls from the Standing Position." *Journal of Trauma Injury, Infection, and Critical Care* 67, no. 5 (November 2009): 954–58.

Sharma, Sunjay, David Gomez, Charles de Mestral, Marvin Hsiao, James Rutka, and Avery B. Nathens. "Emergency Access to Neurosurgical Care for Patients with Traumatic Brain Injury." *Journal of the American College of Surgeons* 218, no. 1 (January 2014): 51–57.

Shelden, C. Hunter. "Prevention, the Only Cure for Head Injuries Resulting from Automobile Accidents." *Journal of the American Medical Association* 159, no. 10 (November 1955): 981–86.

Sowell, Mike. *The Pitch That Killed: The Story of Carl Mays, Ray Chapman, and the Pennant Race of 1920.* Guilford, CT: Lyons Press, 2016.

Stone, James L., Vimal Patel, and Julian E. Bailes. "Sir Hugh Cairns and World War II British Advances in Head Injury Management, Diffuse Brain Injury, and Concussion: An Oxford Tale." *Journal of Neurosurgery* 125, no. 5 (November 2016): 1301–14.

Tailor, J., and A. Handa. "Hugh Cairns and the Origin of British Neurosurgery." *British Journal of Neurosurgery* 21, no. 2 (April 2007), 190–96.

Taylor, Colman B., Kate Curtis, Stephen Jan, and Mark Newcombe. "Helicopter Emergency Medical Services (HEMS) Over-Triage and the Financial Implications for Major Trauma Centres in NSW, Australia." *BMC Emergency Medicine* 13 (July 2013): 1–8.

Tew, John M. "Frank H. Mayfield, M.D., 1908–1991." *Journal of Neurosurgery* 75, no. 3 (1991): 347–48.

Uscinski, Ronald H. "Shaken Baby Syndrome: An Odyssey." *Neurologia Medico-Chirurgica* 46, no. 2 (February 2006): 57–61.

———. "Shaken Baby Syndrome: Fundamental Questions." *British Journal of Neurosurgery* 16, no. 3 (June 2002): 217–19.

Chapter 5. Sports Neurosurgery

Boden, Barry P., Robin L. Tacchetti, Robert C. Cantu, Sarah B. Knowles, and Frederick O. Mueller. "Catastrophic Head Injuries in High School and College Football Players." *American Journal of Sports Medicine* 35, no. 7 (July 2007): 1075–81.

Cantu, Robert C. "Chronic Traumatic Encephalopathy in the National Football League." *Neurosurgery* 61, no. 2 (August 2007): 223–25.

Casson, Ira R., Elliot J. Pellman, and David C. Viano. "Chronic Traumatic Encephalopathy in a National Football League Player." *Neurosurgery* 58, no. 5 (May 2006): 1–4.

Corsellis, J. A. N., C. J. Bruton, and Dorothy Freeman-Browne. "The Aftermath of Boxing." *Psychological Medicine* 3, no. 3 (August 1973): 270–303.

Dunn, Ian F., Gavin Dunn, and Arthur L. Day. "Neurosurgeons and Their Contributions to Modern-Day Athletics: Richard C. Schneider Memorial Lecture." *Neurosurgical Focus* 21, no. 4 (October 2006): 1–6.

Goldfinger, Marc H., Helen Ling, Bension S. Tilley, Alan K. L. Liu, Karen Davey, Janice L. Holton, Tamas Revesz, and Steve M. Gentleman. "The Aftermath of Boxing Revisited: Identifying Chronic Traumatic Encephalopathy Pathology in the Original Corsellis Boxer Series." *Acta Neuropathologica* 136, no. 6 (2018): 973–74.

Guskiewicz, Kevin M., Stephen W. Marshall, Julian Bailes, Michael McCrea, Robert C. Cantu, Christopher Randolph, and Barry D. Jordan. "Association Between Recurrent Concussion and Late-Life Cognitive Impairment in Retired Professional Football Players." *Neurosurgery* 57, no. 4 (October 2005): 719–26.

Kucera, Kristen L., David Klossner, Bob Colgate, and Robert C. Cantu. Annual Survey of Football Injury Research. NCCSIR, March 27, 2023. https://nccsir.unc.edu/wp-content/uploads/sites/5614/2023/04/Annual-Football-2022-Fatalities-FINAL-web.pdf.

McKee, Ann C., Christopher J. Nowinski, Robert A. Stern, Thor D. Stein, Victor E. Alvarez, Daniel H. Daneshvar, Hyo-Soon Lee et al. "The Spectrum of Disease in Chronic Traumatic Encephalopathy." *Brain* 136 (part 1) (January 2013): 43–64.

McLendon, Loren A., Stephen F. Kralik, Patricia A. Grayson, and Meredith R. Golomb. "The Controversial Second Impact Syndrome: A Review of the Literature." *Pediatric Neurology* 62 (2016): 9–17.

Omalu, Bennet I., Steven T. DeKosky, Ryan L. Minster, M. Ilyas Kamboh, Ronald L. Hamilton, and Cyril H. Wecht. "Chronic Traumatic Encephalopathy in a National Football League Player." *Neurosurgery* 57, no. 1 (July 2005): 128–34.

Omalu, Bennet I., Steven T. DeKosky, Ronald L. Hamilton, Ryan L. Minster, M. Ilyas Kamboh, Abdulrezak N. Shakir, and Cyril H. Wecht. "Chronic Traumatic Encephalopathy in a National Football League Player: Part II." *Neurosurgery* 59, no. 5 (November 2006): 1086–93.

Pellman, Elliot J. "Background on the National Football League's Research on Concussion in Professional Football." *Neurosurgery* 53, no. 4 (October 2003): 797–98.

——, Mark R. Lovell, David C. Viano, and Ira R. Casson. "Concussion in Professional Football: Recovery of NFL and High School Athletes Assessed by Computerized Neuropsychological Testing—Part 12." *Neurosurgery* 58, no. 2 (February 2006): 263–74.

——, Mark R. Lovell, David C. Viano, Ira R. Casson, and Andrew M. Tucker. "Concussion in Professional Football: Neuropsychological Testing—Part 6." *Neurosurgery* 55, no. 6 (December 2004): 1290–1305.

——, John W. Powell, David C. Viano, Ira R. Casson, Andrew M. Tucker, Henry Feuer, Mark Lovell et al. "Concussion in Professional Epidemiological Features of Game Injuries and Review of the Literature—Part 3." *Neurosurgery* 54, no. 1 (January 2004): 81–96.

——, David C. Viano, Ira R. Casson, Cynthia Arfken, and Henry Feuer. "Concussion in Professional Football: Players Returning to the Same Game—Part 7." *Neurosurgery* 56, no. 1 (January 2005): 79–92.

——, David C. Viano, Ira R. Casson, Cynthia Arfken, and John W. Powell. "Concussion in Professional Football: Injuries Involving 7 or More Days Out—Part 5." *Neurosurgery* 55, no. 5 (December 2004): 1100–19.

——, David C. Viano, Ira R. Casson, Andrew M. Tucker, Joe F. Waeckerle, John W. Powell, and Henry Feuer. "Concussion in Professional Football: Repeat Injuries—Part 4." *Neurosurgery* 55, no. 4 (November 2004): 860–76.

——, David C. Viano, Andrew M. Tucker, and Ira R. Casson. "Concussion in Professional Football: Location and Direction of Helmet Impacts—Part 2." *Neurosurgery* 53, no. 6 (December 2003): 1328–41.

——, David C. Viano, Andrew M. Tucker, Ira R. Casson, and Joe F. Waeckerle. "Concussion in Professional Football: Reconstruction of Game Impacts and Injuries." *Neurosurgery* 53, no. 4 (October 2003): 799–814.

Schneider, Richard C., Edward Reifel, Herbert O. Crisler, and Bennie G. Oosterbaan. "Serious and Fatal Football Injuries Involving the Head and Spinal Cord." *JAMA* 177, no. 6 (1961): 106–111.

Sills, Allen K. "The Sports Neurosurgeon." *AANS Neurosurgical Education* 28, no. 3 (2019): 1–4.

Tagliabue, Paul. "Tackling Concussions in Sports." *Neurosurgery* 53, no. 4 (October 2003): 796.

Tator, Charles, Jill Starkes, Gillian Dolansky, Julie Quet, Jean Michaud, and Michael Vassilyadi. "Fatal Second Impact Syndrome in Rowan Stringer, a 17-Year-Old Rugby Player." *Canadian Journal of Neurological Sciences* 46, no. 3 (May 2019): 351–54.

Viano, David C., Ira R. Casson, and Elliot J. Pellman. "Concussion in Professional Football: Biomechanics of the Struck Player—Part 14." *Neurosurgery* 61 (2007): 313–28.

——, Ira R. Casson, Elliot J. Pellman, Cynthia A. Bir, Liying Zhang, Donald C. Sherman, and Marilyn A. Boitano. "Concussion in Professional Football: Comparison with Boxing Head Impacts—Part 10." *Neurosurgery* 57, no. 6 (January 2006): 1154–72.

——, Ira R. Casson, Elliot J. Pellman, Liying Zhang, Albert I. King, and King H. Yang. "Concussion in Professional Football: Brain Responses by Finite Element Analysis: Part 9." *Neurosurgery* 57, no. 5 (November 2005): 891–916.

Yengo-Kahn, Aaron M., Ryan M. Gardner, Andrew W. Kuhn, Gary S. Solomon, Christopher M. Bonfield, and Scott L. Zuckerman. "Sport-Related Structural Brain Injury: 3 Cases of Subdural Hemorrhage in American High School Football." *World Neurosurgery* 106 (October 2017): 5–11.

Zuckerman, Scott L., Andrew Kuhn, Michael C. Dewan, Peter J. Morone, Jonathan A. Forbes, Gary S. Solomon, and Allen K. Sills. "Structural Brain Injury in Sports-Related Concussion." *Neurosurgical Focus* 33, no. 6 (December 2012): 1–12.

Chapter 6. Weighing the Risks

Ansari, Shaheryar F., Nicholas G. Gianaris, and Aaron A. Cohen-Gadol. "A Meningioma and Its Consequences for American History and the Rise of Neurosurgery." *Journal of Neurosurgery* 115, no. 6 (December 2011): 1067–71.

Gildenberg, Philip L. "Spiegel and Wycis—The Early Years." *Stereotactic and Functional Neurosurgery* 77, nos. 1–4 (2001): 11–16.

Goffaux, Philippe, and David Fortin. "Brain Tumor Headaches: From Bedside to Bench." *Neurosurgery* 67, no. 2 (August 2010): 459–66.

Grunert, Peter, Sr., Doerthe Keiner, and Joachim Oertal. "Remarks upon the Term Stereotaxy: A Linguistic and Historical Note." *Stereotactic Functional Neurosurgery* 93, no. 1 (January 2015): 42–49.

Ljunggren, Bengt. "The Case of General Wood." *Journal of Neurosurgery* 56, no. 4 (April 1982): 471–74.

Lunsford, L. Dade. "Lars Leksell: Notes at the Side of a Raconteur." *Stereotactic and Functional Neurosurgery* 67, nos. 3–4 (1997): 153–68.

Rzesnitzek, Lara, Marwan Hariz, and Joachim K. Krauss. "The Origins of Human Functional Stereotaxis: A Reappraisal." *Stereotactic and Functional Neurosurgery* 97, no. 1 (2019): 49–54.

——, Marwan Hariz, and Joachim K. Krauss. "Psychosurgery in the History of Stereotactic Functional Neurosurgery." *Stereotactic and Functional Neurosurgery* 98, no. 4 (August 2020): 241–47.

Trifiletti, Daniel M., Henry Ruiz-Garcia, Alfredo Quinones-Hinojosa, Rohan Ramakrishna, and Jason P. Sheehan. "The Evolution of Stereotactic Radiosurgery in Neurosurgical Practice." *Journal of Neuro-Oncology* 151 (February 2021): 451–59.

Chapter 7. Where to Begin?

Bahuleyan, Biji, Shenandoah Robinson, Ajith Rajappan Nair, Jyothish L. Sivandandapanicker, and Alan R. Cohen. "Anatomic Hemispherectomy: Historical Perspective." *World Neurosurgery* 80, nos. 1–4 (September–October 2013): 396–98.

Biden, Joe. *Promise Me, Dad: A Year of Hope, Hardship, and Purpose.* New York: Flatiron Books, 2017.

Groopman, Jerome. *The Anatomy of Hope: How People Prevail in the Face of Illness.* New York: Random House, 2003.

Harris, Lauren Julius, and Jason B. Almerigi. "Probing the Human Brain with Stimulating Electrodes: The Story of Roberts Bartholow's (1874) Experiment on Mary Rafferty." *Brain and Cognition* 70, no. 1 (June 2009): 92–115.

Isitan, Cigdem, Qi Yan, Dennis D. Spender, and Rafeed Alkawadri. "Brief History of Electrical Cortical Stimulation: A Journey in Time from Volta to Penfield." *Epilepsy Research* 166 (October 2020): 1–7.

Jusue-Torres, Ignacio, Vikram C. Prabhu, and G. Alexander Jones. "Dandy's Hemispherectomies: Historical Vignette." *Journal of Neurosurgery* 135, no. 6 (May 2021): 1836–42.

Ojemann, George A. "A 'Triple Threat' Career in Epilepsy Surgery." *Epilepsy & Behavior* 55 (February 2016): 189–92.

——, "In Memoriam: Ettore 'Hector' Lettich." *American Journal of Electroneurodiagnostic Technology* 50, no. 1 (2010): 2–3.

Parent, André. "Giovanni Aldini: From Animal Electricity to Human Brain Stimulation." *Canadian Journal of Neurological Sciences* 31, no. 4 (November 2004): 576–84.

Penfield, Wilder. *No Man Alone: A Neurosurgeon's Life*. Boston: Little, Brown, 1977.

——, and Edwin Boldrey. "Somatic Motor and Sensory Representation in the Cerebral Cortex of Man as Studied by Electrical Stimulation." *Brain* 60, no. 4 (December 1937): 389–443.

——, and Lamar Roberts. *Speech and Brain-Mechanisms*. Princeton, NJ: Princeton University Press, 1959

Razmara, Ashkaun. "Commentary: 3 Senators, 3 Votes—Glioblastoma's Uncanny Historical Parallels." *Neurosurgery* 82, no. 2 (February 2018): 55–57.

Son, Colin. "Clair Engle and the Brain Tumor That Almost Derailed the Civil Rights Act." *Neurosurgical Focus* 39, no. 1 (July 2015): 1–4.

Chapter 8. The Hardest Part Is Knowing When to Stop

Elsamadicy, Aladine A., Ranjith Babu, John P. Kirkpatrick, and David Cory Adamson. "Radiation-Induced Malignant Gliomas: A Current Review." *World Neurosurgery* 83, no. 4 (April 2015): 530–42.

Flaherty, Michael R., Alexander M. Kim, Michael D. Salt, and Lois K. Lee. "Distracted Driving Laws and Motor Vehicle Crash Fatalities." *Pediatrics* 145, no. 6 (2020): 1–9.

Giantini-Larsen, Alexandra M., Whitney E. Parker, Steven S. Cho, Jacob L. Goldberg, Joseph A. Carnevale, Alex P. Michael, Clara W. Teng et al. "The Evolution of 5-Aminolevulinic Acid Fluorescence Visualization: Time for a Headlamp/Loupe Combination." *World Neurosurgery* 159 (March 2022): 136–43.

Kahn, Christopher A., Victor Cisneros, Shahram Loftipour, Ghasem Imani, and Bharath Chakravarthy. "Distracted Driving, A Major Preventable Cause of Motor Vehicle Collisions: 'Just Hang Up and Drive.'" *Western Journal of Emergency Medicine* 16, no. 7 (December 2015): 1033–36.

O'Kelly, Eugene. *Chasing Daylight: How My Forthcoming Death Transformed My Life*. New York: McGraw Hill, 2005.

Ostrom, Quinn T., Patil Nirav, Gino Cioffi, Kristin Waite, Carol Kruchko, and Jill S. Barnholtz-Sloan. "CBTRUS Statistical Report: Primary Brain and Other Central

Nervous System Tumors Diagnosed in the United States in 2013–2017." *Neuro-Oncology* 22, suppl. 1 (2020): 1–96.

Preston, Dale L., Elaine Ron, Shuji Yonehara, Toshihiro Kobuke, Hideharu Fujii, Masao Kishikawa, Masayoshi Tokunaga, Shoji Tokuoka, and Kiyohiko Mabuchi. "Tumors of the Nervous System and Pituitary Gland Associated with Atomic Bomb Radiation Exposure." *Journal of the National Cancer Institute* 94, no. 20 (October 2002): 1555–63.

Proctor, Robert N. "The History of the Discovery of the Cigarette–Lung Cancer Link: Evidentiary Traditions, Corporate Denial, Global Toll." *Tobacco Control* 21, no. 2 (March 2012): 87–91.

Sadetzki, Siegal, Angela Chetrit, Laurence Freedman, Marilyn Stovall, Baruch Modan, and Ilya Novikov. "Long-Term Follow-Up for Brain Tumor Development After Childhood Exposure to Ionizing Radiation for Tinea Capitis." *Radiation Research* 163, no. 4 (April 2005): 424–32.

Umansky, Felix, Yigal Shoshan, Guy Rosenthal, Shifra Fraifeld, and Sergey Spektor. "Radiation-Induced Meningioma." *Neurosurgical Focus* 24, no. 5 (2008): 1–8.

Wilson, Fernando A., and Jim P. Stimpson. "Trends in Fatalities from Distracted Driving in the United States, 1999–2008." *American Journal of Public Health* 100, no. 11 (2010): 2213–19.

Yamanaka, Ryuya, Azusa Hayano, and Tomohiko Kanayama. "Radiation-Induced Gliomas: A Comprehensive Review and Meta-Analysis." *Neurosurgical Review* 41, no. 3 (July 2018): 719–31.

Zamstein, Omri, Aya Biderman, Michael Sherf, Ran Ben David, and Jacob Dreiher. "Cardiovascular Morbidity and Risk Factors in Holocaust Survivors in Israel." *Journal of the American Geriatrics Society* 66, no. 9 (September 2018): 1684–91.

Chapter 9. Journey to the Center of the Brain

Apuzzo, Michael L. J. *Surgery of the Third Ventricle.* Philadelphia: William and Wilkins, 1987.

Bergland, Richard M. "New Information Concerning the Irish Giant." *Journal of Neurosurgery* 23, no. 3 (1965): 265–69.

Bhattacharyya, Kalyan B. "Walter Edward Dandy (1886-1946): The Epitome of Adroitness and Dexterity in Neurosurgery." *Neurology India* 66, no. 2 (2018): 304–7.

Campbell, Eldridge. "Walter E. Dandy—Surgeon 1886-1946." *Journal of Neurosurgery* 8, no. 3 (1950): 249–62.

Carney, J. Aidan. "The Search for Harvey Cushing's Patient, Minnie G., and the Cause of Her Hypercortisolism." *American Journal of Surgical Pathology* 19, no. 1 (January 1995): 100–108.

Cavallo, Luigi M., Teresa Somma, Domenico Solari, Gianpiero Iannuzzo, Federico Frio, Cinzia Baiano, and Paolo Cappabianca. "Endoscopic Endonasal Transsphenoidal Surgery: History and Evolution." *World Neurosurgery* 127 (July 2019): 686–94.

Dandy, Walter E. *Benign Tumors of the Third Ventricle of the Brain: Diagnosis and Treatment.* Springfield, IL: Charles C. Thomas, 1933.

de Divitiis, Enrico. "Endoscopic Transsphenoidal Surgery: Strone-in-the-Pond Effect." *Neurosurgery* 59, no. 3 (September 2006): 512–20.

Du, Fengzhou, Qiao Chen, Xiaojun Wang, Xiaopeng Guo, Zihao Wang, Lu Gao, Xiao Long, and Bing Xing. "Long-Term Facial Changes and Clinical Correlations in Patients with Treated Acromegaly: A Cohort Study." *European Journal of Endocrinology* 184, no. 2 (February 2021): 231–41.

Gladwell, Malcolm. *David and Goliath: Underdogs, Misfits, and the Art of Battling Giants.* New York: Little, Brown, 2013.

Goodrich, James Tait. "The Cushing-Dandy Conflict—Two Powerful Personalities That Were Best Not to Collide!" *World Neurosurgery* 83, no. 1 (January 2015): 11–12.

Grauer, Neil A. *The Special Field: A History of Neurosurgery at Johns Hopkins.* Baltimore: Johns Hopkins Medicine, 2015.

Hutchinson, Robert. *Henry VIII: The Decline and Fall of a Tyrant.* London: Weidenfeld & Nicolson, 2019.

Kelsall, Alan, and John Newell-Price. "Cushing's Disease—From Minnie G to Key Issues in the Early 21st Century." *Lancet Diabetes & Endocrinology* 7, no. 12 (December 2019): 959–64.

Lanzino, Giuseppe, Niki F. Maartens, and Edward R. Laws. "Cushing's Case XLV: Minnie G." *Journal of Neurosurgery* 97, no. 1 (July 2002): 231–34.

Laws, Edward R., Jr. "The Evolution of Cushing's Surgical Treatment of Pituitary Lesions." *World Neurosurgery* 79, no. 2 (February 2013): 290–91.

Meng, Tian, Xiaopeng Guo, Wei Lian, Kan Deng, Lu Gao, Zihao Wang, Jiuzuo Huang et al. "Identifying Facial Features and Predicting Patients of Acromegaly Using Three-Dimensional Imaging Techniques and Machine Learning." *Frontiers in Endocrinology* 11 (July 2020): 1–12.

Patz, Michael D., Edward R. Laws, and Ajith J. Thomas. "The Cushing-Dandy Conflict—The Dandy Family Perception of the Discord." *World Neurosurgery* 83, no. 1 (January 2015): 69–73.

Pendleton, Courtney, Hadie Adams, Edward R. Laws, and Alfredo Quiñones-Hinojosa. "The Elusive Minnie G.: Revisiting Cushing's Case XLV, and His Early Attempts at Improving Quality of Life." *Pituitary* 13, no. 4 (December 2010): 361–66.

———, Hadie Adams, Nestoras Mathioudakis, and Alfredo Quiñones-Hinojosa. "Sellar Door: Harvey Cushing's Entry into the Pituitary Gland, the Unabridged Johns Hopkins Experience 1896–1912." *World Neurosurgery* 79, no. 2 (February 2013): 394–403.

———, Hadie Adams, Roberto Salvatori, Gary Wand, and Alfredo Quiñones-Hinojosa. "On the Shoulders of Giants: Harvey Cushing's Experience with Acromegaly and Gigantism at the John Hopkins Hospital, 1896–1912." *Pituitary* 14, no. 1 (March 2011): 53–60.

Rabin, David, and Pauline L. Rabin. "David, Goliath, and Smiley's People." *New England Journal of Medicine* 309 (1983): 1–2.

Sherman, Irving J., Ryan M. Kretzer, and Rafael J. Tamargo. "Personal Recollections of Walter E. Dandy and His Brain Team." *Journal of Neurosurgery* 105, no. 3 (September 2006): 487–93.

Shilts, Randy. *And The Band Played On: Politics, People and the AIDS Epidemic.* New York: St. Martin's Press, 1987.

Wei, Ren, Chendan Jiang, Jun Gao, Ping Xu, Debing Zhang, Zhicheng Sun, Xiaohai Liu et al. "Deep-Learning Approach to Automatic Identification of Facial Anomalies in Endocrine Disorders." *Neuroendocrinology* 110, no. 5 (2020): 328–37.

Zada, Gabriel, Charles Liu, and Michael L. J. Apuzzo. "'Through the Looking Glass': Optical Physics, Issues, and the Evolution of Neuroendoscopy." *World Neurosurgery* 77, no. 1 (January 2012): 92–102.

Chapter 10. A Time Bomb in the Brain

Abecassis, Isaac Josh, Qzi Zeeshan, Basavaraj V. Ghodke, Michael R. Levitt, Richard G. Ellenbogen, and Laligam N. Sekhar. "Surgical Versus Endovascular Management of Ruptured and Unruptured Intracranial Aneurysms: Emergent Issues and Future Directions." *World Neurosurgery* 136 (April 2020): 17–27.

Biden, Joe. *Promises to Keep: On Life and Politics.* New York: Random House, 2007.

Byrne, J. V. "The Aneurysm 'Clip or Coil' Debate." *Acta Neurochirurgica* 148, no. 2 (February 2006): 115–20.

Clarke, Emilia. "A Battle for My Life." *New Yorker,* March 21, 2019.

Cohen-Gadol, Aaron A., and Dennis D. Spencer. "Harvey W. Cushing and Cerebrovascular Surgery: Part l, Aneurysms." *Journal of Neurosurgery* 101, no. 3 (September 2004): 547–52.

Daly, Michael. "Surgeon Who Saved Biden's Life Recalls Fateful Prediction." *Daily Beast*, November 8, 2020. https://www.thedailybeast.com/dr-neal-kassell -surgeon-who-saved-bidens-life-recalls-fateful-prediction.

Donaghy, R. M. Peardon. "The History of Microsurgery in Neurosurgery." *Clinical Neurosurgery* 26 (January 1979): 619–25.

Frazer, Duncan, Abha Ahuja, Laurence Watkins, and Lisa Cipolotti. "Coiling Versus Clipping for the Treatment of Aneurysmal Subarachnoid Hemorrhage: A Longitudinal Investigation into Cognitive Outcome." *Neurosurgery* 60, no. 3 (March 2007): 434–42.

Jumah, Fareed, Travis Quinoa, Omar Akel, Smit Shah, Vinayak Narayan, Nimer Adeeb, Gaurav Gupta, and Anil Nanda. "The Origins of Eponymous Aneurysm Clips: A Review." *World Neurosurgery* 134 (February 2020): 518–31.

Kretzer, Ryan M., Alexander L. Coon, and Rafael J. Tamargo. "Walter E. Dandy's Contributions to Vascular Neurosurgery." *Journal of Neurosurgery* 112, no. 6 (June 2010): 1182–91.

Kriss, Timothy C., and Vesna Martich Kriss. "History of the Operating Microscope: From Magnifying Glass to Microneurosurgery." *Neurosurgery* 42, no. 4 (April 1998): 899–907

Latimer, Sophie F., F. Colin Wilson, Chris G. McCusker, Sheena B. Caldwell, and Ian Rennie. "Subarachnoid Haemorrhage (SAH): Long-Term Cognitive Outcome in Patients Treated with Surgical Clipping or Endovascular Coiling." *Disability & Rehabilitation* 35, no. 10 (2013): 845–50.

Ligon, B. Lee. "History of Developments in Imaging Techniques: Egas Moniz and Angiography." *Seminars in Pediatric Infectious Diseases* 14, no. 2 (April 2003): 173–81.

Link, Timothy E., Erica Bisson, Michael A. Horgan, and Bruce I. Tranmer. "Raymond M. P. Donaghy: A Pioneer in Microneurosurgery." *Journal of Neurosurgery* 112, no. 6 (June 2010): 1176–81.

Lovato, Renan Maximilian, João Luiz Vitorino Araujo, Vinícius Monteiro de Paula Guirado, and José Carlos Esteves Veiga. "The Legacy of Yaşargil: The Father of Modern Neurosurgery." *Indian Journal of Surgery* 78, no. 1 (February 2016): 77–78.

Rogers, L. M. *Gazi Yaşargil: Father of Modern Neurosurgery*. Virginia Beach, VA: Koehler Books, 2015.

Savitz, Martin H. "History of the Operating Microscope: From Magnifying Glass to Microneurosurgery." *Neurosurgery* 45, no. 2 (August 1999): 418.

Schwartz, Theodore H., and Robert A. Solomon. "Perimesencephalic Subarachnoid Hemorrhage: Review of the Literature." *Neurosurgery* 39 (1996): 433–44.

Tew, John M., Jr. "M. Gazi Yaşargil: Neurosurgery's Man of the Century." *Neurosurgery* 45, (1999): 1010–14.

Wang, Huan, Kenneth Fraser, David Wang, and Giuseppe Lanzino. "The Evolution of Endovascular Therapy for Neurosurgical Disease." *Neurosurgery Clinics of North America* 16, no. 2 (April 2005): 223–29.

Yaşargil, Mahmut Gazi. *Microsurgery Applied to Neurosurgery.* Stuttgart: Thieme, 1969.

——, "Personal Considerations of the History of Microneurosurgery." *Journal of Neurosurgery* 112, no. 6 (June 2010): 1163–75.

Chapter 11. Too Close for Comfort

Boyle, Karl, Raed A. Joundi, and Richard I. Aviv. "An Historical and Contemporary Review of Endovascular Therapy for Acute Ischemic Stroke." *Neurovascular Imaging* 3, no. 1 (2017): 1–12.

Campbell, Bruce C. V., Atte Meretoja, Geoffrey A. Donnan, and Stephen M. Davis. "Twenty-Year History of the Evolution of Stroke Thrombolysis with Intravenous Alteplase to Reduce Long-Term Disability." *Stroke* 46, no. 8 (August 2015): 2341–46.

Caplan, Louis R. *C. Miller Fisher: Stroke in the 20th Century.* New York: Oxford University Press, 2020.

Chartrain, Alexander G., Hazem Shoirah, Edward C. Jauch, and J. Mocco. "A Review of Acute Ischemic Stroke Triage Protocol Evidence: A Context for Discussion." *Journal of NeuroInterventional Surgery* 10, no. 11 (November 2018): 1047–52.

Easton, J. Donald. "History of Carotid Endarterectomy Then and Now: Personal Perspective." *Stroke* 45, no. 6 (June 2014): 101–3.

Friedman, Steven G. "The First Carotid Endarterectomy." *Journal of Vascular Surgery* 60, no. 6 (December 2014): 1703–8.

Goldstein, David S., and Irwin J. Kopin. "Evolution of Concepts of Stress." *International Journal on the Biology of Stress* 10, no. 2 (June 2007): 109–20.

Inoue, Nobutaka. "Stress and Atherosclerotic Cardiovascular Disease." *Journal of Atherosclerosis and Thrombosis* 21, no. 5 (2014): 391–401.

Min, W. David, and Christopher M. Loftus. "History of Carotid Surgery." *Neurosurgery Clinics of North America* 12, no. 1 (January 2001): 167–72.

Mohammed, Nasser, Vinayak Narayan, Devi Prasad Patra, and Anil Nanda. "Louis Victor Leborgne ('Tan')." *World Neurosurgery* 114 (June 2018): 121–25.

Naylor, A. Ross. "A Surgeon's View on Endarterectomy and Stenting in 2011: Lest We Forget, It's All About Preventing Stroke." *Cardiovascular Interventional Radiological Society of Europe* 35, no. 2 (April 2012): 225–33.

——, "Endarterectomy Versus Stenting for Stroke Prevention." *Stroke and Vascular Neurology* 3, no. 2 (June 2018): 101–6.

Pearce, J. M. S. "Marie-Jean-Pierre Flourens (1794–1867) and Cortical Localization." *European Neurology* 61, no. 5 (2009): 311–14.

Sarraj, Amrou, Sean Savitz, Deep Pujara, Haris Kamal, Kirsten Carroll, Faris Shaker, Sujan Reddy et al. "Endovascular Thrombectomy for Acute Ischemic Strokes: Current US Access Paradigms and Optimization Methodology." *Stroke* 51, no. 4 (April 2020): 1207–17.

Stein, Laura K., Stanley Tuhrim, Nathalie Jette, Johanna Fifi, J. Mocco, and Mandip S. Dhamoon. "Nationwide Analysis of Endovascular Thrombectomy Provider Specialization for Acute Stroke." *Stroke* 51, no. 12 (December 2020): 3651–57.

Vincent, Sophie, Maria Eberg, Mark J. Eisenberg, and Kristian B. Filion. "Meta-Analysis of Randomized Controlled Trials Comparing the Long-Term Outcomes of Carotid Artery Stenting Versus Endarterectomy." *Circulation Cardiovascular Quality and Outcomes* 8, no. 6., suppl. 3 (October 2015): 99–108.

Chapter 12. Psychosurgery or Psycho Surgeon?

Bertolote, José Manoel. "Egas Moniz: Twice a Double Life." *Arqivos de Neuro-Psiquiatria* 73, no. 10 (October 2015): 885–86.

Caruso, James P., and Jason P. Sheehan. "Psychosurgery, Ethics, and Media: A History of Walter Freeman and the Lobotomy." *Neurosurgical Focus* 43, no. 3 (September 2017): 1–8.

Crawford, M., J. F. Fulton, C. F. Jacobsen, and J. B. Wolfe. "Frontal Lobe Ablation in Chimpanzee: A Resume of Becky and Lucy." *Research Publications—Association for Research in Nervous and Mental Disease* 27 (1948): 3–58.

Delgado, Jose M. R. *Physical Control of the Mind: Toward a Psychocivilized Society.* New York: Harper & Row, 1969.

El-Hai, Jack. *The Lobotomist: The Maverick Medical Genius and His Tragic Quest to Rid the World of Mental Illness.* New York: John Wiley & Sons, 2005.

Freeman, Walter, and James W. Watts. "Prefrontal Lobotomy in Agitated Depression." *Medical Annals of the District of Columbia* 5 (1936): 326–28.

——, and James W. Watts. "Prefrontal Lobotomy in the Treatment of Mental Disorders." *Southern Medical Journal* 30 (1937): 23–31.

Greenblatt M., R. E. Arnot, J. L. Poppen, and W. P. Chapman. "Report on Lobotomy Studies at the Boston Psychopathic Hospital." *American Journal of Psychiatry* 104, no. 6 (December 1947): 361–68.

Heller, A. Chris, Arun P. Amar, Charles Y. Liu, and Michael L. J. Apuzzo. "Surgery of the Mind and Mood: A Mosaic of Issues in Time and Evolution." *Neurosurgery* 62, no. 6, suppl. 3 (June 2008): 921–40.

Holland, Ryan, David Kopel, Peter W. Carmel, and Charles J. Prestigiacomo. "Topectomy Versus Leukotomy: J. Lawrence Pool's Contribution to Psychosurgery." *Neurosurgical Focus* 43, no. 3 (September 2017): 1–7.

Koehler-Pentacoff, Elizabeth. *The Missing Kennedy: Rosemary Kennedy and the Secret Bonds of Four Women.* Baltimore: Bancroft Press, 2015.

Leblanc, Richard. "Against the Current: Wilder Penfield, the Frontal Lobes and Psychosurgery." *Canadian Journal of Neurological Sciences* 46, (2019): 585–90.

Lynn, John G., and Tracy J. Putnam. "Histology of Cerebral Lesions Produced by Focused Ultrasound." *American Journal of Pathology* 20, no. 3 (May 1943): 637–49.

Meyers, Russell, William J. Fry, Frank J. Fry, Leroy L. Dreyer, Donald F. Schultz, and Robert F. Noyes. "Early Experiences with Ultrasonic Irradiation of the Pallidofugal and Nigral Complexes in Hyperkinetic and Hypertonic Disorders." *Journal of Neurosurgery* 15, no. 1 (January 1959): 32–54.

Michaleas, Spyros N., Gregory Tsoucalas, Elias Tzavellas, George Stranjalis, and Marianna Karamanou. "Gottlieb Burckhardt (1836–1907): 19th-Century Pioneer of Psychosurgery." *Surgical Innovation* 28, no. 3 (June 2021): 381–38.

Nijensohn, Daniel E. "Prefrontal Lobotomy on Evita Was Done for Behavior/Personality Modification, Not Just for Pain Control." *Neurosurgical Focus* 39, no. 1 (July 2015): 1–6.

——, Luis E. Savastano, Alberto D. Kaplan, and Edward R. Laws Jr. "New Evidence of Prefrontal Lobotomy in the Last Months of the Illness of Eva Perón." *World Neurosurgery* 77, nos. 3–4 (March–April 2012): 583–90.

Poppen, James L. "Technic of Prefrontal Lobotomy." *Journal of Neurosurgery* 5, no. 6 (1948): 514–20.

Pool, J. Lawrence. "Neurosurgical Treatment of Disorders of the Affect." *Journal of Chronic Diseases* 2, no. 1 (July 1955): 1–10.

——, "Topectomy: The Treatment of Mental Illness by Frontal Gyrectomy or Bilateral Subtotal Ablation of Frontal Cortex." *Lancet* 254, no. 6583 (October 1949): 776–81.

Schiff, Nicholas D., Joseph T. Giacino, Christopher R. Butson, Eun Young Choi, Jonathan L. Baker et al. "Thalamic Deep Brain Stimulation in Traumatic Brain Injury: A Phase 1, Randomized Feasibility Study." *Nature Medicine* 29 (December 2023): 3162–74.

Sheth, Sameer A., Kelly R. Bijanki, Brian Metzger, Anush Allawala, Victoria Pirtle, Joshua A. Adkinson, John Myers et al. "Deep Brain Stimulation for Depression Informed by Intracranial Recordings." *Biological Psychiatry* 92, no. 3 (August 2021): 246–51.

Tan, Siang Yong, and Angela Yip. "António Egas Moniz (1874–1955): Lobotomy Pioneer and Nobel Laureate." *Singapore Medical Journal* 55, no. 4 (April 2014): 175–76.

Wu, Hemmings, Marwan Hariz, Veerle Visser-Vandewalle, Ludvic Zrinzo, Volker A. Coenen, Sameer A. Sheth, Chris Bervoets et al. "Deep Brain Stimulation for Refractory Obsessive-Compulsive Disorder (OCD): Emerging or Established Therapy?" *Molecular Psychiatry* 26 (2021): 60–65.

Young, Grace J., Wenya Linda Bi, Timothy R. Smith, Ryan Brewster, William B. Gormley, Ian F. Dunn, Edward R. Laws et al. "Evita's Lobotomy." *Journal of Clinical Neuroscience* 22, no. 12 (December 2015): 1883–88.

Chapter 13. Luck Favors the Prepared Mind

Abel, Taylor J., Timothy Walch, and Matthew A. Howard III. "Russell Meyers (1905–1999): Pioneer of Functional and Ultrasonic Neurosurgery." *Journal of Neurosurgery* 125, no. 6 (December 2016): 1589–95.

Bucy, Paul C., and Theodore J. Case. "Tremor: Physiologic Mechanism and Abolition by Surgical Means." *Archives of Neurology and Psychiatry* 41, no. 4 (1939): 721–46.

Campbell, Peter G., Olatilewa O. Awe, Mitchell G. Maltenfort, Darius M. Moshfeghi, Theodore Leng, Andrew A. Moshfeghi, and John K. Ratliff. "Medical School and Residency Influence on Choice of Academic Career and Academic Productivity Among Neurosurgery Faculty in the United States." *Journal of Neurosurgery* 115, no. 2 (August 2011): 380–6.

Christian, Eisha, Cheng Yu, and Michael L. J. Apuzzo. "Focused Ultrasound: Relevant History and Prospects for the Addition of Mechanical Energy to the Neurosurgical Armamentarium." *World Neurosurgery* 82, nos. 3–4 (September–October 2014): 354–65.

Ciric, Ivan. "Paul C. Bucy, M.D., 1904–1992." *Journal of Neurosurgery* 78, no. 5 (1993): 693–94.

Cooper, Irving S. "Intracerebral Injection of Procaine into the Globus Pallidus in Hyperkinetic Disorders." *Science* 119, no. 3091 (March 1954): 417–18.

———, "Neurosurgical Alleviation of Parkinsonism." *Bulletin of the New York Academy of Medicine* 32, no. 10 (October 1956): 713–24.

———, *The Vital Probe: My Life as a Brain Surgeon*. New York: W. W. Norton, 1981.

Corsellis, J. A. N., C. J. Bruton, and Dorothy Freeman-Browne. "The Aftermath of Boxing." *Psychological Medicine* 3, no. 3 (August 1973): 270–303.

Das, Kaushik, Deborah L. Benzil, Richard L. Rovit, Raj Murali, and William T. Couldwell. "Irving S. Cooper (1922–1985): A Pioneer in Functional Neurosurgery." *Journal of Neurosurgery* 89 (1998): 865–73.

Fox, Michael J. *Lucky Man: A Memoir*. New York: Hyperion, 2002.

Fry, W. J., W. H. Mosberg Jr., J. W. Barnard, and F. J. Fry. "Production of Focal Destructive Lesions in the Central Nervous System with Ultrasound." *Journal of Neurosurgery* 11, no. 5 (September 1954): 471–78.

Giammalva, Giuseppe Roberto, Cesare Gagliardo, Salvatore Marrone, Federica Paolini, Rosa Maria Gerardi, Giuseppe Emmanuele Umana, Kaan Yağmurlu et al. "Focused Ultrasound in Neuroscience: State of the Art and Future Perspectives." *Brain Sciences* 11, no. 1 (January 2021): 1–12.

Gildenberg, Philip L. "The History of Surgery for Movement Disorders." *Neurosurgery Clinics of North America* 9, no. 2 (April 1998): 283–93.

Goetz, Christopher G. "The History of Parkinson's Disease: Early Clinical Descriptions and Neurological Therapies." *Cold Spring Harbor Perspectives in Medicine* 1, no. 1 (September 2011): 1–15.

Harary, Maya, David J. Segar, Kevin T. Huang, Ian J. Tafel, Pablo A. Valdes, and G. Rees Cosgrove. "Focused Ultrasound in Neurosurgery: A Historical Perspective." *Neurosurgical Focus* 44, no. 2 (February 2018): 1–9.

Jagannathan, Jay, Narendra T. Sanghvi, Lawrence A. Crum, Chun-Po Yen, Ricky Medel, Aaron S. Dumont, Jason P. Sheehan et al. "High-Intensity Focused Ultrasound Surgery of the Brain: Part 1—A Historical Perspective with Modern Applications." *Neurosurgery* 64, no. 2 (February 2009): 201–11.

Kahn, Lora, Brianne Sutton, Helena R. Winston, Aviva Abosch, John A. Thompson, and Rachel A. Davis. "Deep Brain Stimulation for Obsessive-Compulsive Disorder: Real World Experience Post-FDA-Humanitarian Use Device Approval." *Frontiers in Psychiatry* 12 (March 2021): 1–13.

Lang, Min, John Tsiang, Nina Z. Moore, Mark D. Bain, and Michael P. Steinmetz. "A Tribute to Dr. Robert J. White." *Neurosurgery* 85, no. 2 (August 2019): 366–73.

Mantione, Mariska, Martijn Figee, and Damiaan Denys. "A Case of Musical Preference for Johnny Cash Following Deep Brain Stimulation of the Nucleus Accumbens." *Frontiers in Behavioral Neuroscience* 8 (2014): 1–4.

O'Brien, William D., Jr., and Floyd Dunn. "An Early History of High-Intensity Focused Ultrasound." *Physics Today* 68, no. 10 (October 2015): 40–45.

Parkinson, James. *An Essay on the Shaking Palsy*. London: Sherwood, Neely, and Jones, 1817.

Quadri, Syed A., Muhammad Waqas, Inamullah Khan, Muhammad Adnan Khan, Sajid S. Suriya, Mudassir Forooqi, and Brian Fiani. "High-Intensity Focused Ultrasound: Past, Present, and Future in Neurosurgery." *Neurosurgical Focus* 44, no. 2 (February 2018): 1–9.

Revah, Omer, Felicity Gore, Kevin W. Kelly, Jimena Andersen, Noriaki Sakai, Xiaoyu Chen, Min-Yin Li et al. "Maturation and Circuit Integration of Transplanted Human Cortical Organoids." *Nature* 610 (2022): 319–26.

Roberts, Anthony Herber. *Brain Damage in Boxers: A Study of the Prevalence of Traumatic Encephalopathy Among Ex-Professional Boxers.* London: Pitman Medical & Scientific Publishing Company, 1969.

Ropper, Allan H., and Brian David Burrell. *Reaching Down the Rabbit Hole: A Renowned Neurologist Explains the Mystery and Drama of Brain Disease.* New York: St. Martin's Press, 2014.

Rowland, Lewis P. *The Legacy of Tracy J. Putnam and H. Houston Merritt: Modern Neurology in the United States.* New York: Oxford University Press, 2009.

Samra, Khairy, Joseph M. Waltz, Manuel Riklan, Maxim Koslow, and Irving S. Cooper. "Relief of Intention Tremor by Thalamic Surgery." *Journal of Neurology, Neurosurgery and Psychiatry* 33, no. 1 (February 1970): 7–15.

van Grootheest, Daniël S., Daniëlle C. Cath, Aartjan T. Beekman, and Dorret I. Boomsma. "Twin Studies on Obsessive-Compulsive Disorder: A Review." *Twin Research and Human Genetics* 8, no. 5 (October 2005): 450–58.

White, Robert J., Maurice S. Albin, and Javier Verdura. "Preservation of Viability in the Isolated Monkey Brain Utilizing a Mechanical Extracorporeal Circulation." *Nature* 202 (June 1964): 1082–83.

Chapter 14. What Is It Like to Be a Brain?

Alajouanine, T. "Dostoiewski's Epilepsy." *Brain* 86 (June 1963): 209–18.

Burton, Adrian. "How Far Away the Cornfield: Dennis Spencer's Journey." *Lancet* 18, no. 3 (2019): 236.

Corkin, Suzanne. "What's New with the Amnesic Patient H.M.?" *Nature Reviews Neuroscience* 3 (February 2002): 153–60.

Dittrich, Luke. *Patient H.M.: A Story of Memory, Madness, and Family Secrets.* New York: Random House, 2016.

Fried, Itzhak, Firas Fahoum, Andrew Frew, Fani Andelman, Michal M. Andelman-Gur, and Noriko Salamon. "Laser Ablation of Human Guilt." *Brain Stimulation* 15, no. 1 (January–February 2002): 164–66.

——, Roy Mukamel, and Gabriel Kreiman. "Internally Generated Preactivation of Single Neurons in Human Medial Frontal Cortex Predicts Volition." *Neuron* 69, no. 3 (February 2011): 548–62.

Gasenzer, Elena, and Edmund A. M. Neugebauer. "George Gershwin: A Case of New Ways in Neurosurgery as Well as in the History of Western Music." *Acta Neurochirurgica* 156, no. 6 (March 2014): 1251–58.

Gelbard-Sagiv, Hagar, Liad Mudrik, Michael R. Hill, Christof Koch, and Itzhak Fried. "Human Single Neuron Activity Precedes Emergence of Conscious Perception." *Nature Communications* 9 (2018): 1–13.

Gross, Robert A. "A Brief History of Epilepsy and Its Therapy in the Western Hemisphere." *Epilepsy Research* 12, no. 2 (July 1992): 65–74.

Hawkins, Jeff. *A Thousand Brains: A New Theory of Intelligence.* New York: Basic Books, 2021.

Hermann, Bruce P. "Comments on Devinsky O, Lai G. Spirituality and Religion in Epilepsy." *Epilepsy & Behavior* 40 (2014): 49–51.

Kliemann, Dorit, Ralph Adolphs, Lynn K. Paul, J. Michael Tyszka, and Daniel Tranel. "Reorganization of the Social Brain in Individuals with Only One Intact Cerebral Hemisphere." *Brain Sciences* 11, no. 8 (August 2021): 1–20.

Ladino, Lady Diana, Syed Rizvi, and José Francisco Téllez-Zenteno. "The Montreal Procedure: The Legacy of the Great Wilder Penfield." *Epilepsy & Behavior* 83, (June 2018): 151–61.

Ljunggren, Bengt. "The Case of George Gershwin." *Neurosurgery* 10, no. 6 (June 1982): 733–36.

Mauguière, F., and S. Corkin. "H.M. Never Again!: An Analysis of H.M.'s Epilepsy and Treatment." *Revue Neurologique* 171, no. 3 (March 2015): 273–81.

Nagel, Thomas. "What Is It Like to Be a Bat?" *Philosophical Review* 83, no. 4 (October 1974): 435–50.

Penfield, Wilder. *No Man Alone: A Neurosurgeon's Life.* New York: Little, Brown, 1977.

Richards, Whitman. "Time Reproductions by H.M." *Acta Psychologica* 37, no. 4 (August 1973): 279–82.

Scoville, William Beecher. "Psychosurgery." *Journal of Neurosurgery* 38, no. 4 (1973): 535.

——, "Selective Cortical Undercutting as a Means of Modifying and Studying Frontal Lobe Function in Man: Preliminary Report of 43 Operative Cases." *Journal of Neurosurgery* 6, no. 1 (January 1949): 65–73.

——, and Brenda Milner. "Loss of Recent Memory After Bilateral Hippocampal Lesions." *Journal of Neurology, Neurosurgery and Psychiatry* 20, no. 1 (February 1957): 11–21.

Sporns, Olaf. "The Human Connectome: A Complex Network." *Annals of the New York Academy of Sciences* 1224 (April 2011): 109–25.

Squire, Larry R. "The Legacy of Patient H.M. for Neuroscience." *Neuron* 61, no. 1 (January 2009): 6–9.

Taylor, David C. "One Hundred Years of Epilepsy Surgery: Sir Victor Horsley's

Contribution." *Journal of Neurology, Neurosurgery and Psychiatry* 49, no. 5 (May 1986): 485–88.

Thiebaut de Schotten, M., F. Dell'Acqua, P. Ratiu, A. Leslie, H. Howells, E. Cabanis, M. T. Iba-Zizen et al. "From Phineas Gage and Monsieur Leborgne to H.M.: Revisiting Disconnection Syndromes." *Cerebral Cortex* 25, no. 12 (December 2015): 4812–27.

Uddin, Lucina Q. "Stability and Plasticity of Functional Brain Networks After Hemispherectomy: Implications for Consciousness Research." *Quantitative Imaging in Medicine and Surgery* 10, no. 6 (June 2020): 1408–12.

Whitcomb, Benjamin B. "William Beecher Scoville." *Surgical Neurology* 12, no. 2 (August 1979): 109–10.

Chapter 15. We Tell Ourselves Stories in Order to Live

Beier, Alexandra D., and James T. Rutka. "Hemispherectomy: Historical Review and Recent Technical Advances." *Neurosurgical Focus* 34, no. 6 (2013): 1–5.

Bogen, J. E., and M. S. Gazzaniga. "Cerebral Commissurotomy in Man: Minor Hemisphere Dominance for Certain Visuospatial Functions." *Journal of Neurosurgery* 23, no. 394 (1965): 394–99.

Bowren, Mark, Jr., Daniel Tranel, and Aaron D. Boes. "Preserved Cognition After Right Hemispherectomy." *Neurology: Clinical Practice* 11, no. 6 (December 2021): 906–8.

de Jong, Bauke M. "Neurology of Widely Embedded Free Will." *Cortex* 47, no. 10 (November–December 2011): 1160–65.

Delgado, José M., Vernon Mark, William Sweet, Frank Ervin Gerhard Weiss, George Bach-Y-Rita, and Rioji Hagiwara. "Intracerebral Radio Stimulation and Recording in Completely Free Patients." *Journal of Nervous and Mental Disease* 147, no. 4 (October 1968): 329–40.

Desmurget, Michel, Karen T. Reilly, Nathalie Richard, Alexandru Sathmari, Carmine Mottolese, and Angela Sirigu. "Movement Intention After Parietal Cortex Stimulation in Humans." *Science* 324, no. 5928 (May 2009): 811–13.

Fried, Itzhak. "Neurosurgery as a Window to the Human Mind: Free Will and the Sense of Self." *Acta Neurochirurgica* 163 (2021): 1211–12.

——, Patrick Haggard, Biyu J. He, and Aaron Schurger. "Volition and Action in the Human Brain: Processes, Pathologies, and Reasons." *Journal of Neuroscience* 37, no. 45 (November 2017): 10842–47.

Gazzaniga, Michael S. "Cerebral Specialization and Interhemispheric Communication: Does the Corpus Callosum Enable the Human Condition?" *Brain* 123, no. 7 (July 2000): 1293–1326.

——, *Tales from Both Sides of the Brain: A Life in Neuroscience.* New York: HarperCollins, 2015.

——, *The Social Brain: Discovering the Networks of the Mind.* New York: Basic Books, 1969.

Libet, Benjamin. "Cortical Activation in Conscious and Unconscious Experience." *Perspectives in Biology and Medicine* 9, no. 1 (Autumn 1965): 77–86.

——, W. W. Alberts, E. W. Wright, L. D. Delattre, G. Levin, and B. Feinstein. "Production of Threshold Levels of Conscious Sensation by Electrical Stimulation of Human Somatosensory Cortex." *Journal of Neurophysiology* 27 (July 1964): 546–78.

——, Curtis A. Gleason, Elwood W. Wright, and Dennis K. Pearl. "Time of Conscious Intention to Act in Relation to Onset of Cerebral Activity (Readiness-Potential): The Unconscious Initiation of a Freely Voluntary Act." *Brain* 106, part 3 (September 1983): 623–42.

——, Elwood W. Wright Jr., Bertram Feinstein, and Dennis K. Pearl. "Subjective Referral of the Timing for a Conscious Sensory Experience: A Functional Role for the Somatosensory Specific Projection System in Man." *Brain* 102, no. 1 (March 1979): 193–224.

Mathews, Marlon S., Mark E. Linskey, and Devin K. Binder. "William P. van Wagenen and the First Corpus Callosotomies for Epilepsy." *Journal of Neurosurgery* 108, no. 3 (March 2008): 608–13.

McGilchrist, Iain. *The Master and His Emissary: The Divided Brain and the Making of the Western World.* New Haven, CT: Yale University Press, 2009.

Park, Hae-Jeong, and Karl Friston. "Structural and Functional Brain Networks: From Connections to Cognition." *Science* 342, no. 6158 (November 2013): 579–87.

Perez, Omri, Roy Mukamel, Ariel Tankus, Jonathan D. Rosenblatt, Yehezkel Yeshurun, and Itzhak Fried. "Preconscious Prediction of a Driver's Decision Using Intracranial Recordings." *Journal of Cognitive Neuroscience* 27, no. 8 (August 2015): 1492–1502.

Pilcher, Webster H. *Dedication.* Rochester, NY: University of Rochester Press, 2022.

Quiroga, R. Quian, G. Kreiman, C. Koch, and I. Fried. "Sparse but Not 'Grandmother-Cell' Coding in the Medial Temporal Lobe." *Trends in Cognitive Sciences* 12, no. 3 (March 2008): 87–91.

——, L. Reddy, G. Kreiman, C. Koch, and I. Fried. "Invariant Visual Representation by Single Neurons in the Human Brain." *Nature* 435, no. 7045 (June 2005): 1102–7.

Rahimpour, Shervin, Michael M. Haglund, Allan H. Friedman, and Hugues Duffau. "History of Awake Mapping and Speech and Language Localization: From Modules to Networks." *Neurosurgical Focus* 47, no. 3 (September 2019): 1–6.

Ramachandran, V. S. *The Tell-Tale Brain: A Neuroscientist's Quest for What Makes Us Human.* New York: W. W. Norton, 2011.

Schaller, Karl, Giannina Rita Iannotti, Pavo Orepic, Sophie Betka, Julien Haemmerli, Colette Boex, Sixto Alcoba-Banqueri et al. "The Perspective of Mapping and Monitoring of the Sense of Self in Neurosurgical Patients." *Acta Neurochirurgica* 163, no. 5 (May 2021): 1213–26.

Sjöberg, Rickard L. "Free Will and Neurosurgical Resections of the Supplementary Motor Area: A Critical Review." *Acta Neurochirurgica* 163, no. 5 (May 2021): 1229–37.

Suthana, Nanthia, and Itzhak Fried. "Percepts to Recollections: Insights from Single Neuron Recordings in the Human Brain." *Trends in Cognitive Sciences* 16, no. 8 (August 2012): 427–36.

Vaddiparti, Aparna, Richard Huang, David Blihar, Maira Du Plessis, Michael J. Montalbano, R. Shane Tubbs, and Mario Loukas. "The Evolution of Corpus Callosotomy for Epilepsy Management." *World Neurosurgery* 145 (January 2021): 455–61.

Vaz, Alex P., Sara K. Inati, Nicolas Brunel, and Kareem A. Zaghloul. "Coupled Ripple Oscillations Between the Medial Temporal Lobe and Neocortex Retrieve Human Memory." *Science* 363, no. 6430 (March 2019): 975–78.

——, John H. Wittig Jr., Sara K. Inati, and Kareem A. Zaghloul. "Replay of Cortical Spiking Sequences During Human Memory Retrieval." *Science* 367, no. 6482 (March 2020): 1131–34.

Chapter 16. The Terminal Man

Anumanchipalli, Gopala K., Josh Chartier, and Edward F. Chang. "Speech Synthesis from Neural Decoding of Spoken Sentences." *Nature* 568, no. 7753 (April 2019): 493–512

Bouton, Chad. E., Ammar Shaikhouni, Nicholas V. Annetta, Marcia A. Bockbrader, David A. Friedenberg, Dylan M. Nielson, Gaurav Sharma et al. "Restoring Cortical Control of Functioning Movement in a Human with Quadriplegia." *Nature* 533, no. 7602 (May 2016): 247–59.

Button, John, and Tracy Putnam. "Visual Responses to Cortical Stimulation in the Blind." *Journal of the Iowa Medical Society* 52 (1962): 17–21.

Chen, Spencer C., Gregg J. Suaning, John W. Morley, and Nigel H. Lovell. "Stimulating Prosthetic Vision: l. Visual Models of Phosphenes." *Vision Research* 49, no. 12 (June 2009): 1493–1506.

Collinger, Jennifer L., Brian Wodlinger, John E. Downey, Wei Wang, Elizabeth C. Tyler-Kabara, Douglas J. Weber, Angus J. C. McMorland et al. "High-Performance Neuroprosthetic Control by an Individual with Tetraplegia." *Lancet* 381, no. 9866 (February 2013): 557–64.

Dietrich, Susanne, Ingo Hertrich, and Hermann Ackermann. "Ultra-Fast Speech Comprehension in Blind Subjects Engages Primary Visual Cortex, Fusiform Gyrus, and Pulvinar: A Functional Magnetic Resonance Imaging (fMRI) Study." *BioMed Central Neuroscience* 14, no. 1 (2013): 1–15.

Dobelle, William H. "Artificial Vision for the Blind by Connecting a Television Camera to the Visual Cortex." *ASAIO Journal* 46, no. 1 (January–February 2000): 3–9.

———. "Artificial Vision for the Blind: The Summit May Be Closer Than You Think." *ASAIO Journal* 40, no. 4 (October–December 1994): 919–22.

———, M. G. Mladejovsky, and J. P. Girvin. "Artificial Vision for the Blind: Electrical Stimulation of Visual Cortex Offers Hope for a Functional Prosthesis." *Science* 183, no. 4123 (February 1974): 440–444.

———, Michael G. Mladejovsky, Jerald R. Evans, T. S. Roberts, and J. P. Girvin. "'Braille' Reading by a Blind Volunteer by Visual Cortex Stimulation." *Nature* 259, no. 5539 (January 1976): 111–112.

———, Donald O. Quest, João L. Antunes, Theodore S. Roberts, and John P. Girvin. "Artificial Vision for the Blind by Electrical Stimulation of the Visual Cortex." *Neurosurgery* 5, no. 4 (October 1979): 521–27.

Fernández, Eduardo, Arantxa Alfaro, and Pablo González-López. "Toward Long-Term Communication with the Brain in the Blind by Intracortical Stimulation: Challenges and Future Prospects." *Frontiers in Neuroscience* 14 (2020): 1–8.

Foroushani, Armin Najarpour, Christopher C. Pack, and Mohamad Sawan. "Cortical Visual Prostheses: From Microstimulation to Functional Percept." *Journal of Neural Engineering* 15, no. 2 (April 2018): 1–23.

Gearing, Marla, and Philip Kennedy. "Histological Confirmation of Myelinated Neural Filaments Within the Tip of the Neurotrophic Electrode After a Decade of Neural Recordings." *Frontiers in Human Neuroscience* 14 (April 2020): 1–8.

Gilja, Vikash, Chethan Pandarinath, Christine H. Blabe, Paul Nuyujukian, John D. Simeral, Anish A. Sarma, Brittany L. Sorice et al. "Clinical Translation of a High-Performance Neural Prosthesis." *Nature Medicine* 21, no. 10 (October 2015): 1142–47.

Hochberg, Leigh R., Daniel Bacher, Beata Jarosiewicz, Nicolas Y. Masse, John D. Simeral, Joern Vogel, Sami Haddadin et al. "Reach and Grasp by People with

Tretraplegia Using a Neurally Controlled Robotic Arm." *Nature* 485, no. 7398 (May 2012): 372–77.

Kawala-Sterniuk, Aleksandra, Natalia Browarska, Amir Al-Bakri, Mariusz Pelc, Jaroslaw Zygarlicki, Michaela Sidikova, Radek Martinek et al. "Summary of Over Fifty Years with Brain-Computer Interfaces: A Review." *Brain Sciences* 11, no. 1 (January 2021): 1–41.

Leuthardt, Eric C., Daniel W. Moran, and Tim R. Mullen. "Defining Surgical Terminology and Risk for Brain Computer Interface Technologies." *Frontiers in Neuroscience* 15 (March 2021): 1–9.

Lewis, Philip M., and Jeffrey V. Rosenfeld. "Electrical Stimulation of the Brain and the Development of Cortical Visual Prostheses: An Historical Perspective." *Brain Research* 1630 (September 2015): 208–24.

Metzger, Sean L., Kaylo T. Littlejohn, Alexander B. Silva, David A. Moses, Margaret P. Seaton, Ran Wang, Maximilian E. Dougherty et al. "A High-Performance Neuroprosthesis for Speech Decoding and Avatar Control." *Nature* 620, no. 7076 (August 2023): 1–9.

Mirochnik, Rebecca M., and John S. Pezaris. "Contemporary Approaches to Visual Prostheses." *Military Medical Research* 6, no. 1 (June 2019): 1–9.

Mitchell, Peter, Sarah C. M. Lee, Peter E. Yoo, Andrew Morokoff, Rahul P. Sharma, Daryl L. Williams, Christopher MacIsaac et al. "Assessment of Safety of a Fully Implanted Endovascular Brain-Computer Interface for Severe Paralysis in 4 Patients: The Stentrode with Thought-Controlled Digital Switch (SWITCH) Study." *JAMA Neurology* 80, no. 3 (March 2023): 270–78.

Moses, David A., Sean L. Metzger, Jessie R. Liu, Gopala K. Anumanchipalli, Joseph G. Makin, Pengfei F. Sun, Josh Chartier et al. "Neuroprosthesis for Decoding Speech in a Paralyzed Person with Anarthria." *New England Journal of Medicine* 385 (July 2021): 217–27.

Naumann, Jens. *Search for Paradise: A Patient's Account of the Artificial Vision Experiment.* Xlibris Corporation, 2012.

Niketeghad, Soroush, and Nader Pouratian. "Brain Machine Interfaces for Vision Restoration: The Current State of Cortical Visual Prosthetics." *Neurotherapeutics* 16, no. 1 (January 2019): 134–43.

Normann, Richard A., and Eduardo Fernandez. "Clinical Applications of Penetrating Neural Interfaces and Utah Electrode Array Technologies." *Journal of Neural Engineering* 13, no. 6 (December 2016): 1–16.

——, Edwin M. Maynard, Patrick J. Rousche, and David J. Warren. "A Neural Interface for a Cortical Vision Prosthesis." *Vision Research* 39, no. 15 (July 1999): 2577–87.

Oxley, Thomas J., Peter E. Yoo, Gil S. Rind, Stephen M. Ronayne, C. M. Sarah Lee, Christin Bird, Victoria Hampshire et al. "Motor Neuroprosthesis Implanted with Neurointerventional Surgery Improves Capacity for Activities of Daily Living Tasks in Severe Paralysis: First In-Human Experience." *Journal of NeuroInterventional Surgery* 13, no. 2 (February 2021): 102–8.

Pandarinath, Chethan, Paul Nuyujukian, Christine H. Blabe, Brittany L. Sorice, Jad Saab, Francis R. Willett, Leigh R. Hochberg et al. "High Performance Communication by People with Paralysis Using an Intracortical Brain-Computer Interface." *eLIFE* 6 (February 2017): 1–27.

Ryu, Stephen I., and Krishna V. Shenoy. "Human Cortical Prostheses: Lost in Translation?" *Neurosurgical Focus* 27, no. 1 (July 2009): 1–11.

Saha, Simanto, Khondaker A. Mamun, Khawza Ahmed, Raqibul Mostafa, Ganesh R. Naik, Sam Darvishi, Ahsan H. Khandoker et al. "Progress in Brain Computer Interface: Challenges and Opportunities." *Frontiers in Systems Neuroscience* 15 (February 2021): 1–20.

Schütz, Stefan, Bernhard Weissbecker, Hans E. Hummel, Karl-Heinz Apel, Helmut Schmitz, and Horst Bleckmann. "A Spelling Device for the Paralyzed." *Nature* 398, no. 6725 (March 1999): 297–98.

Soldozy, Sauson, Steven Young, Jeyan S. Kumar, Stepan Capek, Daniel R. Felbaum, Walter C. Jean, Min S. Park et al. "A Systematic Review of Endovascular Stent-Electrode Arrays, a Minimally Invasive Approach to Brain-Machine Interfaces." *Neurosurgical Focus* 49, no. 1 (July 2020): 1–9.

Vansteensel, Mariska J., Elmar G. M. Pels, Martin G. Bleichner, Mariana P. Branco, Timothy Denison, Zachary V. Freudenburg, Peter Gosselaar et al. "Fully Implanted Brain-Computer Interface in a Locked-In Patient with ALS." *New England Journal of Medicine* 375 (2016): 2060–66.

Willett, Francis R., Donald T. Avansino, Leigh R. Hochberg, Jaimie M. Henderson, and Krishna V. Shenoy. "High-Performance Brain-to-Text Communication via Handwriting." *Nature* 593, no. 7858 (May 2021): 249–64.

Wilson, Guy H., Sergey D. Stavisky, Francis R. Willett, Donald T. Avansino, Jessica N. Kelemen, Leigh R. Hochberg, Jaimie M. Henderson et al. "Decoding Spoken English from Intracortical Electrode Arrays in Dorsal Precentral Gyrus." *Journal of Neural Engineering* 17, no. 6 (November 2020): 1–22.

ACKNOWLEDGMENTS

I would like to acknowledge the many patients who have trusted me with the health of their brains. I do not take this monumental responsibility lightly. Without your faith in my ability, I wouldn't have had the opportunity to hone the skills I needed to become the neurosurgeon I am today. Every patient operated on by a surgeon owes a debt of gratitude to the patients who came before. I also want to dedicate this book to the families of my patients, with whom I have spent countless hours discussing the care of their loved ones. These conversations, motivated by your curiosity, helped me to organize my thoughts on how to make the most complex organ in the body more comprehensible.

I also want to thank my family. To my wife, Nancy, whose patience, wisdom, limitless EQ, beauty, grace, and support have allowed me to lead the richest and most productive life I could ever imagine. She is an Ivy League–educated, sharp, capable lawyer who decided to devote her time to raising our children, not out of necessity or reluctant acceptance that she "couldn't have it all," but out of choice. Nancy is a rare combination of beauty, grace, and style combined with warmth, modesty, sensitivity, and empathy, in equal proportions. She puts everyone else's needs before her own, works tirelessly to make every aspect of our family life run smoothly, and makes it all look effortless—like Ginger Rogers zipping along with Fred Astaire, backward and in high heels.

To my four perfect and unique children, Jonathan, Benjamin, Jenna, and Ali, who put up with the "dumbest smart person" they know and suffer through my often absurd discussions of esoteric topics at the dinner table.

I hope this book gives you a clearer vision of who I am, why I do what I do, and why I may have missed a few of your games or events when you were growing up. You never gave me a hard time and always let me know you understood why my work sometimes took precedent. And to my brother, Ralph, with whom I shared an upbringing by two remarkable parents. Perhaps no one understands me quite as well as you.

As Cushing once said, "The pen is more difficult than the scalpel." Special thanks are deserved by those who read and greatly helped me with earlier versions of this manuscript: Abby Pogrebin, who managed to get through it faster than I thought humanly possible and provided me with that first, critically important injection of positive feedback. Jim Solomon and Mitch Elkind, two of my college roommates, whose friendship and wisdom have always been reliable North Stars, should my compass ever misalign. Deb Copaken and Beth Rashbaum for their editorial assistance. John Schwartz, who reminded me, so rightfully, that a reader craves an experience and not a lecture. Charlie Melcher and Chris Godsick for convincing me to start this project in the first place, and Charlie for encouraging me to "think big." Rick Landgarten and Jeff and Susan Goldenberg for the layperson's perspective. Jenna Schwartz for help with the bibliography, and Matt Holt for his illustrations.

I also want to especially thank my agent, Kristine Dahl, who saw something in my story that she thought was worth sharing with the world and has had my back at every turn. You were a calming force that never let an email go unanswered.

I was lucky enough to have a team of editors at Dutton. Special thanks first to Stephen Morrow, who gave me the green light and then provided the first set of needed trimming shears, which he wielded with insight and sensitivity. Additionally, I am grateful to Lexy Cassola, John Parsley, and Maya Ziv for picking up the baton and bringing the manuscript over the finish line.

Certain individuals who have supported my work over the years deserve mention, most notably David and Ursel Barnes, Tim and Michele

Barakett, Leonard and Eleanor Udolf, Jeff and Susan Goldenberg, David Adelson, Phil and Tina Vasan, Ralph and Victoria Schwartz, Robert and Danielle Udolf, and Elise Udolf.

I want to give special thanks to all my neurosurgeon friends and colleagues. Only a small few could be mentioned in this book. Please forgive me for all the subjects and people that have been omitted. I could easily have written dozens more chapters and profiled many more of the neurosurgical pioneers and innovators who created and then transformed the field. Alas, the book would have gone on far too long. Each of you has your own stories to tell. I hope you take up the challenge. I look forward to reading your books.

A few of you provided advice, were sent parts of this manuscript, or participated in interviews. These include Rich Ellenbogen, Itzhak Fried, Eddie Chang, Michael Apuzzo, Dennis Spencer, Marty Weiss, Neal Kassell, Art Lyons, Phil Weinstein, Joseph Madsen, Ed Tarlov, Michael Schulder, John Jane Jr., Jacques Morcos, Kareem Zaghloul, Jay Wellons, Sameer Sheth, Michael Lawton, and Dan Yoshor. Others uniquely provided me with the inspiration, knowledge, skills, and motivation that spurred my own career interests. These include Giorgio Frank, Paolo Cappabianca, Dan Kelly, Aldo Stamm, Charlie Teo, Paolo Castelnuovo, Phil Stieg, Kris Moe, Axel Perneczky, Takanori Fukushima, Kyle Godfrey, and Doo-Sik Kong.

A special mention to Chuck Rich, my co-resident and close friend, whose support, warmth, and wry sense of humor made my training tolerable and even, dare I say, enjoyable at times.

Neurosurgery requires mentorship. I have benefited from many over the years. On the research side, Rafael Yuste and Tobias Bonhoeffer, you both allowed a naive but motivated MD to spend time in your labs, learning how to ask thoughtful questions, design scientific experiments, and engage in basic science research at its highest level. On the clinical side, two mentors deserve mention. George Ojemann agreed to host a wide-eyed medical student for a year of neurosurgical research. I was looking for inspiration and you delivered. Your passion for neurosurgery and unending curiosity continue to inspire me to this day. While it's unusual to have a mentor outside your field of expertise, Vijay Anand, the rhinologist who taught me how to operate through the nose, opened my eyes to the possibilities of minimally invasive skull base surgery. Our fortuitous collaboration completely changed the course of my career.

INDEX

Note: Italicized page numbers indicate material in photographs or illustrations.

ABOUT THE AUTHOR

THEODORE H. SCHWARTZ, MD, is the David and Ursel Barnes Endowed Professor of Minimally Invasive Neurosurgery at Weill Cornell Medical Center at NewYork-Presbyterian Hospital, one of the busiest and highest-ranked neurosurgery centers in the world. He has published over five hundred scientific articles and chapters on neurosurgery and has lectured around the world—from Bogotá to Vienna to Mumbai—on new, minimally invasive surgical techniques that he helped develop. He also runs a basic science laboratory devoted to epilepsy research. He studied philosophy and literature at Harvard.